HORIZONS IN MEDICINE 4

Horizons in Medicine

Edited by
Carol A Seymour
PhD FRCP
St George's Hospital Medical School

Anthony M Heagerty
MD FRCP
University Hospital of South Manchester

*Royal College
of Physicians
of London*

No. 4

McGRAW-HILL BOOK COMPANY

London · New York · St Louis · San Francisco · Auckland
Bogotá · Caracas · Hamburg · Lisbon · Madrid · Mexico
Milan · Montreal · New Delhi · Panama · Paris · San Juan
São Paulo · Singapore · Sydney · Tokyo · Toronto

Published by
McGRAW-HILL Book Company Europe
Shoppenhangers Road, Maidenhead, Berkshire, SL6 2QL, England
Tel 0628 23432; Fax 0628 770224

British Library Cataloguing in Publication Data
Horizons in Medicine. – No. 4
  I. Seymour, Carol A.
  II. Heagerty, Anthony M.
  610

ISBN 0-07-707511-0

Admission copies presented by
The New England Journal of Medicine
EMD GmbH, Zeitschriftenvertrieb,
Hohenzollernring 96,
1000 Berlin 20,
Germany
Fax: 49(30) 336 9236

Copyright © 1993 McGraw-Hill International (UK) Limited.
All rights reserved. No part of this publication may be reproduced,
stored in a retrieval system, or transmitted, in any form or by
any means, electronic, mechanical, photocopying, recording, or
otherwise, without the prior permission of the authors.

12345 CUP 96543

Typeset by BookEns Limited, Baldock, Herts.
and printed and bound in Great Britain at the University Press, Cambridge.

FOREWORD

Every branch of medicine is currently experiencing rapid change involving therapeutic advances and the way in which we employ our scarce resources. We are having to look at how we provide health care for our patients with an eye on both current management and how it may be influenced in the future, by both cost and research developments. As a result, the 1992 Advanced Medicine Conference was designed to present a programme to highlight the most recent innovations in a number of fields, as well as challenging speakers in the audience to examine whether some of our current practices are appropriate. Developments in the fields of cardiology, hepatology and gastroenterology were examined with an additional perspective on audit. Dermatology and metabolic disease were also considered in separate sessions as were recent innovations in nephrology and hypertension. The way ahead was indicated by recent developments in immunology, molecular biology and clinical genetics.

The Goulstonian Lecture was delivered by Professor Turnbull and dealt with the diseases caused by mitochondrial dysfunction, whilst Professor Hales, in his Croonian Lecture, examined new theories about the aetiology of diabetes.

All of the subjects have been expansively discussed by the speakers in their contributions to this fourth volume in the *Horizons in Medicine* series. For us it has been an immense pleasure to have been involved in the organisation of the meeting and subsequently the preparation of this volume. We are particularly grateful for the immense efforts made by the College staff, initially under the guidance of Miss Gillian Andrew, in regard to the running of the Advanced Medicine Conference itself.

Carol A Seymour, London
Anthony M Heagerty, Manchester
August 1992

LIST OF CONTRIBUTORS

Peter L Amlot
FRCP
Senior Lecturer in Clinical Immunology, Academic Department of Clinical Immunology, Royal Free Hospital School of Medicine, Pond Street, London NW3 2QG

Alexander R Attard
FRCS
Surgical Registrar, Queen Elizabeth Medical Centre, Edgbaston, Birmingham B15 2TH

Paul JR Barton
PhD
Senior Lecturer, Department of Cardiothoracic Surgery, National Heart and Lung Institute, Dovehouse Street, London SW3 6LY

David H Bennett
MD FRCP FACC
Consultant Cardiologist, Wythenshawe Hospital, Southmoor Road, Manchester M23 9LT

Laurence A Bindoff
BSc MD MRCP
Division of Clinical Neuroscience, The School of Neurosciences, The Medical School, University of Newcastle upon Tyne NE2 4HH

Lindsey A Brawn
MB ChB MRCP
Research Registrar, University Department of Medicine and Pharmacology, Royal Hallamshire Hospital, Glossop Road, Sheffield S10 2JF

Martin J Brodie
MD FRCP (Glasg, Edin)
Consultant Clinical Pharmacologist, Epilepsy Research Unit, University Department of Medicine and Therapeutics, Western Infirmary, Glasgow G11 6NT

David C Brooks
MD FACS
Division of GI Surgery, Brigham and Women's Hospital, Boston, Massachusetts 02115, USA

David A Burns
FRCP
Consultant Dermatologist, Leicester Royal Infirmary, Leicester LE1 5WW

Andrew K Burroughs
MB ChB(Hons) FRCP

Senior Lecturer in Medicine and Honorary Consultant Physician, Hepatobiliary and Liver Transplantation Unit, University Department of Medicine, Royal Free Hospital and School of Medicine, Pond Street, London NW3 2QG

Hamish A Cameron
MB ChB MRCP

Research Registrar, University Department of Medicine and Pharmacology, Royal Hallamshire Hospital, Glossop Road, Sheffield S10 2JF

Ronald WF Campbell
MB ChB FRCP

British Heart Foundation Professor of Cardiology, University Department of Academic Cardiology, Freeman Hospital, Newcastle upon Tyne NE7 7DN

David L Carr-Locke
MD FRCP FACG

Director of Endoscopy, Brigham and Women's Hospital, Boston, Massachusetts 02115, USA

Richard M Clayton
MD FRCP

Department of Endocrinology and Diabetes Mellitus, North Staffordshire Royal Infirmary, Princes Road, Hartshill, Stoke-on-Trent ST4 7LN

Colin F Close
MB ChB MRCP

Senior Medical Registrar (Diabetes and Endocrinology), General Hospital, Steelhouse Lane, Birmingham B4 6NH

John MC Connell
MD FRCP

Honorary Clinical Senior Lecturer and Consultant Physician, MRC Blood Pressure Unit, Western Infirmary, Glasgow G11 6NT

Gareth S Cross
MA PhD

Head Clinical Scientist, Molecular Genetics Department, Interdisciplinary Centre for Medical Genetics, City Hospital, Nottingham NG5 1PB

John Cunningham
DM FRCP

Consultant and Senior Lecturer in Nephrology, Royal London Hospital and Medical College, London E1 1BB

Katharine L Dalziel
MD MRCP

Department of Dermatology, University Hospital, Queen's Medical Centre, Nottingham NG7 2UH

Martin Dennis
MD MRCP

Senior Lecturer in Stroke Medicine, Department of Clinical Neurosciences, Western General Hospital, Crewe Road, Edinburgh EH4 2XU

Malcolm G Dunlop
MD FRCS(Ed)

MRC Clinical Scientist, MRC Human Genetics Unit, Western General Hospital, Crewe Road, Edinburgh EH4 2XU

Geoffrey M Dusheiko
MB BCh FCP(SA) FRCP

Reader in Medicine, Royal Free Hospital and School of Medicine, Pond Street, London NW3 2QG

Glyn R Evans
MB ChB MRCP(UK)

Occupational Health Department, Dudley Road Hospital, Dudley Road, Birmingham B18 7QH

Alexander M Farrell
MB ChB MRCPath

Senior Registrar, Department of Immunopathology, University Hospital, Queen's Medical Centre, Nottingham NG7 2UH

M John R Feehally
DM FRCP

Department of Nephrology, Leicester General Hospital, Gwendolen Road, Leicester LE5 4PW

Andrew Y Finlay
MB BS FRCP

Consultant Dermatologist and Honorary Senior Lecturer, Department of Dermatology, University of Wales College of Medicine, Heath Park, Cardiff CF4 4XN

Peter S Friedmann
MD FRCP

Professor of Dermatology, Department of Dermatology, PO Box 147, Royal Liverpool University Hospital, Prescott Street, Liverpool L69 3BX

Mansel Haeney
MB BCh MSc FRCP FRCPath

Consultant Immunologist, Department of Immunology, Clinical Sciences Building, Hope Hospital (University of Manchester School of Medicine), Salford M6 8HD

C Nick Hales
FRS FRCP

Professor of Clinical Biochemistry, Addenbrooke's Hospital, Hills Road, Cambridge CB2 2QR

Steven J Harper
MB MRCP

Research Fellow, Department of Nephrology, Leicester General Hospital, Gwendolen Road, Leicester LE5 4PW

Julian Hopkin
MD MSc FRCP

Consultant Physician, Osler Chest Unit, Churchill Hospital, Old Road, Headington, Oxford OX3 7LJ

Peter R Jackson
MB ChB PhD MRCP

Senior Lecturer, University Department of Medicine and Pharmacology, Royal Hallamshire Hospital, Glossop Road, Sheffield S10 2JF

Sandra Jackson
BSc

Division of Clinical Neuroscience, School of Neurosciences, The Medical School, University of Newcastle upon Tyne, Framlington Place, Newcastle upon Tyne NE2 4HH

Alan G Jardine
MD FRCP

Senior Registrar, MRC Blood Pressure Unit, Western Infirmary, Glasgow G11 6NT

Derek P Jewell
MA BM BCh FRCP

Senior Registrar, Radcliffe Infirmary, Oxford OX2 6HE

Alastair J MacGilchrist
MD MRCP

Senior Registrar, Liver Unit, Queen Elizabeth Hospital, Edgbaston, Birmingham B15 2TH

Rona M MacKie
MD FRCP FRCPath FRSE FIBiol

Professor of Dermatology, Department of Dermatology, University of Glasgow, Glasgow G12 8QQ

Paul McMaster
MA MB ChM

Consultant Surgeon, Queen Elizabeth Medical Centre, Edgbaston, Birmingham B15 2TH

David H Miller
MB ChB MD FRACP

Senior Lecturer in Clinical Neurology, Institute of Neurology, National Hospital for Neurology and Neurosurgery, Queen Square, London WC1 3BG

James M Neuberger
DM FRCP

Consultant Physician, Liver Unit, Queen Elizabeth Hospital, Edgbaston, Birmingham B15 2TH

Philip A Poole-Wilson
MD FRCP

Department of Cardiac Medicine, National Heart and Lung Institute, Dovehouse Street, London SW3 6LY

Anthony EG Raine
BA BMedSc DPhil FRCP

Professor of Renal Medicine, Department of Nephrology, Royal Hospital of St Bartholomew, London EC1A 7BE

Lawrence E Ramsay
MB ChB FRCP FFPM

Professor, University Department of Medicine and Pharmacology, Royal Hallamshire Hospital, Glossop Road, Sheffield S10 2JF

Neville R Rowell
MD FRCP

Emeritus Professor of Dermatology, University of Leeds, Nuffield Hospital, Outward Lane, Horsforth, Leeds LS18 4HP

Herb F Sewell
MB ChB BDS MSc PhD FRCP FRCPath

Professor of Immunology/Consultant Immunologist, University Hospital, Queen's Medical Centre, Nottingham NG7 2UH

Roger Smith
MD PhD FRCP

Consultant Physician, Nuffield Orthopaedic Centre, Headington, Oxford OX3 7LD

C Mark Taylor
FRCP DCH

Consultant Paediatric Nephrologist, The Children's Hospital, Ladywood, Birmingham B16 8ET

Stephen Tomlinson
MD FRCP

Professor of Medicine, University of Manchester; Consultant Physician, The Manchester Diabetes Centre, Manchester M13 0HZ

Douglass M Turnbull
PhD MD FRCP

Division of Clinical Neuroscience, School of Neurosciences, The Medical School, University of Newcastle upon Tyne, Framlington Place, Newcastle upon Tyne NE2 4HH

Patrick C Waller
MB ChB MRCP

Medicine Controls Agency, Business C, Market Towers, 1 Nine Elms Lane, London SW8 5NQ

Gordon K Wilcock
BSc DM(Oxon) FRCP

Professor in Care of the Elderly, Frenchay Hospital, Bristol BS16 1LE

Wilfred W Yeo
MB ChB MRCP

Lecturer, University Department of Medicine and Pharmacology, Floor L, Royal Hallamshire Hospital, Glossop Road, Sheffield S10 2JF

Ian D Young
MSc MD FRCP

Consultant Clinical Geneticist, Interdisciplinary Centre for Medical Genetics, City Hospital, Nottingham NG5 1PB

CONTENTS

Foreword — v

List of Contributors — vi

Part I – LECTURES

The Goulstonian Lecture — 1
Diseases due to mitochondrial dysfunction
S Jackson, LA Bindoff, DM Turnbull

The Croonian Lecture — 19
The aetiology of non-insulin-dependent diabetes
CN Hales

Part II – CARDIOLOGY, NEEDS, DIRECTIONS AND COST

Coronary angioplasty – how much and how much? — 30
David H Bennett

Cardiac failure – size, cost and implications — 38
Philip A Poole-Wilson

Lipid clinics – do we need them? — 47
Glyn R Evans

Life-threatening arrhythmias in the district general hospital – what can we afford? — 54
Ronald WF Campbell

Part III – IMMUNOLOGY AND THE CLINICIAN

New tests in immunology for the clinician — 60
HF Sewell, AM Farrell

The therapy of primary immunodeficiency   69
Mansel Haeney

Antibodies as killers   80
PL Amlot

Part IV – HEPATOLOGY AND GASTROENTEROLOGY

Hepatitis C   89
Geoffrey M Dusheiko

Management of portal hypertension with beta-blockers   103
Andrew K Burroughs

Laparoscopic cholecystectomy   119
David L Carr-Locke, David C Brooks

Liver transplantation   130
P McMaster, AR Attard

Update on the management of ulcerative colitis   141
DP Jewell

Primary biliary cirrhosis and sclerosing cholangitis   154
Alastair J MacGilchrist, James M Neuberger

Part V – DERMATOLOGY

Malignant melanoma   166
Rona M MacKie

Psychological impact of skin disease   172
AY Finlay

Immunology and the skin   180
PS Friedmann

Connective tissue diseases and the skin   188
Neville R Rowell

Ageing and the skin   194
Katharine L Dalziel

Infestations – recognition and management   202
DA Burns

Part VI – MOLECULAR BIOLOGY AND CLINICAL GENETICS

Molecular biology – new insights into genetic disease   213
ID Young, GS Cross

Genetics and the heart   225
Paul JR Barton

Clinical genetics applied to asthma Julian Hopkin	232
Genetic markers for polyposis coli MG Dunlop	240

Part VII – METABOLIC DISEASE

Diabetes: are we doing better than 10 years ago? Stephen Tomlinson	249
Neutral endopeptidase – therapeutic possibilities of atrial natriuretic factor John MC Connell, Alan G Jardine	257
Osteoporosis: advances and controversies Roger Smith	263
Octreotide: the somatostatin analogue with diverse therapeutic potential RN Clayton	272

Part VIII – NEUROLOGY

Transient ischaemic attacks and stroke: prognosis and management Martin Dennis	285
Pharmacological management of epilepsy in adolescents and adults Martin J Brodie	293
The use of MRI in diagnostic neurology DH Miller	304
Recent advances in dementia GK Wilcock	314

Part IX – THE KIDNEY

IgA nephropathy SJ Harper, MJR Feehally	322
The management of bone disease in renal failure John Cunningham	330
The haemolytic uraemic syndromes CM Taylor	339
Hypertension and renal failure AEG Raine	348
Clinical aspects of renal artery stenosis LE Ramsay, WW Yeo, LA Brawn, HA Cameron, CF Close, PC Waller, PR Jackson	359
Index	369

The Goulstonian Lecture

DISEASES DUE TO MITOCHONDRIAL DYSFUNCTION

S Jackson, LA Bindoff, DM Turnbull
The Medical School, University of Newcastle upon Tyne

Mitochondria are essential organelles in all aerobic cells and their main function is to generate energy, in the form of ATP, from the metabolic fuels. This is a complex process requiring several enzyme systems and the genetic information for these proteins comes from two genomes, nuclear and mitochondrial. Whilst these oxidative pathways have been known for many years, it has only been recognized over the last decade that defects of these metabolic processes are an important cause of disease. This chapter reviews the important clinical, biochemical and molecular features of defects involving two of these pathways, mitochondrial fatty acid oxidation and the mitochondrial respiratory chain.

MITOCHONDRIAL FATTY ACID OXIDATION

Biochemistry
Mitochondrial fatty acid oxidation results in the formation of acetyl-CoA with the production of reduced nicotinamide dinucleotide (NADH) and reduced flavin adenine dinucleotide ($FADH_2$). The subsequent oxidation of these moieties and the associated transport of electrons along the respiratory chain is tightly coupled to ATP formation (see below). The acetyl-CoA generated by β-oxidation may then be converted to ketone bodies in the liver or completely oxidized to CO_2 by the tricarboxylic acid cycle in other tissues.

Before mitochondrial β-oxidation can occur, fatty acids first have to be converted to their CoA-thiosters catalysed by long-chain, medium-chain and short-chain acyl-CoA synthetases [1]. The long-chain enzyme is present on the outer mitochondrial membrane whilst the other two are in the mitochondrial matrix. Long-chain acyl-CoA esters cannot cross the inner mitochondrial membrane directly. They are transferred into the matrix associated with carnitine. Acyl-groups are transferred from CoA to carnitine by carnitine palmitoyltransferase I (CPT I) which is located on the outer mitochondrial membrane [2]. The acylcarnitines cross the mitochondrial inner membrane in exchange for carnitine in a reaction catalysed by the carnitine:acylcarnitine translocase [3]. Long-chain acyl-CoA esters reformed by the action of CPT II are then substrates for the enzymes of mitochondrial β-oxidation. Short-chain and medium-chain fatty acids are activated to their acyl-CoA esters in the matrix.

Once inside the matrix the acyl-CoA esters undergo the repeated sequence of four reactions which comprise mitochondrial β-oxidation (Figure 1). The first reaction is catalysed by the acyl-CoA dehydrogenases and involves the dehydrogenation of the acyl-CoA to form a 2-*trans*-enoyl-CoA. There were thought to be only three acyl-CoA dehydrogenases in mammalian tissue – short-chain, medium-chain and long-chain enzymes and that these had different but overlapping chain length specificities [4]. Recently, however, a very long-chain acyl-CoA dehydrogenase has been purified from rat liver [5]; it is not yet known if this enzyme is present in human tissues. All these acyl-CoA dehydrogenases contain a flavin adenine dinucleotide (FAD) which functions as an electron acceptor for the dehydrogenation reaction. Electrons from the prosthetic group of the enzymes are transferred to the respiratory chain via two additional flavoproteins, electron transfer flavoprotein (ETF) and ETF:ubiquinone oxidoreductase. The latter enzyme is situated in the mitochondrial inner membrane and transfers the electrons via ubiquinone to complex III of the respiratory chain (see section on the mitochondrial respiratory chain, below) [6].

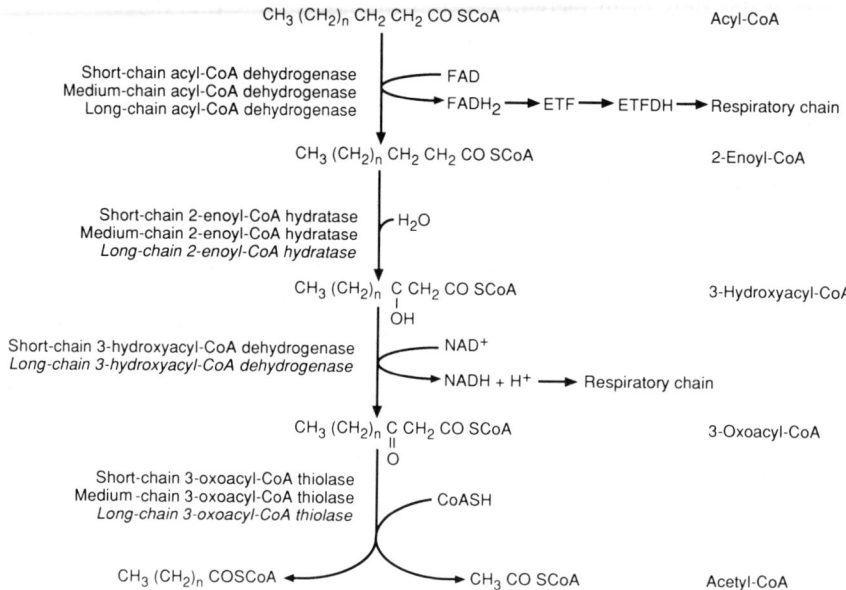

Figure 1. Mitochondrial β-oxidation of saturated fatty acids. The long-chain 2-enoyl-CoA hydratase, long-chain 3-hydroxyacyl-CoA dehydrogenase and long-chain 3-oxoacyl-CoA thiolase activities all form part of the trifunctional enzyme of β-oxidation. The presence of a medium-chain 2-enoyl-CoA hydratase is presumed from studies of patients with defects of the trifunctional enzyme (see reference 12).

Hydration of 2-*trans*-enoyl-CoA to L-3-hydroxyacyl-CoA is the second reaction of β-oxidation and is catalysed by the 2-enoyl-CoA hydratases [7]. Again there is uncertainty as to the number of enzymes catalysing this reaction in human tissues (see below). The third reaction is the dehydrogenation of L-3-hydroxyacyl-CoA esters to 3-oxoacyl-CoA esters and this is catalysed by the 3-hydroxyacyl-CoA dehydrogenases [8]. This dehydrogenation reaction is associated with the formation of NADH from NAD^+. The fourth and final reaction of mitochondrial β-oxidation is the thiolytic cleavage of 3-oxoacyl-CoA by 3-oxoacyl-CoA thiolase to generate acetyl-CoA and an acyl-CoA ester which is chain shortened by two carbon atoms [9]. This chain-shortened acyl-CoA is then a substrate for the acyl-CoA dehydrogenases. The number of enzymes involved in each of these final three steps of mitochondrial β-oxidation is uncertain. A trifunctional enzyme, which catalyses the 3-hydroxyacyl-CoA dehydrogenation, 2-enoyl-CoA hydration and 3-oxoacyl-CoA thiolysis of long-chain acyl-CoA esters, has recently been identified [10, 11] and it is now thought that there are, in addition to this enzyme, two 2-enoyl-CoA hydratases, one 3-hydroxyacyl-CoA dehydrogenase and two 3-oxoacyl-CoA thiolases [12].

Clinical features of defects of fatty acid oxidation
The clinical features of defects of mitochondrial fatty acid oxidation fall into two main groups: those in which systemic symptoms predominate and those in which there seems to be isolated organ involvement. Symptoms are likely to be induced by a number of metabolic changes which result from the defect of fatty acid oxidation. These include:

1. An impaired ability to withstand fasting or stress; since these patients cannot generate energy from fat they depend upon glycogen stores and circulating carbohydrate. Energy depletion will follow consumption of these fuels.
2. During fasting there is a stimulation of lipolysis with a concomitant increase in the concentration of free fatty acids. Free fatty acids entering the tissues are diverted to triacylglycerol synthesis resulting in deposition of lipid.
3. The generation of potentially toxic acyl-CoA ester intermediates resulting from the continuing partial β-oxidation of fatty acids.

The predominant systemic manifestations of fatty acid oxidation defects are sudden infant death [13] and hypoketotic hypoglycaemic episodes. The incidence of fatty acid oxidation defects in sudden infant death is still uncertain, although it is probably less than first thought [14]. Non-ketotic hypoglycaemia is a relatively common finding particularly in young children. These episodes can lead to death or permanent brain damage and must therefore be treated aggressively. Isolated organ involvement most commonly involves muscle, heart or liver. The myopathy associated with these disorders is often painful, particularly following prolonged exertion, and may be associated with myoglobinuria. The cardiomyopathy may be hypertrophic and associated with cardiac failure. Liver dysfunction is a common finding in patients with fatty acid oxidation defects and may be severe causing liver failure.

Clinical features associated with specific defects

Carnitine palmitoyltransferase (CPT) deficiency. CPT deficiency was the first defect of fatty acid oxidation to be described [15]. Patients with CPT II deficiency usually present in early adult life with muscle pain [15]. This pain may be associated with myoglobinuria and is usually precipitated by prolonged exercise, fasting or a combination of both. The myoglobinuria may be severe and lead to renal failure. CPT I deficiency presents in early infancy with severe hypoglycaemia [16].

Primary carnitine deficiency. Whilst secondary carnitine deficiency is a common finding in patients with β-oxidation disorders [17], primary carnitine deficiency is rare and due to an abnormality of carnitine transport across the plasma membrane [18]. Most patients present in childhood (2–7 years old) with progressive muscle weakness and hypertrophic cardiomyopathy [19]. Some patients may present somewhat younger (1–2 years) with hypoglycaemic episodes [19].

Acyl-CoA dehydrogenase deficiency. Defects of the acyl-CoA dehydrogenases are the most frequently identified abnormalities of fatty acid oxidation. Short-chain acyl-CoA dehydrogenase may present as a severe illness in infancy with hypoglycaemic episodes and hepatomegaly [20], or as a proximal myopathy in adult life [21]. Medium-chain acyl-CoA dehydrogenase deficiency may be one of the most commonly inherited metabolic disorders with an incidence of approximately 1 in 6500 in the UK [22]. Usually it presents in early life with hypoglycaemic episodes but sudden infant death and Reye's syndrome are also described [23]. Some cases present later with exercise-induced muscle pain whilst others are asymptomatic and are only detected after the disorder is diagnosed in another family member. Long-chain acyl-CoA dehydrogenase may present in the first 6 months with cardiac failure and hypoglycaemic episodes [24]. Another group of patients present later in childhood with muscle pain and myoglobinuria when the patient is stressed or following prolonged exercise [24].

Trifunctional enzyme deficiency. Defects of this enzyme have been described [12, 25] although in most cases only the activity of the long-chain 3-hydroxyacyl-CoA dehydrogenase has been measured [26]. The clinical features include recurrent non-ketotic hypoglycaemia, sudden infant death, hepatic dysfunction, cardiomyopathy, myopathy, pigmentary retinopathy and sensorimotor polyneuropathy.

Investigation of defects of fatty acid oxidation

Concentration of metabolic fuels and intermediary metabolites in blood. In normal subjects under fasting or stressed conditions, lipolysis is stimulated and free fatty acids are released into the circulation and taken up by tissues. The fatty acids undergo β-oxidation to generate acetyl-CoA, which is converted in the liver to the alternative metabolic fuel, ketone bodies. Circulating ketone bodies may then be oxidized by extrahepatic tissues, notably the brain, which is unable to oxidize fatty acids directly. In addition, glycogen stores are mobilized to release glucose, the blood concentration of which must be maintained for normal cerebral metabolism. Studies of these metabolic interrelationships under different conditions give important clues as to the presence of a defect of β-oxidation; for example, hypoketotic hypoglycaemia in the presence of a normal insulin concentration is strongly suggestive of a β-oxidation defect.

Measurement of plasma, urine and tissue carnitine concentrations. In patients with β-oxidation defects, abnormalities of carnitine metabolism are common [17] since there is an intramitochondrial accumulation of acyl-CoA esters. These acyl-CoA esters combine with carnitine in a reaction catalysed by the acyltransferases and the acylcarnitines are transported out of the mitochondria. Thus a higher percentage of carnitine is present in the acylated form which leads to the excretion of specific acylcarnitines in the urine and to secondary carnitine deficiency. Since carnitine metabolism is altered in all defects of intramitochondrial β-oxidation, measurement of total or free acylcarnitine is only of help in alerting one to the possibility of a defect of fatty acid oxidation and in the diagnosis of primary carnitine deficiency. However, sophisticated spectrophotometric techniques have been developed which measure the individual acylcarnitines in the blood and urine and are of great value in the diagnosis of β-oxidation defects [27].

Measurement of dicarboxylic acids and acylglycines in urine. When mitochondrial β-oxidation is impaired fatty acids are partially oxidized by ω-oxidation in the endoplasmic reticulum and by β-oxidation in peroxisomes. These oxidations generate dicarboxylic acids which are excreted in the urine. The pattern of the organic aciduria may be helpful in the diagnosis of a defect of fatty acid oxidation; e.g. hydroxydicarboxylic aciduria is seen in the majority of patients with trifunctional enzyme deficiency. When acyl-CoA esters accumulate in liver mitochondria due to a β-oxidation defect they combine with glycine. This reaction is catalysed by glycine-*N*-acylase and the acylglycines are subsequently excreted in the urine. The excretion of specific acylglycines can be valuable in the diagnosis of β-oxidation defects; e.g. excretion of suberylglycine in medium-chain acyl-CoA dehydrogenase deficiency.

Measurement of carnitine transport and enzyme activity. In many patients the definitive diagnosis depends on the measurement of enzyme activity using either radiochemical, spectrophotometric or fluorometric techniques. Primary carnitine deficiency is due to a defect of carnitine transport which is measured by studying the uptake of radio-labelled carnitine into fibroblasts [18]. The measurement of the carnitine palmitoyltransferases and the intramitochondrial enzymes of β-oxidation is described in detail elsewhere [28].

Molecular studies. Genetic studies are only available for a few of the enzymes of β-oxidation, since some of the enzymes have not been purified and neither the cDNA nor gene has been sequenced. In medium-chain acyl-CoA dehydrogenase deficiency the point mutation responsible for about 90% of cases has been identified [29, 30]. This is an A to G transition at position 985 of the coding sequence and results in a lysine to glutamic acid substitution. This point mutation may be rapidly identified by amplification of genomic DNA by the polymerase chain reaction (PCR) followed by restriction digestion or allele specific oligonucleotide probing. Very recently a point mutation has been identified in four cases of long-chain acyl-CoA dehydrogenase deficiency [31].

Treatment

The treatment of patients with fatty acid oxidation disorders is often successful and consists of three main approaches.

Diet. It is essential in all patients with β-oxidation disorders that sufficient calories, in the form of carbohydrate, are provided to ensure that prolonged fasting does not occur. This is particularly important in infants and young children who may die suddenly during fasting. Episodes of illness with hypoglycaemia must be treated promptly and aggressively with intravenous glucose infusions aimed at completely suppressing lipolysis. A low fat, high carbohydrate diet is recommended for most patients, although medium-chain triglycerides may be helpful for patients with defects of long-chain specific enzymes.

Carnitine. Carnitine therapy (100mg/kg in children) is effective in the treatment of primary carnitine deficiency [19] but the benefit of carnitine in patients with other β-oxidation defects is uncertain.

Riboflavine. Riboflavine is a precursor of FAD, the coenzyme essential as a prosthetic group for the acyl-CoA dehydrogenases, ETF and ETF:ubiquinone oxidoreductases. Some patients with deficiencies of these enzymes have responded to pharmacological doses of riboflavine (100–300mg per day) [32, 33].

MITOCHONDRIAL RESPIRATORY CHAIN

Biochemistry

The mitochondrial respiratory chain is a series of five multi-subunit complexes situated within the inner mitochondrial membrane: complex I – NADH ubiquinone oxidoreductase; complex II – succinate ubiquinone oxidoreductase; complex III – ubiquinol-cytochrome c oxidoreductase; complex IV – cytochrome c oxidase; and complex V – ATP synthase. Their function is to reoxidize reduced cofactors (NADH and reduced flavoproteins) and generate ATP. Reoxidization of reduced cofactors is associated with the transfer of reducing equivalents (electrons) from cofactors to the respiratory chain. NADH, generated by several dehydrogenase reactions within the mitochondria, is reoxidized by complex I with the formation of NAD+; electrons are then transferred to the mobile electron carrier ubiquinone. The reduced flavoprotein (FADH$_2$) generated during succinate oxidation transfers electrons to ubiquinone via complex II, whilst the FADH$_2$ generated during β-oxidation at the acyl-CoA dehydrogenase step is transferred to ubiquinone by ETF and ETF:ubiquinone oxidoreductase. The electrons are transferred from the reduced ubiquinone (ubiquinol) to complex III, and from complex III to complex IV via cytochrome c. Cytochrome c oxidase donates electrons directly to molecular oxygen. Sufficient energy is generated at three steps (complexes I, III and IV) to drive the extrusion of protons (H+) out of the mitochondrial matrix and across the inner mitochondrial membrane [34]. Because of the insulating properties of the inner mitochondrial membrane an electrochemical or proton gradient is created and the discharge of this gradient through complex V (ATP synthase) is associated with the conversion of ADP to ATP.

The respiratory chain complexes each contain several protein subunits ranging from four for complex II to >25 for complex I. In addition, the complexes all contain redox centres to allow the transfer of electrons. These redox centres are either iron-sulphur groups, copper atoms or iron-porphyrin groups (cytochromes) but the exact pathway of electron flow through the complexes is still being investigated.

Two genomes are involved in the synthesis of respiratory chain proteins, the nuclear genome and a separate cytoplasmic DNA found within the mitochondria. Mitochondrial DNA (mtDNA) is a circular 16.5kb molecule [35] that encodes 13 polypeptides, 22 transfer RNA (tRNA) and two ribosomal RNA (rRNA). The 13 proteins are all subunits of respiratory chain complexes: seven are complex I proteins, one is the apocytochrome b protein of complex III, three are cytochrome c oxidase subunits, and two are subunits of complex V. These proteins are synthesized within the mitochondria using the tRNA and rRNA encoded by mtDNA. As well as being the only extra chromosomal DNA in mammalian cells, mtDNA has several unique features: (a) it is predominantly inherited maternally (less than 0.1% of the mtDNAs are contributed by the sperm); (b) there is more than one copy of mtDNA per mitochondrion; and (c) transcription generates a large polycistronic message which has to be subsequently processed into its component RNA.

All the other protein subunits of the respiratory chain are encoded by nuclear DNA. They are synthesized on cytosolic ribosomes and are post-translationally imported into mitochondria [36]. The proteins have to be targeted to the mitochondria and for the majority of proteins this targeting information is contained within an N-terminal presequence. Proteins are imported into the mitochondria where this presequence is cleaved by specific proteases. The mature protein then combines with the mitochondrially encoded proteins (for complexes I, III, IV and V) with the formation of the complex within the inner mitochondrial membrane.

Investigation of defects of the respiratory chain

Clinical
Respiratory chain defects are associated with a wide variety of clinical features and a crucial factor is a high index of suspicion by clinicians. The initial clinical investigation is the measurement of lactate concentrations in the blood and cerebrospinal fluid (CSF). In some cases basal blood lactate concentrations are not increased, whilst in many patients elevation of blood lactate concentration is provoked by fasting or a carbohydrate load. In patients with predominantly central nervous system (CNS) symptoms, only CSF lactate may be elevated. Computerized tomographic (CT) scanning and nuclear magnetic resonance (NMR) imaging are both useful methods of detecting disease within the CNS. NMR spectroscopy will detect abnormalities in skeletal muscle, low phosphocreatine and impaired conversion of ADP to ATP, but these are fairly non-specific [37]. Positron emission tomographic (PET) scanning may be helpful since it is possible to show uncoupling of the normal ratio of oxygen consumed per molecule of glucose metabolized [38]. Both these latter two techniques are only available in specialized research centres.

Morphological studies
Owing to the frequency with which it is involved, the tissue most commonly studied is skeletal muscle. Historically, morphological abnormalities in skeletal muscle have provided one of the earliest indications that disease may be caused by altered respiratory chain function. Quantitative and qualitative changes in mitochondria have been found, the most well known finding being the 'ragged red fibre' [39]. This describes the accumulation of mitochondria beneath the muscle cell membrane giving it a ragged edge. When stained by the Gomori trichrome technique the accumulated mitochondria are stained red. This abnormality is more specifically detected by the use of a mitochondrial specific stain such as succinate dehydrogenase. Qualitative differences in mitochondria are best seen using electron microscopy.

In addition, several other important observations can be made on tissue section. Direct enzyme measurement of succinate dehydrogenase activity, part of complex II, and cytochrome c oxidase activity may be made. The amount and localization of mitochondrial proteins can be determined using immunocytochemistry [40] and finally, in situ hybridization using single-stranded RNA or DNA probes can detect the presence/absence of mRNA for the proteins of the respiratory chain [41]. This technique can also be used to detect mtDNA and demonstrate the site and concentration of any abnormal population of this genome.

Biochemical studies
The biochemical assessment of respiratory chain activity involves several possible studies, all of which help to give an understanding of the biochemical defect. Not all studies are possible for each patient because the majority of these investigations require the preparation of a mitochondrial

fraction, usually from skeletal muscle, and the amount of mitochondria obtained will depend upon the size of the biopsy. Overall flux through the pathway can be measured polarographically and this has the additional advantage that the coupling of substrate oxidation to the amount of ADP and oxygen is also measured [42]. Polarographic studies have the disadvantage that they use relatively large amounts of mitochondria, and spectrophotometric methods to measure overall flux are more sensitive [42]. Measurements of flux through a pathway are not specific and will not necessarily detect defects of individual components. The measurement of individual respiratory chain complexes is now possible and is an important component in the investi-gation of these disorders [28]. In addition to measuring enzyme activity, it is possible to determine the steady state concentration of the individual protein subunits by the technique of immunoblotting. This involves the separation of the proteins on the basis of molecular weight and their detection using antibodies specific to individual subunits [43]. The concentration of the important redox proteins, the cytochromes, can be determined since they contain iron-porphyrin rings which absorb light in a characteristic manner. This enables them to be detected in the mitochondrial membranes using the technique of difference spectroscopy [42].

Molecular studies
The molecular investigation of respiratory chain disease has concentrated on finding abnormalities of the mitochondrial genome. Nuclear gene mutations must occur because of an autosomal pattern of inheritance in some patients, but the precise defect has not been established in any patient. The major abnormalities of mtDNA are rearrangements (either deletions or duplication) and point mutations. Deletions and duplications may be detected by either Southern blotting, using purified mtDNA as a probe, or by the polymerase chain reaction (PCR) [44, 45]. Although the latter is extremely sensitive, quantitation is difficult. Known point mutations can be detected either by sequencing the region of interest or, if the mutation creates or destroys a restriction endonuclease site, by PCR amplification and restriction digest [46, 47]. Since mtDNA exists in multiple copies and not all may be involved, the appearance of two populations, one normal and one abnormal, is possible. This situation is termed heteroplasmy.

Clinical features
The clinical features associated with respiratory chain defects are extremely variable and different clinical presentations are being recognized. This makes the classification of respiratory chain defects extremely difficult. A clinical classification is limited because different clinical features are seen with the same apparent molecular defect. Biochemical classification is even more difficult, in part because the biochemical evaluation is so difficult. Also, defects of the mtDNA which involve either a deletion or a tRNA mutation induce multiple respiratory chain defects due to impaired synthesis of all mtDNA encoded proteins. A classification based upon the apparent molecular

defect may be the most satisfactory in the long-term, but at present there are many patients in whom the molecular defect has not been identified.

Clinical syndromes

Isolated myopathy
Despite the frequent involvement of muscle in patients with respiratory chain defects, isolated myopathy is uncommon. These patients present with non-specific symptoms such as cramp-like pain, burning discomfort in muscles, weakness and fatigue. The distribution of the weakness is proximal/axial and may involve the face. These patients often have multiple respiratory chain complex defects and usually mutations involving tRNAs.

Chronic progressive external ophthalmoplegia
Chronic progressive external ophthalmoplegia (CPEO) is one of the commonest presentations in adults of respiratory chain dysfunction. It may occur as an isolated finding or in association with myopathy and pigmentary retinopathy and/or CNS disease. The concentration of lactate in blood is either normal or mildly elevated. Muscle biopsy shows subsarcolemmal accumulation of mitochondria and cytochrome oxidase negative fibres [48]. The biochemical abnormality is usually a deficiency of several complexes and genetic analysis shows that the majority of patients have a deletion of mtDNA [44, 49]. Deletions vary from approximately 1kb to over 7kb and are invariably heteroplasmic (that is, a mixture of wild-type and mutant mtDNA). Between 40 and 60% of these patients have what is termed the 'common' deletion [50]. The use of mtDNA screening looking for deletions is an important adjunct to diagnosis in these patients [51]; however, their absence does not exclude a diagnosis.

Encephalopathies

Kearns–Sayre syndrome (KSS). This syndrome could be regarded as a severe form of the CPEO syndrome with an onset before the age of 20. Whilst the eye movement disorder is similar to CPEO, deafness, ataxia and cardiac conduction defects are common. In these patients lactate concentration is usually elevated in blood and/or CSF and the CSF protein concentration is also often elevated. The muscle histology and biochemical findings are similar to those in CPEO which is not surprising since almost all patients with KSS have major rearrangement of mtDNA. In the majority this is a deletion [49], often the so-called 'common' deletion. In rare cases, a duplication of mtDNA has been documented [52].

Myoclonus epilepsy with ragged red fibres (MERRF). In this disorder myoclonus is a major clinical feature. Weakness, ataxia, deafness and dementia are also found. Morphological abnormalities in skeletal muscle (ragged red fibres) gave the initial clue that this disorder may be due to mitochondrial dysfunction. In addition, maternal transmission of this disorder was found.

The biochemical abnormality in those patients investigated is usually multiple respiratory chain defects. In a high proportion of patients, but not all cases, there is a point mutation in the tRNA^{Lys} [53].

Myopathy, encephalopathy, lactic acidosis and stroke-like episodes (MELAS). This clinical syndrome is associated with the occurrence of stroke-like episodes, so-called because they mimic stroke clinically. They are thought to be due to metabolic insufficiency rather than an impaired vascular supply. Characteristic lesions are seen on CT and magnetic resonance imaging (MRI); these lesions may resolve rapidly or proceed to an established neurological defect. The onset of symptoms is before the age of 15 in most patients. Cortical blindness or hemianopia is present in virtually all patients and stroke-like episodes may be preceded by a migraine-like headache together with nausea and vomiting [54]. Focal or generalized seizures are common as is dementia. There may be an overlap between MELAS and other mitochondrial encephalopathies with some patients having myoclonus, ophthalmoplegia, retinopathy and ptosis [54]. Lactate levels in blood and especially CSF are often high. The MELAS syndrome has been associated with different biochemical findings, including multiple respiratory chain defects, although complex I deficiency appears to be by far the most common. The majority of patients with this syndrome have a point mutation within the tRNA$^{Leu(UUR)}$ [55], but a mutation in the tRNA^{Ile} [56] has also been associated with this phenotype. As expected the family history is compatible with maternal inheritance although other family members may be asymptomatic.

Neurogenic weakness, ataxia and retinitis pigmentosa. This maternally inherited syndrome is one of progressive weakness, ataxia and pigmentary retinopathy [46]. No morphological abnormality is detected in skeletal muscle from these patients. There is a point mutation involving the ATPase 6 gene but no biochemical abnormality has been reported.

Leigh's syndrome
Leigh's syndrome (subacute necrotizing encephalomyelopathy) is a syndrome essentially diagnosed on the neuropathological findings of spongy necrosis, glial reaction and vascular proliferation of the brain. It may present in a variety of different ways and different ages, although it is commonest in infants from 6 months to around 4 years. The major clinical problems are failure to thrive, vomiting, motor delay, intellectual retardation and respiratory problems, especially irregularity in the pattern of respiration with hyper- and hypoventilation. No single biochemical defect has been linked to Leigh's syndrome and whilst defects of the respiratory chain are probably the most common, abnormalities of the pyruvate dehydrogenase complex have also been described [57]. Lactate and pyruvate concentrations in the CSF are usually elevated but may be normal in blood; CT and MRI scans show very characteristic (but not pathognomonic) low density areas within the basal ganglia and less commonly the cerebellum. In patients with respiratory chain defects the most common abnormality is an isolated defect of complex IV [58]. This

is associated with an autosomal pattern of inheritance in many patients suggesting the defect is within the nuclear genome. However, defects of mtDNA may cause this clinical phenotype and can be associated with the typical neuropathological findings [59].

Leber's optic atrophy
This disorder is one of the most common inherited causes of blindness in young men and is clearly maternally inherited suggesting that it is due to a disorder of mtDNA. In addition to blindness, several members of Leber's pedigrees manifest non-ophthalmological features including encephalopathy, deafness, dystonia and cardiac conduction defects. Mutations in several mitochondrial protein encoding genes have been identified, the commonest involving ND4 and ND1 [60, 61]. Biochemical studies have shown a biochemical defect of complex I in individuals with the ND1 mutation [61]; a more subtle abnormality in those patients with the ND4 mutation and has been found [62].

Syndromes with non-neuromuscular presentation

Gastrointestinal involvement. Gastrointestinal symptoms are fairly common in patients with respiratory chain defects and are probably under-reported. The most common symptoms are vomiting, anorexia and abdominal pain. Occasionally, liver dysfunction has been reported and may be the major organ involved, although it may be that respiratory chain defects are not considered in many patients with so-called idiopathic liver disease.

Cardiomyopathy. Heart involvement occurs in patients with Kearns–Sayre/CPEO phenotype. The cardiac conductive system is predominantly affected and may lead to complete heart block. This is thought to be a significant cause of mortality and should be actively sought and treated by insertion of a pacemaker. In other patients there is involvement of cardiac muscle leading to cardiac failure [63]. In many of these patients there is also involvement of skeletal muscle.

Renal disease. Generalized aminoaciduria (deToni–Fanconi–Debré syndrome) has been described in several patients with respiratory chain disease. In the majority of patients the renal component was only part of a systemic syndrome usually with lactic acidosis and muscle involvement. It is not known if respiratory chain defects can present with renal disease alone.

Haematological. Haematological disease is a rare presentation of respiratory chain dysfunction. Abnormalities of mtDNA are frequently sought and identified in white blood cells in patients with Kearns–Sayre syndrome or MELAS [51], although they are often at lower frequency (i.e. a greater percentage of wild-type mtDNA) in these cells compared to muscle. One haematological presentation is that of Pearson's syndrome, a disorder that presents at birth or in early infancy with refractory sideroblastic anaemia, thrombocytopenia, neutropenia, metabolic acidosis, pancreatic insufficiency and hepatic dysfunction. Children usually die due to liver failure. Deletions of mtDNA have now been identified in a significant proportion of children with this syndome [64]. Interestingly, there are recorded cases of children presenting initially with Pearson's syndrome that later develop a disease identical to the Kearns-Sayre syndrome [65].

Lactic acidosis in infancy
Whilst many of the above syndromes may present early in life, there are a few conditions which appear to be confined to infants, often, but not always, associated with severe lactic acidosis and death in the first few months. The most severe presentation is of a profound lactic acidosis presenting from birth to around 3 months of age. Hypotonia, vomiting and ventilatory distress are all commonly associated features and death from respiratory failure is the usual outcome, often before the age of 6 months. This presentation occurs with a severe systemic defect of the respiratory chain and has been associated with defects of complexes I, III and IV [66].

An important condition to differentiate from the fatal lactic acidosis is a benign condition associated with cytochrome c oxidase deficiency [67]. Failure to thrive, hypotonia and ventilatory difficulties are all features of this condition and lactic acid concentration in plasma may be as high as in the fatal form. Despite this, the condition gradually improves and by 12-18 months the children are often normal. Biochemical studies have shown that all reported cases have been due to a severe defect of cytochrome c oxidase, and that the defect involves a foetal isoform of a nuclear encoded subunit of complex IV, the switch to the adult form being associated with the clinical improvement.

mtDNA depletion syndrome
A recently described molecular defect is that of mtDNA depletion which is associated with a severe presentation in infancy or early childhood [68, 69]. Weakness, hypotonia and ventilatory difficulty are once again common. The degree of mtDNA depletion may vary between tissues in the same individual and may lead to clinical presentations outside the nervous system, e.g. with liver disease. The condition appears to be inherited in an autosomal recessive pattern indicating the involvement of a nuclear gene defect. Biochemical studies have shown that complexes I, III and IV are affected and that the condition is fatal in the majority of patients before the age of 12 months.

Neurodegenerative disease
There is considerable debate as to the possible involvement of defects of the respiratory chain in neurodegenerative disease. The link between neurodegenerative disease and the respiratory chain was provided by the finding that 1-methyl-4-phenyl-1,2,3,6-tetrahydrapyridine (MPTP) caused a condition identical to Parkinson's disease [70]. A metabolite of MPTP was subsequently shown to be a profound inhibitor of complex I [71]. Since this discovery a variety of respiratory chain defects have been identified in a number of tissues from

patients with Parkinson's disease [72–74]. At this stage it is not possible to be certain which defects are primary or secondary, or whether mtDNA abnormalities are involved.

Following the findings in Parkinson's disease, the role of respiratory chain dysfunction has been investigated in other neurodegenerative disorders. In both Alzheimer's disease and Huntington's chorea respiratory chain abnormalities have been reported [75, 76]. However, the role of these defects in these neurodegenerative diseases is even more controversial.

Ageing
Studies have shown an age-related decline in mitochondrial respiratory chain activity [77]. It has been suggested that mtDNA mutations are important in the decline and that these mutations are important in the ageing process [78]. The initial damage to mtDNA may be caused by free radical damage to the mtDNA, known to occur at a much greater frequency than nuclear DNA [79]. Since most mitochondria have a half-life of days to a few weeks, the mitochondrial population may reproduce itself several hundred times during the lifetime of an individual. If this abnormality also has a selective advantage, for example a deletion would give rise to a smaller genome which replicates faster than the larger, normal one, then it may become the dominant form in the cell. There is some evidence to support the theory of increasing mtDNA mutations with age. Low levels of a specific mtDNA deletion, previously only found in patients with mitochondrial encephalomyopathies, have been found in normal heart, muscle and brain from adult humans [80] but not in foetal brain or liver. Similar findings have been reported in heart and liver from adult human tissues [81, 82].

Treatment
The treatment of patients with respiratory chain defects is more difficult than that of fatty acid oxidation because the biochemical defect affects the final common pathway of energy metabolism. Therefore, unlike fatty acid oxidation, it is impossible to bypass the block by providing alternative metabolic fuels. Most success has been achieved with substances that act as artificial electron acceptors, e.g. vitamin C, vitamin K_3 [83] and ubiquinone [84]. Objective increases in muscle strength have been reported and improvements in electron transfer have been demonstrated by **NMR** studies [83]. There have been suggestions that riboflavine, carnitine, thiamine and free radical scavengers may be of value but none of these have been proven to be of value.

REFERENCES
1. Londesborough JC, Webster JR. Fatty acyl-CoA synthetases. In Boyer PD, ed. *The Enzymes*, 3rd edn, Vol 10. New York: Academic Press. 1974: 469–488
2. Murthy MR, Pande SV. Malonoyl-CoA binding site and overt carnitine palmitoyltransferase activity reside on opposite sides of the outer mitochondrial membrane. *Proc Natl Acad Sci USA* 1987; *84*: 378–382
3. Pande SV. A mitochondrial carnitine acyltransferase translocase system. *Proc Natl Acad Sci USA* 1075; 72: 883–887

4 Finocchiaro G, Ito M, Tanaka K. Purification and properties of short-chain acyl-CoA, medium-chain acyl-CoA, and isovaleryl-CoA dehydrogenases from human liver. *J Biol Chem* 1987; *262*: 7982-7989
5 Izai K, Uchida Y, Orii T et al. Novel fatty acid β-oxidation enzymes in rat liver mitochondria. I. Purification and properties of very long-chain acyl-coenzyme A dehydrogenase. *J Biol Chem* 1992; *267*: 1027-1033
6 Beckmann JD, Frerman FE. Electron transfer oxidoreductase from pig liver: Purification and molecular, redox, and catalytic properties. *Biochemistry* 1985; *24*: 3913-3921
7 Fong JC, Schulz H. Short-chain and long-chain enoyl-CoA hydratases from pig heart muscle. *Methods Enzymol* 1981; *71*: 390-398
8 Noyes BE, Bradshaw RA. L-3 Hydroxyacyl CoA dehydrogenase from pig heart muscle: subunit structure. *J Biol Chem* 1973; *248*: 3060-3066
9 Middleton B. The oxoacyl-coenzyme A thiolases of animal tissues. *Biochem J* 1973; *132*: 717-730
10 Uchida Y, Izai K, Orii T, Hashimoto T. Novel fatty acid β-oxidation enzymes in rat liver mitochondria. II Purification and properties of enoyl-coenzyme A (CoA) hydratase/3-hydroxyacyl-CoA dehydrogenase/3-ketoacyl-CoA thiolase trifunctional protein. *J Biol Chem* 1992; *267*: 1034-1041
11 Carpenter K, Pollitt RJ, Middleton B. Human liver long-chain 3-hydroxyacyl-coenzyme A dehydrogenase is a multifunctional membrane-bound beta-oxidation enzyme of mitochondria. *Biochem Biophys Res Commun* 1992; *183*: 443-448
12 Jackson S, Singh Kler R, Bartlett K et al. Combined enzyme defect of mitochondrial fatty acid oxidation. *J Clin Invest* 1992 (in press)
13 Howat AJ, Bennett MJ, Variend S et al. Defects of metabolism of fatty acids in the sudden infant death syndrome. *Br Med J* 1985; *290*: 1771-1773
14 Miller ME, Brooks JG, Forkes N, Insel R. Frequency of medium-chain acyl-CoA dehydrogenase deficiency G-985 mutation in sudden infant death syndrome. *Pediatr Res* 1992; *31*: 305-307
15 DiMauro S, DiMauro PP. Muscle carnitine palmitoyltransferase deficiency and myoglobinuria. *Science* 1973; *182*: 929-931
16 Bougnères PF, Saudubray JM, Marsac C et al. Fasting hypoglycaemia resulting from hepatic carnitine palmitoyltransferase deficiency. *J Pediatr* 1981; *98*: 742-746
17 Turnbull DM, Sherratt HSA. Mitochondrial myopathies: defects in β-oxidation. *Biochem Soc Trans* 1985; *13*: 645-647
18 Treem WR, Stanley CA, Finegold DN et al. Primary carnitine deficiency due to a failure of carnitine transport in kidney, muscle and fibroblasts. *N Engl J Med* 1988; *319*: 1331-1336
19 Stanley CA, Treem WR, Hale DE, Coates PM. A genetic defect in carnitine transport causing primary carnitine deficiency. In Tanaka K, Coates PM, eds. *Fatty Acid Oxidation: Clinical, Biochemical, and Molecular Aspects*. New York: Alan R. Liss. 1990: 457-464
20 Amendt BA, Green C, Sweetman L et al. Short-chain acyl-coenzyme A dehydrogenase deficiency: Clinical and biochemical studies in two patients. *J Clin Invest* 1987; *79*: 1303-1309
21 Turnbull DM, Bartlett K, Stevens DL et al. Short-chain acyl-CoA dehydrogenase deficiency associated with a lipid-storage myopathy and secondary carnitine deficiency. *N Engl J Med* 1984; *311*: 1232-1236
22 Editorial. Medium-chain acyl-CoA dehydrogenase deficiency. *Lancet* 1991; *i*: 544-545
23 Roe CR, Coates PM. Acyl-CoA dehydrogenase deficiencies. In Scriver CR, Beaudet AL, Sly WS, Valle D, eds. *The Metabolic Basis of Inherited Disease*. New York: McGraw Hill. 1989: 889-914
24 Hale DE, Stanley CA, Coates PM. The long-chain acyl-CoA dehydrogenase deficiency. In Tanaka K, Coates PM, eds. *Fatty Acid Oxidation: Clinical, Biochemical and Molecular Aspects*. New York: Alan R Liss. 1990: 303-311
25 Jackson S, Bartlett K, Land J et al. Long-chain 3-hydroxyacyl-CoA dehydrogenase deficiency. *Pediatr Res* 1991; *29*: 406-411
26 Rocchiccioli F, Wanders RJA, Aubourg P et al. Deficiency of long-chain 3-hydroxyacyl-CoA dehydrogenase: A cause of lethal myopathy and cardiomyopathy in

early childhood. *Pediatr Res 1990; 28*: 657–662
27 Millington DS, Norwood DK, Kodo N et al. Application of fast atom bombardment with tandem mass spectrometry and liquid chromatography/mass spectrometry to the analysis of acylcarnitines in human urine, blood and tissue. *Anal Biochem 1989; 180*: 331–339
28 Birch-Machin MA, Jackson S, Turnbull DM. Study of skeletal muscle mitochondrial dysfunction. *Methods Toxicol 1992*; in press
29 Kelly DP, Whelan AJ, Ogden ML et al. Molecular characterisation of inherited medium-chain acyl-CoA dehydrogenase deficiency. *Proc Natl Acad Sci USA 1990; 87*: 9236–9240
30 Matsubara Y, Narisawa K, Miyabayashi S et al. Identification of a common mutation in patients with medium-chain acyl-CoA dehydrogenase deficiency. *Biochem Biophys Res Commun 1990; 171*: 498–505
31 Mendelsohn NJ, Kelly DP, Hale DE et al. The molecular basis of human long-chain acyl-CoA dehydrogenase deficiency. *Pediatr Res 1992; 31*: 134A
32 Turnbull DM, Shepherd IM, Ashworth B et al. Lipid storage myopathy associated with low acyl-CoA dehydrogenase activities. *Brain 1988; 111*: 815–828
33 DiDonato S, Gellera C, Peluchetti D et al. Normalization of short-chain acyl-coenzyme A dehydrogenase after riboflavin treatment in a girl with multiple acylcoenzyme A dehydrogenase-deficient myopathy. *Ann Neurol 1989; 25*: 479–484
34 Sherratt HSA, Turnbull DM. Mitochondrial oxidation and ATP synthesis in muscle. In Harris JB, Turnbull DM, eds. *Metabolic Myopathies*. London: Baillière-Tindall. 1990: 523–560
35 Anderson S, Bankier AT, Barrell BG et al. Sequence organisation of the human mitochondrial genome. *Nature 1981; 290*: 457–465
36 Hartl F-U, Neupert W. Protein sorting to mitochondria: evolutionary conservations of folding and assembly. *Science 1990; 247*: 930–938
37 Arnold DL, Taylor DJ, Radda GK. Investigation of human mitochondrial myopathies by phosphorous magnetic resonance spectroscopy. *Ann Neurol 1985; 18*: 189–196
38 Frackowiak RSJ, Herold S, Petty RKH, Morgan-Hughes JA. The cerebral metabolism of glucose and oxygen measured with positron tomography in patients with mitochondrial diseases. *Brain 1988; 111*: 1009–1024
39 Olsen W, King-Engel W, Walsh GO, Einangler R. Oculocraniosomatic neuromuscular disease with 'ragged-red' fibres. *Arch Neurol 1972; 26*: 192–211
40 Johnson MA, Kadenbach B, Droste M et al. Immunocytochemical studies of cytochrome oxidase subunits in skeletal muscle of patients with partial cytochrome oxidase deficiencies. *J Neurol Sci 1988; 87*: 75–90
41 Mita S, Schmidt B, Schon EA et al. Detections of deleted mitochondrial genomes in cytochrome c oxidase deficient muscle fibres of a patient with Kearns-Sayre syndrome. *Proc Natl Acad Sci USA 1989; 95*: 1345–1350
42 Sherratt HSA, Watmough NJ, Johnson M, Turnbull DM. Methods used for the study of normal and abnormal skeletal muscle mitochondria. *Meth Biochem Anal 1988; 33*: 243–335
43 Schapira AHU, Cooper JM, Morgan-Hughes JA et al. Molecular basis of mitochondrial myopathies: polypeptide analysis of complex I deficiency. *Lancet 1988; i*: 500–503
44 Holt IJ, Harding AE, Morgan-Hughes JA. Deletions of muscle mitochondrial DNA in patients with mitochondrial myopathies. *Nature 1988; 331*: 717–719
45 Holt IJ, Harding AE, Morgan-Hughes JA. Deletions of muscle mitochondrial DNA in mitochondrial myopathies: sequence analysis and possible mechanisms. *Nucl Acid Res 1989; 12*: 4465–4469
46 Holt IJ, Harding AE, Petty RKH, Morgan-Hughes JA. A new mitochondrial disease associated with mitochondrial DNA heteroplasmy. *Am J Hum Genet 1990; 46*: 428–433
47 Zeviani M, Amati P, Bresolin N et al. Rapid detection of A-G$^{(8344)}$ mutation of mtDNA in Italian families with myoclonus epilepsy and ragged-red fibres (MERRF). *Am J Hum Genet 1991; 48*: 203–211
48 Johnson MA, Turnbull DM, Dick DJ, Sherratt HSA. A partial deficiency of cytochrome c oxidase in chronic progressive external ophthalmoplegia. *J Neurol Sci*

1983; 60: 31-53
49 Moraes CT, DiMauro S, Zeviani M et al. Mitochondrial DNA deletions in progressive external ophthalmoplegia and Kearns-Sayre syndrome. *N Engl J Med 1989; 320*: 1293-1299
50 Schon EA, Rizzuto R, Moraes CT et al. A direct repeat is a hot spot for large-scale deletion of human mitochondrial DNA. *Science 1989; 244*: 346-349
51 Hammans SR, Sweeney MG, Brockington M et al. Mitochondrial encephalomyopathies: molecular genetic diagnosis from blood samples. *Lancet 1991; 337*: 1311-1313
52 Poulton J, Deadman ME, Gardner RM. Duplications of mitochondrial DNA in mitochondrial myopathy. *Lancet 1989; i*: 236-240
53 Shoffner JM, Lott MT, Lezza AMS et al. Myoclonic epilepsy and ragged-red fibre disease (MERRF) is associated with a mitochondrial DNA tRNA^{Lys} mutation. *Cell 1990; 61*: 931-937
54 Ciataloni E, Ricci E, Shansker S et al. MELAS: clinical features, biochemistry, and molecular genetics. *Ann Neurol 1992; 31*: 391-398
55 Goto Y-I, Nonaka I, Horai S. A mutation in the tRNA$^{Leu(UUR)}$ gene associated with the MELAS subgroup of mitochondrial encephalopathies. *Nature 1990; 348*: 651-653
56 Tanaka M, Ino H, Ohno K et al. Mitochondrial mutation in fatal infantile cardiomyopathy. *Lancet 1992; ii*: 1452
57 Kretzchmar JA, DeArmond SJ, Koch TK et al. Pyruvate dehydrogenase complex deficiency as a cause of subacute necrotising encephalopathy (Leigh Disease). *Pediatrics 1987; 79*: 370-373
58 DiMauro S, Lombes A, Nakas H et al. Cytochrome c oxidase deficiency. *Pediatr Res 1990; 28*: 536-541
59 Tatuch Y, Christodoulou J, Feigenbaum A et al. Heteroplasmic mtDNA mutation (T-G) at 8993 can cause Leigh Disease when the percentage of abnormal mtDNA is high. *Am J Hum Genet 1992; 50*: 842-848
60 Wallace DC, Singh G, Lott MT et al. Mitochondrial DNA mutation associated with Leber's hereditary optic neuropathy. *Science 1988; 242*: 1427-1430
61 Howell N, Bindoff LA, McCullough DA et al. Leber's hereditary optic neuropathy: identification of the same ND1 mutation in six pedigrees. *Am J Hum Genet 1991; 49*: 939-950
62 Majander A, Huoponen K, Savontaus ML et al. Electron transfer properties of NADH:ubiquinone reductase in the ND1/3460 and the ND4/1178 mutations of the Leber hereditary optic neuroretinopathy (LHON). *FEBS Lett 1991; 292*: 289-292
63 Zeviani M, Gellera C, Antozzi C et al. Maternally inherited myopathy and cardiomyopathy: association with a mutation in mitochondrial DNA tRNA$^{Leu(UUR)}$. *Lancet 1991; 338*: 143-147
64 Rotig A, Colonna M, Bonnefont JP et al. Mitochondrial DNA deletion in Pearson's marrow/pancreas syndrome. *Lancet 1989; i*: 902-903
65 McShane MA, Hammans SR, Sweeney M et al. Pearson syndrome and mitochondrial encephalomyopathy in a patient with a deletion of mtDNA. *Am J Hum Genet 1991; 48*: 39-42
66 Birch-Machin MA, Shepherd IM, Cartlidge NEF et al. Mitochondrial function in Parkinson's disease. *Lancet 1989; i*: 49
67 DiMauro S, Nicholson JF, Hays AP et al. Benign infantile mitochondrial myopathy due to reversible cytochrome c oxidase deficiency. *Ann Neurol 1983; 14*: 226-234
68 Moraes CT, Shanske S, Tritschler H-J et al. Mitochondrial DNA depletion with variable tissue specificity: a novel genetic abnormality in mitochondrial diseases. *Am J Hum Genet 1991; 48*: 492-501
69 Tritschler H-J, Andreetta F, Moraes CT et al. Mitochondrial myopathy of childhood associated with depletion of mitochondrial DNA. *Neurology 1992; 42*: 209-217
70 Langston JW, Ballard P, Tetrud JW, Irwin I. Chronic parkinsonism in humans due to a product of meperidine-analog synthesis. *Science 1983; 219*: 979-980
71 Ramsay RR, Salach JI, Dadger J, Singer TP. Inhibition of mitochondrial NADH dehydrogenase by pyridine derivatives and its possible relation to experimental and idiopathic parkinsonism. *Biochem Biophys Res Commun 1986; 135*: 269-275

72 Shapira AHV, Mann VM, Cooper JM et al. Anatomic and disease specificity of NADH CoQ$_1$ reductase (complex I) deficiency in Parkinson's disease. *J Neurochem 1990; 55*: 2142-2145
73 Bindoff LA, Birch-Machin MA, Cartlidge NEF et al. Respiratory chain abnormalities in skeletal muscle from patients with Parkinson's disease. *J Neurol Sci 1991; 104*: 203-208
74 Shoffner JM, Watts RL, Juncos JL et al. Mitochondrial oxidative phosphorylation defects in Parkinson's disease. *Am Neurol 1991; 30*: 332-339
75 Parker WD, Filley CM, Parks JK. Cytochrome oxidase deficiency in Alzheimer's disease. *Neurology 1990; 40*: 1302-1303
76 Parker WD, Boyson SJ, Luder AS, Parks JK. Huntington's disease. *Neurology 1990; 40*: 1231-1233
77 Trounce I, Byrne E, Marzuki S. Decline in skeletal muscle mitochondrial respiratory chain function: possible factor in ageing. *Lancet 1989; i*: 637-639
78 Linnane AW, Marzuki S, Ozawa T, Tanaka M. Mitochondrial DNA mutations as an important contributor to ageing and degenerative disease. *Lancet 1989; i*: 642-645
79 Richter C, Park J-W, Ames BN. Normal oxidative damage to mitochondrial and nuclear DNA is extensive. *Proc Natl Acad Sci USA 1988; 85*: 6465-6467
80 Cortopassi GA, Arnheim N. Detection of a specific mitochondrial DNA deletion in tissues of older humans. *Nucl Acid Res 1990; 18*: 6927-6933
81 Yen T-C, Su J-H, King K-L, Wei Y-H. Ageing-associated 5kb deletion in human liver mitochondrial DNA. *Biochem Biophys Res Commun 1991; 178*: 124-131
82 Ozawa T, Tanaka M, Sugiyama S et al. Multiple mitochondrial DNA deletions exist in cardiomyocytes of patients with hypertrophic or dilated cardiomyopathy. *Biochem Biophys Res Commun 1990; 170*: 830-836
83 Argov Z, Bank WJ, Maris J et al. Treatment of mitochondrial myopathy due to complex III deficiency with vitamins K$_3$ and C: a ^{31}P-NMR follow-up study. *Ann of Neurol 1986; 19*: 598-602
84 Ogasahara S, Nihikawa Y, Yoritugi S et al. Treatment of Kearns-Sayre syndrome with coenzyme Q$_{10}$. *Neurology 1986; 36*: 45-53

The Croonian Lecture

THE AETIOLOGY OF NON-INSULIN-DEPENDENT DIABETES

CN Hales
Addenbrooke's Hospital, Cambridge

Looking back over the titles of the Croonian Lectures given in this century I was surprised to find that the lectures have been concerned with diabetes only once. This was in 1940 when Dr George Graham gave two lectures [1, 2]. However, in the last quarter of last century Dr Frederick Pavy gave no less than seven Croonian Lectures on the subject, the last in 1897 being a supplementary Croonian Lecture [3-5].

The decline from seven to two to one (the present) lecture over two intervals of fifty years prompts me to wonder whether there will be a lecture on diabetes at all in another fifty years' time. In some ways one would be only too pleased to believe this as it would surely mean that the subject was no longer one of pressing medical importance. In fact I do not believe that it would be wildly over-optimistic to suspect that in fifty years' time this might be the case. Advances in the understanding and control of immunological processes are very likely to have led to the prevention of insulin-dependent diabetes by then. The other 80% of diabetes, the so-called non-insulin-dependent diabetes which is my topic, may be reduced to a group of diverse but rare genetically determined abnormalities which, if advances in gene therapy have not rendered them innocuous, will be considered under their own specific title rather than as 'diabetes'.

What I am going to propose below is that the vast majority of non-insulin-dependent diabetes, affecting an estimated 100 million people worldwide, is within sight of becoming a preventable disease – at least in theory. The sobering fact is that if these ideas are correct it will be 50 years before they have a major impact on the incidence of the condition.

In reviewing the problems which are posed by diabetes let me start by quoting what Pavy said at the beginning of his first lecture in 1878 [3]:

> From time immemorial diabetes has been one of the most inscrutable of diseases. All sorts of vague notions have existed regarding the nature of the affection and at the present day it must be said that opinions are by no means settled upon the fundamental points to be dealt with.

I doubt whether my colleagues in the field would have any qualms if in introducing my topic I simply plagiarized Pavy. Diabetes continues to present fascinating problems and is indeed a microcosm of medicine. There is virtually no organ or system in the body which is not involved in some way in its aetiology, control or complications. Many advances in biomedical science have sprung directly or indirectly from attempts to understand diabetes and to improve its control. Despite all this it is true to say that current opinions are sharply divided as to where to even start looking for the fundamental mechanisms leading to the disease. In discussing non-insulin-dependent diabetes I want first of all to outline our own attempts to learn something of the aetiology of this disorder. Then from our data I shall propose a novel hypothesis which may explain at least one major mechanism leading to diabetes and which also may help to explain some of its puzzling features. Finally, based upon these ideas, I want to consider the wider implications for future research, and for improving health more generally.

There are a number of features of non-insulin-dependent diabetes which need to be explained in any theory of the aetiology of the condition. It is generally agreed that non-insulin-dependent diabetes is strongly familial although the role of genetic factors is less clear-cut. There are pronounced and unexplained differences in the geographical prevalence which in extremes varies from 1% or less up to 40%. Socio-economic factors appear to influence the incidence [6] and finally non-insulin-dependent diabetes is found in association with other so-called degenerative or age-related conditions.

The exact role of genetic factors and inheritance remains elusive. Certainly unlike insulin-dependent diabetes there does not appear to be an HLA association or an involvement of autoimmunity. High concordance rates for identical twins have suggested that there is strong genetic determination of the condition. On the other hand the concordance rates reported for non-identical twins vary widely and in some studies approach those of identical twins [7]. The pattern of inheritance, if so it is, is very odd – certainly not simply Mendelian. For example, it has been shown that people with two diabetic siblings are more likely to develop diabetes than they are if they have two diabetic parents [8]. It has also been observed that an offspring is twice as likely to develop diabetes if the mother is diabetic rather than the father [9].

North American Indian populations often have a very high prevalence of diabetes, most notably the Pima Indians who have the highest prevalence worldwide of some 30–40% of the adult population [10]. This population represents one of many in which a rapid move from subsistence living to relative affluence and inactivity with a consequent high frequency of gross obesity leads to diabetes. Another example of a population with an almost equal prevalence of diabetes is that on the Pacific island of Nauru [11]. This population went from virtual starvation under Japanese occupation during the war to post-war affluence resulting from the mining of phosphate. Examples of migration-associated higher incidences of diabetes include rural to urban migration in many countries [12], removal of starving Ethiopian Jews to Israel [13] and immigrants from the Indian subcontinent in the UK [14].

Several years ago Neal proposed the thrifty genotype hypothesis [15] in an attempt to explain the persistence in the population of genes causing diabetes and the effect of adequate or over nutrition on its prevalence. The essence of this hypothesis is that genes which predispose to diabetes in an affluent society are beneficial to survival in conditions of poor nutrition. Hence the thrifty genotype is one which is best constituted to survive conditions of semi-starvation. However, recognizing the detrimental influence on populations of recent affluence it is puzzling to note that a study of nine UK towns selected to cover a range of socio-economic conditions found an increased incidence of non-insulin-dependent diabetes in towns in a worse socio-economic situation [6].

Lastly, in considering the puzzling features of non-insulin-dependent diabetes, I want to mention the abnormalities which are not necessarily a direct result of diabetes but which are found with high frequency in association with it. These include hypertension, hyperlipidaemia and ischaemic heart disease, a situation which Reaven has described as syndrome X and hypothesized as being due to a common underlying abnormality of insulin resistance [16].

These then are some of the puzzling features of non-insulin-dependent diabetes. I now want to turn to a consideration of the problems and controversies which have confronted attempts to investigate the pathogenesis of the condition. Since all the acute features of the diabetes, but not necessarily of the associated conditions, can be corrected by the administration of insulin the obvious starting point of any investigation of the aetiology of this condition is to establish the role of insulin – is it deficient, inactive or both?

Now it is extraordinary and chastening to have to admit over 30 years after the introduction of the radio-immunoassay of insulin by Yalow and Berson that we are still unable to provide a generally accepted answer to this question. Opinions on the whole are highly polarized into those who favour insulin deficiency as opposed to the other strongly held view that insulin resistance is the most important basic defect.

There are at least three good reasons why we continue to labour under such difficulty. Firstly it is clear that situations in which there is primary insulin deficiency lead secondarily to marked insulin resistance [17]. There are a variety of mechanisms which underlie this. Secondly animals subjected to long-term hyperglycaemia by glucose infusion show reduced insulin secretion [18]. Therefore although it is well established now that non-insulin-dependent diabetics virtually uniformly show a reduced early insulin secretion during a glucose tolerance test, we cannot be sure from this alone that it represents the primary loss of function. Thirdly many insulin radio-immunoassays measure proinsulin-like molecules as if they were insulin [19]. The importance of this is that the proinsulin-like molecules which exist in the circulation have very little biological insulin-like activity [20]. Furthermore their concentration may be very high in the plasma of non-insulin-dependent diabetics [21, 22]. Thus without a specific insulin assay it would be possible to be misled into thinking that a diabetic has in the region of twice as much insulin in the circulation as was really the case. From this one would come to the conclusion, erroneous on these grounds, that the diabetic was insulin resistant.

I should like to briefly illustrate how we have overcome the latter problem as I believe that the approach we have used is more widely applicable to other measurement problems of this nature. Also the ability to measure specifically unprocessed or partially processed proinsulin appears to be capable of revealing early and subtle changes in β-cell function. It is interesting to note in passing that the problems of measuring insulin today are mirrored by earlier problems of measuring glucose. Pavy in 1878 [3] spent most of his two Croonian Lectures describing in great detail how it was that his method of measuring the blood sugar, as it was then described, was superior to that of Claude Bernard and his followers. He describes Bernard's new test as fundamentally fallacious. In reply one of Bernard's school states: 'I will not have the cruelty to state to Dr Pavy that his process is found to have been described a number of years back by Fresenius and Henri Rose whom he could have quoted.' To which Pavy replies 'I will refer to the criticism of it [that is Pavy's method] that has been put forward by the partisans of Bernard's views in Paris. I will not condescend to notice the rancorous remarks which the latter writer has indulged in. I will not have the cruelty to say more than that capacity as an observer, and fidelity as a writer, are needful qualifications for a man who professes to be devoted to science.'

To return to the problem of measuring insulin, several years ago we suggested the use of two antibodies – one on a solid phase and one labelled – as a means of improving assay specificity [23, 24]. The advent of the monoclonal antibody technique [25], and of bioengineered proinsulin [26], greatly aided our attempts to produce highly specific assays for human insulin, intact and the split proinsulins [27].

Having taken such trouble to refine the assay methodology it was at first disappointing to merely confirm what we and the vast majority of other workers over many years have found previously, namely that the rapid release of insulin in response to glucose is deficient in non-insulin-dependent diabetes [28].

The concentrations of intact and partially processed proinsulin are also raised [28]. The simplest explanation of the raised concentrations of the proinsulin-like molecules is that chronic hyperglycaemia accelerates the transit of the insulin precursors through the processing pathway, thereby leading to less complete processing. We do not as yet know whether this is the actual explanation or whether some more basic defect is responsible. Nevertheless these data do show very clearly that the early insulin response virtually completely separates the normal and diabetic subjects [28]. However, for the reasons I have mentioned previously we do not know that this change represents the primary abnormality. To resolve this it is essential to study the prediabetic condition and this we are in the process of doing.

At this stage of our research some 4 years ago I had the great good fortune to become closely acquainted with Professor David Barker, the director of the MRC Environmental Epidemiology Unit in Southampton, and with his research into cardiovascular disease and hypertension. This research had established, amongst many other things, epidemiological links between birth weight and weight at 1 year and adult deaths from cardiovascular disease

[29], and also between birth weight and subsequent adult blood pressure [30]. Mindful of the links between diabetes, hypertension and cardiovascular disease we embarked on a collaborative study of the relationship between birth weight and weight at 1 year and adult onset non-insulin-dependent diabetes (NIDDM).

We recruited men of mean age 64 years in the county of Hertfordshire where from 1911 onwards each birth was notified by the attending midwife. A health visitor then recorded birth weight and again weight at 1 year. Of 468 men of known birth weight and weight at 1 year who attended the clinic fasting, 408 had an oral 75 g glucose tolerance test, and 370 sets of complete data were obtained; 93 men were found to have either impaired glucose tolerance (IGT) or previously undiagnosed NIDDM. The proportion of men having IGT or NIDDM fell consistently from the highest to the lowest birth weight group, as it also did from the highest to the lowest weight at 1 year group. The trends with birth weight or weight at 1 year and glucose intolerance were highly significant with odds ratios for having decreased glucose tolerance of 6.6 or 8.2 going from the highest to the lowest weights at birth or at 1 year respectively. The plasma 32–33 split proinsulin concentration in the fasting state fell with increasing weight at 1 year. Blood pressure was inversely related to birth weight and strongly related to plasma glucose and 32–33 split proinsulin concentrations. It was concluded that impairment of early growth (foetal and infant) is strongly linked to deterioration of glucose tolerance in adult life. The well recognized link between hypertension and impaired glucose tolerance could be explained by reduced intrauterine growth and development [31].

Based upon these results and a review of the related literature we have gone on to develop a 'thrifty phenotype' hypothesis of the aetiology of non-insulin-dependent diabetes [32]. The core feature of this hypothesis is that poor nutrition of the foetus and young infant is detrimental to the development of the structure and function of pancreatic β-cells. The experimental data thus far are limited but it appears that the amino acid supply to the foetus is one key nutritional feature; however, others cannot be excluded. Studies of offspring from pregnant rats fed a protein-deficient diet show substantial changes in islet vasculature as well as the growth of β-cells [33]. If the offspring are maintained on a low protein diet, by 70 days glucose tolerance is impaired with a poorer insulin response to glucose [34]. Thus the detrimental effects of malnutrition may involve more complex changes of islet structure (such as vasculature) as well as simple defects of the β-cells themselves. We have further proposed that more complex interactions of the type and timing of foetal and infant malnutrition may underlie the conjunction of conditions known to associate with impaired glucose tolerance which are sometimes referred to as 'syndrome X'. These have previously been hypothesized to be secondary consequences of insulin resistance [16]. We suggest that they are linked through early malnutrition leading to altered growth and development. The poor development of β-cell structure and function leads to NIDDM at a time in adult life which is determined further by the detrimental effects of obesity and ageing on insulin sensitivity and secretion.

On the basis of these ideas we can offer an explanation of the features of non-insulin-dependent diabetes. High concordance rates between identical twins who commonly share the same placenta and early environment must be reassessed. Whilst currently accepted as the strongest evidence of a genetic determination of the condition it is obviously also consistent with a strong influence of the early environment. Further studies are required to establish the true concordance rates and the concordance rates in non-identical twins. Ideally these should be related to birth weight.

The stronger risk of developing diabetes conferred by having two siblings with diabetes compared with both parents with diabetes is of course consistent with a role for the intrauterine and early postnatal environment, as is the importance of maternal transmission.

The thrifty phenotype hypothesis offers a ready explanation of the oddities of the geographical distribution of non-insulin-dependent diabetes. It proposes that the growth and function of the β-cells is determined by early life nutrition. An infant reared in a malnourished environment is only equipped to survive in such an environment. However, if in later life the individual is exposed to normal or supranormal nutrition and becomes obese then an inadequate ability to produce insulin in the presence of obesity results in diabetes. Similarly the higher incidence of diabetes in towns with a poor socioeconomic situation may be explained by malnutrition during pregnancy. It is well documented that the mean birth weight is lower in populations existing in a poor socio-economic environment. Such populations also have an increased tendency to become obese as adults.

David Barker's work on ischaemic heart disease and hypertension showed them to be linked to early growth failure. Our joint studies of diabetes and impaired glucose tolerance reconfirmed the link of hypertension with small babies and also showed its close link with poor glucose tolerance and β-cell dysfunction. Thus defects of early growth could well explain the association of hypertension and impaired glucose tolerance. Whether hyperlipidaemia and other risk factors for ischaemic heart disease are similarly related is a subject of our current research.

An implication of the thrifty phenotype hypothesis is that if we discover the causes of poor foetal nutrition and can overcome them we can prevent much of this type of diabetes. Worldwide undoubtedly the commonest cause of foetal malnutrition is maternal malnutrition. If this could be prevented could we reduce diabetes? There is one natural experiment which suggests this may be true. On the Pacific island of Nauru, especially during the Second World War, the population existed at the borderline of starvation. Shortly after the war phosphate deposits were found and mined to great economic advantage. The population as a whole became affluent, obese and sedentary. A study of the prevalence of diabetes in the population 20 years after the end of the war in 1975/76 revealed diabetes of epidemic proportions. The population was studied again in 1983 and then in 1987 and the latest survey results have just been published [35].

The prevalence of IGT in 1987 was found to have decreased significantly from 21.1% in 1975/1976 to 8.7% in 1987. The progression from normal to impaired glucose tolerance or NIDDM had decreased dramatically. There were no changes in the recognized risk factors to account for these findings. The authors attributed them to changes in mortality and fertility reducing the frequency of the diabetic genotype in the population.

This seems hard to reconcile with the speed of the effect and the fact that it is limited to the section of the population born post war. To me it seems much more likely that infant growth and development have greatly improved post war and this has been associated with an improvement in β-cell growth and function. Thus it is possible that if we were able to institute appropriate measures now to optimize foetal and infant growth, 50 years from now we could see a dramatic reduction in the incidence of non-insulin-dependent diabetes.

Finally I want to look ahead and consider the implications of these ideas for future research, and the promotion of better health.

As far as future research is concerned I believe that a considerable change in the direction of research and use of resources is required. Much research effort and money has been devoted to trying to find adult diets, life styles and drugs with which to improve the health and longevity of the population. The comparative interest in foetal and infant health is small. Yet basic research has shown very clearly that a failure of cell multiplication in foetal life is never rectified later. In this context I would like to recall for you the rough calculation which indicates that to grow a term infant from a fertilized ovum requires some 42 rounds of cell division, whereas to go from the term infant to the adult only a further 5 rounds [36]. Surely we should be concentrating more effort on optimizing the first 42 rounds than in tinkering with the adult system which has the least plasticity? Our data in relation to diabetes shows that provided an individual reaches the age of 1 year with the highest growth trajectory, a very considerable degree of adult obesity can be tolerated without precipitating even impaired glucose tolerance, let alone diabetes. Furthermore a great deal of work and money is being devoted to sequencing the whole human genome. No amount of sequence data would reveal the mechanism which we propose and which, if correct, relates to a major part of the adult burden of morbidity and mortality. Thirdly in assessing and promoting the health of the population the conclusion must be that we, as medical scientists, must increasingly move away from the wards and outpatients and out into the community. Diabetes provides an excellent model. There is very little, if anything, left to learn of its aetiology by studying the established disease. We must develop methods which allow us to identify developing problems and this is probably true of all the so-called degenerative or age-related diseases. A simple model of these processes is shown in Figure 1.

This model shows diagrammatically the concept that diseases involving the failure of specific organ functions are related to the amount of function provided by early growth and development, the rate of decline of function with age and the demand for the function. In the diagram demand for function is shown as increasing with age but of course this may not be the case in all situations. However, the underlying concept of disease emerging when demand exceeds supply remains applicable.

We have very little idea of what is actually happening in most late onset conditions in relation to even this simple model. Should our main concern be

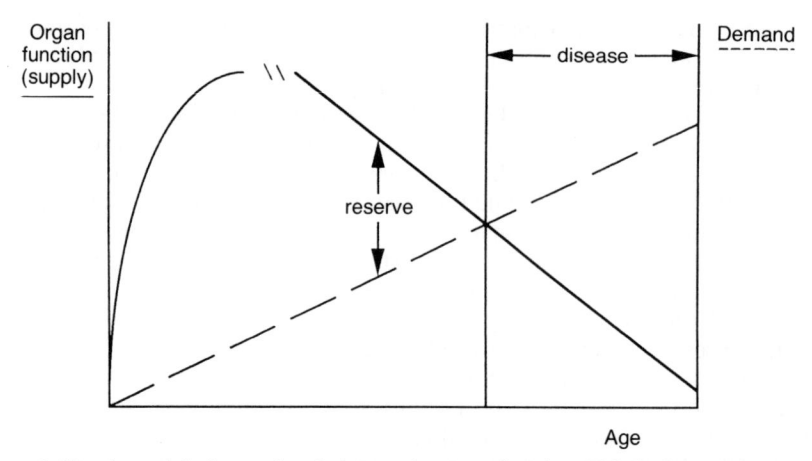

Figure 1. Simple model of age-related changes in organ function. This is shown as reaching a maximum early in life (sometimes at birth) and then, possibly after an interval, declining with age. In this model demand for function is shown as increasing with age but of course this need not be the case in all situations. In order for disease to occur the decline in function of the organ must exceed the demand for that function.

in achieving peak tissue function, delaying decline or reducing demand? In most situations we do not even have techniques for following these processes. Diabetes is unusual in this respect (Figure 2).

Using the oral glucose tolerance test we can identify impaired glucose tolerance which is a prediabetic change and precedes clinical presentation. With new methods for measuring the intermediates of insulin production we may be able to detect still more subtle and early stages of β-cell dysfunction. It is clear that changes in the 32–33 split proinsulin intermediate are providing an early signal of β-cell dysfunction. Further work is required to improve the sensitivity and specificity of this assay. Our hope is that by this means we can push the recognition of dysfunction further back in the natural history of diabetes. It is heartening to see that advances in basic science teach us how to probe into the subcellular processes of small collections of cells hidden both anatomically and physiologically at the back of the abdomen.

Our studies suggest that the intravenous glucose tolerance test is a highly reproducible maximum stimulus with which we may be able to measure the relative functioning mass of β-cells [37], thus defining the peak capacity of the young adult. From here we can and should map the relative decline of function with age. Measurements of obesity and insulin resistance will allow us to plot changes in demand and from all this data with patience and persistence we can unravel the factors leading to clinical disease.

I believe that diabetes again shows the way forward for other degenerative conditions. It is surprising, and I think that those of us who are in clinical biochemistry have been slow to see this, that there are so very few function tests aimed at defining the functional reserve of critical organs. We seem to be content to detect the loss of homeostasis coinciding with a disease and, all too late, to institute treatment of the disease. If we had simple and economical

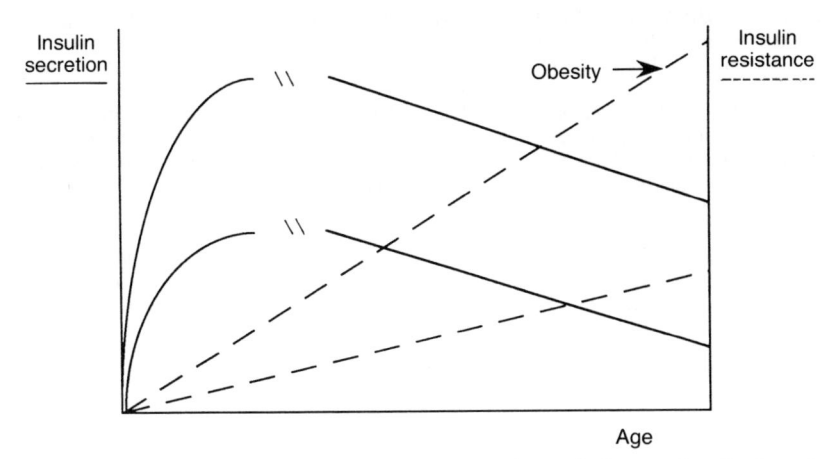

Figure 2. An illustration of how the model in Figure 1 may be applied to non-insulin-dependent diabetes. It depicts the suggestion that the ability to secrete insulin is determined early in life and then declines with age. The diagram also shows insulin resistance increasing with age and the additional increase in resistance due to obesity. Thus an individual with a poor initial development of β-cell function and obesity will develop diabetes relatively early in life.

techniques for defining tissue reserve much earlier in life, we could then initiate preventive measures with a hope of stopping or at least delaying clinical disease by targeting the vulnerable population.

In recognizing the need to optimize foetal and infant health in order to improve adult health we in medicine and the biosciences face once again a humbling admission. This is that the greatest improvements in health result from improvements in the socio-economic circumstances of peoples rather than from scientific and technological advances in medicine. Nevertheless I do think we can hope to elucidate the chain of events which leads from socio-economic deprivation to ill health and disease such that those who make the economic decisions are provided with the evidence from which social priorities can be decided.

I have used this opportunity to digress into broader aspects of medicine and the promotion of health than my title strictly justifies. Despite this the 'underlying message' is very simple and was recognized many years ago, as were so many truths, by Francis Bacon (in his essay 'Of Regiments of Health' 1625): 'For strength of Nature in youth passeth over many excesses which are owing a man till his age.'

REFERENCES
1. Graham G. A review of the causes of diabetes mellitus. *Br Med J 1940; ii*: 479–482
2. Graham G. The role of the liver in diabetes mellitus. *Br Med J 1940; ii*: 513–516
3. Pavy F W. On certain points connected with diabetes. *Lancet 1878; i*: 447–449; 483–485; 557–558; 633–634; 705–707
4. Pavy FW. A new departure in connexion with diabetes. *Lancet 1894; ii*: 1–3; 65–68; 121–125; 177–180
5. Pavy FW. Points connected with the pathology and treatment of diabetes. *Br Med J 1897; ii*: 1494–1496; 1565–1568

6 Barker DJP, Gardner MJ, Power C. Incidence of diabetes amongst people aged 18-50 years in nine British towns. *Diabetologia 1982; 22*: 421-425
7 Newman B, Selby JV, King M-C et al. Concordance for type 2 (non-insulin-dependent) diabetes mellitus in male twins. *Diabetologia 1987; 30*: 763-768
8 Beaty TH, Neel JV, Fajans SS. Identifying risk factors for diabetes in first degree relatives of non-insulin-dependent diabetes patients. *Am J Epidemiol 1982; 115*: 380-397
9 Alcolado JC, Alcolado R. Importance of maternal history of non-insulin-dependent diabetes patients. *Br Med J 1991; 302*: 1178-1180
10 Knowler WC, Savage PJ, Nagulesparan M et al. Obesity, insulin resistance and diabetes mellitus in the Pima Indians. In Köbberling J, Tattersall R, eds. *The Genetics of Diabetes Mellitus*, Serono Symposium No 47. London: Academic Press. 1982: 244-250
11 Zimmet PZ, Kirk RL, Sergeantson SW. Genetic and environmental interactions for non-insulin-dependent diabetes in high prevalence Pacific populations. In Köbberling J, Tattersall R, *The Genetics of Diabetes*, Serono Symposium No 47. London: Academic Press. 1982: 211-224
12 Jarrett RJ. Epidemiology of non-insulin-dependent diabetes mellitus. In Köbberling J, Tattersall R, *The Genetics of Diabetes*, Serono Symposium No 47. London: Academic Press. 1982: 195-199
13 Cohen MP, Stern E, Rusecki Y, Zeidler A. High prevalence of diabetes in young adult Ethiopian immigrants to Israel. *Diabetes 1988; 37*: 824-828
14 McKeigue PM, Marmot MG, Syndercombe Court YD et al. Diabetes, hyperinsulinaemia, and coronary risk factors in Bangladeshis in East London. *Br Heart J 1988; 60*: 390-396
15 Neal JV. Diabetes mellitus: a thrifty genotype rendered detrimental by 'progress'? *Am J Hum Genet 1962; 14*: 353-362
16 Reaven GM. Role of insulin resistance in human disease. *Diabetes 1988; 37*: 1595-1607
17 Weir GC, Leaky JL, Bonner-Weir S. Experimental reduction of β-cell mass: implications for the pathogenesis of diabetes. *Diabetes/Metabolism Reviews 1986; 2*: 125-161
18 Leaky JL, Bonner-Weir S, Weir GC. Minimal chronic hyperglycaemia is a critical determinant of impaired insulin secretion after an incomplete pancreatectomy. *J Clin Invest 1988; 81*: 1407-1414
19 Temple RC, Clark PMS, Nagi DK et al. Radioimmunoassay may overestimate insulin in non-insulin-dependent diabetes. *Clin Endocrinol 1990; 32*: 689-693
20 Peavy DE, Bounner MR, Duckworth WC et al. Receptor binding and biological potency of several split forms (conversion intermediates) of human proinsulin. Studies in cultured IM-9 lymphocytes and in vivo and in vitro in rats. *J Biol Chem 1985; 260*: 13989-13994
21 Gorden P, Hendricks CM, Roth J. Circulating proinsulin-like component in man: increased proportion in hypoinsulinaemic state. *Diabetologia 1974; 10*: 469-474
22 Mako ME, Starr JI, Rubenstein AH. Circulating proinsulin in patients with maturity onset diabetes. *Am J Med 1977; 63*: 865-869
23 Addison GM, Hales CN. The immunoradiometric assay. In Kirkham KE, Hunter WM, eds. *Radioimmunoassay Methods*. Edinburgh: Churchill Livingstone. 1971: 447-461; 481-487
24 Hales CN, Woodhead JS. Labelled antibodies and their use in the immunoradiometric assay. In Van Vunakis H, Lagone JJ, eds. *Methods in Enzymology, Vol 70 of Immunochemical Techniques, Part A*. London: Academic Press. 1980: 334-355
25 Kohler G, Milstein C. Continuous cultures of fused cells secreting antibody of predefined specificity. *Nature 1975; 256*: 495-497
26 Frank BH, Pettee JM, Simmerman RE, Burck PH. The production of human proinsulin and its transformation to human insulin and C-peptide. In Rich DH, Gross E, eds. *Peptides: Synthesis-Structure-Function. Proceedings of the Seventh American Peptide Symposium*. Pierce Chemical Company. 1981: 729-738.
27 Sobey WF, Beer SF, Carrington CA et al. Sensitive and specific two-site immunoradiometric assays for human insulin, proinsulin, 65-66 split and 32-33 split proinsulins. *Biochem J 1989; 260*: 535-541

28 Temple RC, Carrington CA, Luzio SD et al. Insulin deficiency in non-insulin-dependent diabetes. *Lancet 1989; i*: 293–295
29 Barker DJP, Winter PD, Osmond C et al. Weight in infancy and death from ischaemic heart disease. *Lancet 1989; ii*: 577–580
30 Barker DJP, Bull AR, Osmond C, Simmonds SJ. Fetal and placental size and risk of hypertension in adult life. *Br Med J 1990; 301*: 259–262
31 Hales CN, Barker DJP, Clark PMS et al. Foetal and infant growth and impaired glucose tolerance at age 64. *Br Med J 1991; 303*: 1019–1022
32 Hales CN, Barker DJP. Type 2 (non-insulin-dependent) diabetes mellitus: the thrifty phenotype hypothesis. *Diabetologia* 1992; in press
33 Snoeck A, Remacle C, Reusens B, Hoet JJ. Effect of a low protein diet during pregnancy on the foetal rat endocrine pancreas. *Biol Neonate 1990; 57*: 107–118
34 Dahri S, Snoeck A, Reusens-Billen B et al. Islet function in offspring of mothers on low-protein diet during gestation. *Diabetes 1991; 40 (Suppl 2)*: 115–120
35 Dowse GK, Simmet PZ, Finch CF, Collins VR. Decline in incidence of epidemic glucose intolerance in Nauruans: implications for the 'Thrifty Genotype'. *Am J Epidemiol 1991; 133*: 1093–1104
36 Milner RDG. Mechanisms of overgrowth. In Sharp F, Fraser RB, Milner RDG, eds. *Foetal Growth, Proceedings of the twentieth study group of the Royal College of Obstetricians and Gynaecologists*. London: Royal College of Obstetricians and Gynaecologists. 1989: 139–148
37 Rayman G, Clark PMS, Schneider AE, Hales CN. The third phase insulin response to intravenous glucose is highly reproducible. *Diabetologia 1990; 33*: 631–634

CORONARY ANGIOPLASTY – HOW MUCH AND HOW MUCH?

David H Bennett
Wythenshawe Hospital, Manchester

Percutaneous transluminal balloon coronary angioplasty, first performed in 1977 [1], has become a widely accepted method of myocardial revascularization.

The purpose of this paper is to discuss how many patients in the UK may need coronary angioplasty and what resources are required. Before doing this, the current practice of balloon angioplasty is briefly described.

BALLOON ANGIOPLASTY

Technique

The procedure is carried out in a cardiac catheterization laboratory under local anaesthesia. A guiding catheter (approximate diameter 2.7mm) is introduced into a femoral or brachial artery and is advanced to and engaged in the ostium of the left or right coronary artery. Through the guiding catheter, a flexible guide wire (0.25–0.45mm diameter) is passed into the diseased branch of the artery and steered across the stenosis. The guide wire facilitates introduction of the dilatation catheter into the coronary artery. The dilatation catheter consists of a tube of approximate diameter 1.2mm with, at its tip, a 2cm long sausage-shaped balloon which can be inflated to a predetermined transverse diameter (range of sizes: 1.5–4.5mm). The appropriate size dilatation catheter is advanced over the guide wire and the balloon is positioned in the stenosis. The balloon is inflated for a short period (20–300 seconds) to a pressure of 4 to 10 atmospheres and is then withdrawn. The result is assessed by angiography. If necessary, further balloon inflations at higher pressures or with a larger balloon can be carried out.

Progress in technology and, in particular, reduction in the profile of the uninflated balloon and improvements in the flexibility, 'trackability' and 'pushability' of the balloon catheter have now made it possible to reach and cross most stenoses.

Indications
The main clinical indications are the same as for coronary artery bypass surgery: the relief of angina (stable, unstable or post-infarction). In certain situations, angioplasty is preferable to rather than merely an alternative to bypass surgery: in particular, angina in patients who have already undergone or who are not suitable for bypass surgery can often be managed successfully by angioplasty.

Short, discrete stenoses in one or more coronary artery are ideally suited for balloon angioplasty. Long, very tight or tortuous lesions or those with intracoronary thrombus can be dilated but the risk of complication is increased [2, 3]. In a review of a large number of coronary angiograms carried out in a North American centre, approximately half of patients requiring revascularization were found to have lesions suitable for coronary angioplasty [4].

In contrast to surgery, angioplasty necessitates a stay in hospital of only 2 or 3 days, there is no need for convalescence and it is not difficult to undertake repeat procedures should new coronary lesions develop. Angioplasty is somewhat less expensive than bypass surgery [5].

Results
Success rates in excess of 90% for dilating stenosed coronary arteries are being achieved in many centres [3]. The results are less good when the vessel is occluded, and with coronary arteries which have been totally occluded for more than 3 months success rates are in the order of only 70% even in the most experienced hands [6].

The main acute complication of coronary angioplasty is abrupt closure of the dilated segment due to dissection, thrombosis or spasm. The artery can often be reopened by further dilatation but emergency bypass surgery is sometimes required. In a recent review of 1800 procedures, the incidences of acute occlusion and the need for bypass surgery were 6.8% and 2.4%, respectively [2].

In the 2 to 6 months after angioplasty, restenosis, which usually necessitates further dilatation, occurs in at least 30% of patients [7].

The long-term results of angioplasty are good. Any subsequent cardiac events are usually the result of progression of lesions in coronary arteries that have not been dilated or, in the case of multivessel disease, the consequence of incomplete revascularization [8, 9].

CURRENT ACTIVITY IN THE UK
Coronary angioplasty activity in the UK is monitored by the British Cardiovascular Intervention Society. Fifty-three centres, nine of which are in the private sector, currently carry out the procedure. According to data acquired in 1989, the average number of operators per centre able to perform angioplasty without supervision was 3.3 [10].

Number of procedures
A steady increase in the numbers of procedures carried out each year has

been observed (Table I). In 1990, 8459 procedures were carried out: a rate of 148 per million of the population. As with coronary artery bypass surgery, this level of activity is much lower than in most European countries and in North America (Table II). In the USA, more patients are now being treated by coronary angioplasty than by bypass surgery [11].

TABLE I. Number of angioplasties carried out in UK per annum

1984	712	1988	5047
1985	1642	1989	7145
1986	2781	1990	8459
1987	4152		

TABLE II. Revascularization procedures per million population in 1990

	Angioplasty	Bypass surgery
USA	1072	1050
Belgium	569	800
Netherlands	545	733
Canada	453	675
West Germany	543	520
France	400	425
Switzerland	354	400
Australia	229	670
UK	148	240
Italy	79	190
Japan	200	55

Results

In 1990, 83% of procedures were for dilatation of a single vessel. The mortality was 0.62%, success rate 86% and referral rate for emergency bypass surgery 2.0%. For multivessel dilatations, the mortality, success rate and emergency surgical rates were 1.1%, 87% and 2.6%, respectively.

Procedures per centre

There is a marked variation between centres in the number of angioplasties carried out. In 1990, seven centres each performed more than 300 procedures, 28 centres performed 100–300 procedures and 16 centres each carried out less than 100 procedures.

The proportion of patients undergoing coronary angiography in 1990 who were referred for angioplasty also varied from centre to centre, with a range of 2–32% (mean 13%).

Number of cardiologists

Most coronary angiograms and angioplasties are carried out by cardiologists. Assessment of patients in district general hospitals who may require revascularization is best done by a physician trained in cardiology [12].

In 1990, there were only 145 posts in whole-time adult cardiology in the UK. In addition, there were 134 physicians spending more than 40% of their time in adult cardiology [13]. The total number of posts in adult and paediatric cardiology, defined as physicians spending more than 40% of their time in cardiology, was 320, i.e. 5.6 per million of the population. Data published in 1989 [14] showed that European and Scandinavian countries had substantially larger numbers of cardiologists (Table III). As far back as 1974, the American College of Cardiology recommended that there should be 60 cardiologists per million of the population [15]. In 1988, industry estimates indicated that there were no less than 2400 physicians in the USA carrying out coronary angioplasty.

TABLE III. Number of qualified cardiologists in some European and Scandinavian countries

Country	Cardiologists/per million population
Belgium	27
Germany	26
Austria	20
Sweden	46
Norway	37
Finland	10
Netherlands	30
Italy	118
France	65
Switzerland	40
UK	3

COST OF CORONARY ANGIOPLASTY

In calculating the cost of the procedure, it is necessary to incorporate the costs of disposable materials and of keeping a patient in hospital, and also the 'fixed costs' of running cardiac catheterization laboratories, of providing X-ray and other equipment and of general service overheads.

These costings have recently been carried out at Wythenshawe Hospital, a regional cardiothoracic centre which carries out 1000 open heart operations and 3500 catheterization laboratory procedures annually. All procedural details were recorded on a computer database, including equipment used and the times of the start and end of each procedure. Data were acquired from a 12 month period starting in October 1990.

Disposable materials

The most expensive item is the dilatation catheter. On average 1.45 balloon catheters were used per procedure. Table IV shows the cost of disposable items used.

TABLE IV. Disposable items used during coronary angioplasty

Item	Number	Cost (£)
Dilatation catheter	1.45	652
Guiding catheter	1.2	98
Guide wire	1.1	75
Balloon inflation device	1.0	69
Additional equipment		56
Drugs		8
Contrast media		27
Total		985
Total including value added tax		1157

Inpatient stay

Total ward costs including nursing, catering, laundry, medical records, portering, ward consumables, capital charges, general service overheads and electrocardiography were determined:

Stay on cardiology ward (2 days)	£177
Stay on coronary care unit (1 day)	£188
Resting and exercise electrocardiography	£62
Total	£427

Fixed costs

The method used to calculate the 'fixed costs' of running the hospital's two cardiac catheterization laboratories can be applied to all departments to ensure that a hospital's total costs are absorbed. Costing was calculated on a cost per utilized minute basis.

The costs of medical, nursing, technical and radiographic staff, and capital charges on X-ray and other equipment were included in the calculation as were general service overheads such as cleaning, building and engineering maintenance, electricity and water, and capital charges on land and buildings.

The cost of consultant and junior staff was determined as that proportion of the total contracted time which was spent in the catheterization laboratories. The cost of the hospital's general service overheads which was apportioned to the catheterization laboratories was based on floor area occupied by the laboratories as a proportion of the total area occupied by the hospital.

The cost was computed at £4.03 per utilized minute.

Total cost of coronary angioplasty

The total cost of angioplasty can be calculated as the costs of consumables and inpatient treatment plus the product of the fixed costs per minute and length of the procedure (average times spent performing a single and a multivessel coronary angioplasty were 45 and 62 minutes). The cost of repeat angioplasty for restenosis should also be allowed for in the analysis; 26.9% of patients underwent angioplasty for restenosis.

Thus, the total costs for single and multivessel angioplasty were estimated to be £2240 and £2326, respectively. (Using the same methods as described above, the cost of coronary angiography was estimated to be £279.)

HOW MANY PATIENTS NEED CORONARY ANGIOPLASTY?

A precise assessment of the number of patients needing coronary angioplasty is difficult because of insufficient data and because the indications for the procedure are evolving. However, available information strongly suggests that many more patients in the UK would benefit from angioplasty than actually receive it. As shown above, the frequency of angioplasty in France, Germany and the Benelux countries is two- to threefold greater than in the UK whilst in the USA the frequency is seven times greater! A similar situation applies to coronary artery bypass surgery, so the low rates of angioplasty in this country are not a result of patients receiving an alternative form of revascularization. It might be argued that the higher rates elsewhere reflect unnecessary treatment. However, it is improbable that this could be the complete explanation. It is unlikely that cardiological practice throughout Europe and North America could be so inappropriate.

A working group of the British Cardiac Society has recommended a target of 300 to 500 angioplasties per million of the population [16]. A recent report from the Joint Cardiology Committee of the Royal Colleges of Physicians and Surgeons indicated an immediate need for 300 per million angioplasties in the UK [17]. A rate of 500 per million would bring the UK only up to the rates practised in Europe: a modest target, especially in view of the large number of untreated patients currently on surgical waiting lists [16], let alone the very many patients with coronary disease who have not been referred to a cardiac centre.

RESOURCES REQUIRED FOR EXPANSION OF ACTIVITY

As discussed above, cardiac centres vary in the amount of angioplasty that they undertake and in the proportion of patients undergoing coronary angiography who proceed to angioplasty. The number of procedures carried out is increasing each year and it is likely that expertise in and enthusiasm for angioplasty will spread to the less active centres.

If all 53 centres carried out 300 angioplasties each year the annual rate in the UK would rise from the current rate of 148 per million to 279 per million. Clearly, if the numbers are to increase additional funding will be necessary. At the very least, the cost of consumables will have to be met.

Many centres will be unable to increase activity without funding for extra medical and nursing staff. Moreover, whereas some cardiac catheterization laboratories might not be working at full capacity, many are, for it should not be forgotten that there are other demands on catheterization laboratory time including diagnostic angiography, intracardiac electrophysiology and cardiac pacing. In some centres, therefore, the major expense of an additional laboratory (cost at least £600,000) will be necessary. Compared with Europe, there is a paucity of catheterization laboratories in the UK [16] and it is difficult to envisage an expansion to 500 angioplasties per million without a significant increase in the number of laboratories.

FUTURE DEVELOPMENTS

Apart from shortage of resources, the application of angioplasty is currently limited because of its shortcomings: lack of success in dealing with chronically occluded vessels, risk of acute occlusion at the time of the procedure, incomplete revascularization in multivessel disease and high incidence of restenosis. Though the many new transluminal techniques which are being developed such as atherectomy, laser ablation, intracoronary stenting and rotational drills appear to have only a limited role at present [18], further progress may increase the success of and expand the indications for angioplasty.

Several trials in Europe and North America are underway with the purpose of comparing long-term results of angioplasty with coronary artery bypass surgery and medical therapy. The results of these studies may well modify the indications for angioplasty [16].

SUMMARY

Percutaneous coronary balloon angioplasty is an effective method of myocardial revascularization which has considerable advantages over coronary artery bypass grafting for suitable patients though the limitations of current methods should not be forgotten.

The total costs for single and multivessel balloon angioplasty in a UK cardiac centre have been estimated to be £2240 and £2326, respectively.

Despite the high prevalence of coronary artery disease in the UK, rates for angioplasty as well as for bypass grafting are low in comparison with most European countries and North America. A two- to threefold increase in angioplasty activity would seem to be a modest target. This cannot be achieved without additional funding for the disposable equipment used during each procedure and a substantial increase in staff and cardiac catheterization facilities.

ACKNOWLEDGEMENTS

I am grateful to Mr Stephen Tucker, Cost Accountant, Resource Management Unit, Wythenshawe Hospital, Manchester, for carrying out the cost analysis of coronary angioplasty and to Intervention Ltd, Princes Risborough, Buckinghamshire, for data provided.

REFERENCES

1 Gruntzig AR. Transluminal dilatation of coronary-artery stenosis. *Lancet 1978;* i: 263
2 Detre KM, Holmes DR, Holubkov R et al. Incidence and consequences of periprocedural occlusion. The 1985-1986 National Heart, Lung, and Blood Institute Percutaneous Transluminal Coronary Angioplasty Registry. *Circulation 1990; 82*: 729–750

3   Savage MP, Goldberg S, Hirschfield JW et al. Clinical and angiographic determinants of primary coronary angioplasty success. *J Am Coll Cardiol 1991; 17*: 22-28
4   Weintraub BS, Jones EL, King SB III et al. Changing use of coronary angioplasty and coronary bypass surgery in the treatment of chronic coronary artery disease. *Am J Cardiol 1990; 65*: 183-188
5   Van den Brand M, Van Halem F, Van Den Brink et al. Comparison of costs of percutaneous transluminal coronary angioplasty and coronary bypass surgery for patients with angina pectoris. *Eur Heart J 1990; 11*: 765-771
6   Stone GW, Rutherford BD, McConahay DR et al. Procedural outcome of angioplasty for total coronary artery occlusion: an analysis of 971 lesions in 905 patients. *J Am Coll Cardiol 1990; 15*: 849-856
7   Hirschfield JW, Schwartz JS, Jugo R et al. Restenosis after coronary angioplasty: a multivariate statistical model to relate lesion and procedure variables to restenosis. *J Am Coll Cardiol 1991; 18*: 647-656
8   Faxon D, Ruocco N, Jacobs AK. Long-term outcome of patients after percutaneous coronary angioplasty. *Circulation 1990; 81 (supl IV)*: IV9-IV13
9   Talley JD, Hurst JW, King SB III et al. Clinical outcome 5 years after attempted percutaneous transluminal coronary angioplasty in 427 patients. *Circulation 1988; 77*: 820-829
10 Hubner PJ. Cardiac interventional procedures in the United Kingdom in 1989. *Br Heart J 1991; 66*: 469-471
11 Baim DS. Angioplasty as a treatment for coronary artery disease. *N Engl J Med 1992; 326*: 56-58
12 Report of a working group of the British Cardiac society. Cardiology in the district hospital. *Br Heart J 1987; 58*: 537-546
13 Chamberlain D, Pentecost B, Reval K et al. Staffing in cardiology in the United Kingdom 1990. *Br Heart J 1991; 66*: 395-404
14 Chamberlain D, Bailey L, Sowton E et al. Staffing in cardiology in the United Kingdom 1988. *Br Heart J 1989; 62*: 482-487
15 Adams FH, Mendenhall RC. Evaluation of cardiology training and manpower requirements. *Am J Cardiol 1976; 37*: 941-983
16 Sowton E, de Bono D, Gribbin B et al. Coronary angioplasty in the United Kingdom. *Br Heart J 1991; 66*: 325-331
17 Provision of services for the diagnosis and treatment of heart disease. Fourth Report of a Joint Cardiology Committee of the Royal College of Physicians of London and the Royal College of Surgeons of England. *Br Heart J 1992; 67*: 106-116
18 King SB III. Role of new technology in balloon angioplasty. *Circulation 1991; 84*: 2574-2579

CARDIAC FAILURE – SIZE, COST AND IMPLICATIONS

Philip A Poole-Wilson
National Heart and Lung Institute, London

Disease states are of particular importance to the health of the community if they are common, can be detected by simple methods, and have effective remedies. Heart failure fulfils all of these three criteria, but the significance of the condition in general practice, to the community physician and to the hospital physician has not been sufficiently appreciated until recently. Inevitably at a time when the costs of all medical procedures are under close scrutiny and subject to overt or indirect financial limitations, the cost to benefit ratio of treating heart failure must be assessed by comparison with treatments for other common or even uncommon conditions.

DEFINITIONS

A major problem in the study of heart failure is the meaning of the term. Many definitions have been put forward in the past [1]. In general these have been based on selected physiological and biochemical characteristics of heart failure. No single definition has gained wide acceptance, nor can any of the early definitions be applied easily to epidemiological investigations. In general the term heart failure is used by doctors to transfer information between themselves and for this purpose the term is reasonably satisfactory. Heart failure is a syndrome. A pragmatic definition is that heart failure is a condition in which an abnormality of the heart leads to a characteristic patten of renal, neural and hormonal responses [2]. These responses are similar to those activated in a normal person on standing or during exercise when without this reflex response the blood pressure would fall. The body response in heart failure is that of continuous unremitting exercise and is necessary to maintain the perfusion pressure of the body's vital organs [3]. It is important to emphasize that heart failure must be caused initially by an abnormality of the heart itself even if many of the later manifestations or symptoms are a consequence of changes in the peripheral circulation. For example, the retention of salt and water in chronic heart failure is due to abnormal renal function.

Many phrases have been used to describe particular patterns of heart failure.

In general it is sufficient to describe patients in terms of acute heart failure, circulatory collapse, or chronic heart failure. Other terms such as right or left heart failure, forward and backward heart failure, and congestive heart failure are largely redundant and occasionally misleading.

The immediate causes of chronic heart failure are arrhythmias, valve malfunction, pericardial disease or muscle disorders. Abnormalities of the myocardium are much the most common and this is the abnormality to which the term chronic heart failure is usually applied. Chronic heart failure is divided into those patients who have a cardiomyopathy and those who have an abnormality of function due to coronary artery disease. Cardiomyopathy is a loose term and was originally used to refer to reduced myocardial function of unknown cause. More recently cardiomyopathy has come to be used to describe patients in whom ventricular dysfunction is accompanied by normal coronary arteries. There may be many different aetiologies. Alternative classifications [4] of chronic myocardial heart failure have emphasized loss of contracting muscle, incoordinate contraction, cellular abnormalities and extracellular adaptations. Alteration of the architecture and geometry of the heart including shape, size, fibre orientation, cell slippage and fibrosis may be more important in cardiomyopathy than the function of individual myocytes.

EPIDEMIOLOGY

In comparison with other cardiovascular disorders such as hypertension or coronary artery disease there is a dearth of information on the epidemiology of heart failure. Several studies suggest that 0.5–1% of the population have heart failure, 0.2–0.4% develop heart failure each year and 0.2% of the population are admitted to hospital with heart failure each year [5]. At any one time in a district general hospital in the UK approximately 5% of the patients will have heart failure as a major component of their reason for remaining in hospital [6]. Of these patients 30–40% will be re-admitted to hospital within 1 year. Much of the data on the epidemiology of heart failure has been obtained from the Framingham study [7]. Framingham is a small suburb of Boston and the findings do not necessarily apply to the UK. The study, which began in 1948, has now reported a 20 year follow-up of patients with heart failure. The findings do accord with the limited data obtained elsewhere. However, a major problem remains the basis for the diagnosis of heart failure. If that diagnosis is based solely on symptoms and a physical examination then the accuracy of the diagnosis is poor [8]. The diagnosis of definite heart failure is only correct, as judged by follow-up and detailed investigation, in 57% of men or 14% of women. A further problem is that heart failure is particularly difficult to diagnose in the elderly and heart failure is a disease of the elderly. The average age for heart failure in a recent study of patients in a general practice in north London was 73 years [6], whereas the average age of patients admitted with heart failure to my own hospital (the Royal Brompton and National Heart Hospital) is 54 years, and the age of patients in the recent VHeft II (Veterans Administration Cooperative Vasodilator–Heart Failure Trial) [9] and SOLVD (Studies of Left Ventricular Dysfunction) [10] studies was 60 years.

The prevalence of heart failure increases from 0.06% in those under 65 to 3.5% in those over 65. Heart failure is a disease of the elderly [11, 12]. Not only is heart failure more difficult to diagnose in the elderly but often there is a component of diastolic heart failure associated with a small fibrotic and often thickened ventricle.

An important consideration is how the prevalence of heart failure and hospital admissions for heart failure compares with that of myocardial infarction. There is the possibility that in the national statistics deaths attributable to myocardial infarction are falling while deaths due to heart failure are increasing. There could be an undercharged overall mortality as doctors modify the diagnosis in any individual patient. A recent study in a London district hospital [6] serving 155,000 patients found that 5% of admissions were for heart failure. Of these, 21% were under the age of 65 years, 37% had an arrhythmia on admission and 61% had pulmonary oedema, 30% died during the admission and 14% died in the following year. During a 6 month period there were 2877 admissions to medical and geriatric wards; 140 had heart failure of whom 29 were under the age of 65; 89 had acute infarction and 55 (62%) were under the age of 65. Unstable angina was the reason for admission in 52 (1.8%). The total number of patients admitted with heart failure was 169 compared to 141 admitted with acute coronary syndromes. Those with heart failure were in general more elderly. This information suggests that heart failure is almost as important a medical condition as acute coronary artery disease in terms of the need for the provision of medical facilities.

AETIOLOGY OF HEART FAILURE
The data from the Framingham study [7, 12] suggested that a large proportion of patients, up to 70%, had hypertension as a cause of heart failure. This study was begun in 1948 when treatment for hypertension was not as developed as it is now. Recent large trials [13, 14] have indicated a much lower incidence of hypertension as a cause of heart failure. In our own survey in north London [15, 6] only 6% of patients had hypertension as a cause of the heart failure. Much the most common cause was coronary heart disease. The reason for this change may be that patients with hypertension are now treated and no longer go on to heart failure, but develop coronary artery disease. Some of these patients (perhaps one in three) may develop strokes so are never classified as having either heart failure or coronary artery disease. A further factor is that with the success of thrombolytic therapy the number of patients surviving myocardial infarction is increasing and these patients, who do not have hypertension, may go on to develop heart failure. Since heart failure is so common in the elderly, the prevalence of heart failure will increase as the population ages.

PROGNOSIS IN HEART FAILURE
Until the last decade the natural history of heart failure was largely unknown. A 20 year follow-up of patients in the Framingham study [7] shows that half those diagnosed with heart failure are dead at 4 years but 15% of patients are alive at 20 years. The placebo arms of several of the large recent drug trials

also provide important information on prognosis. In the Consensus I study [16] half the patients with severe heart failure were dead within 6 months. The mortality in the placebo arm of the recent SOLVD [10] and VHeft I and II studies [17, 9] was similar to that of the whole population in Framingham. This suggests that the results of those trials do relate to heart failure as seen in the community. However, the average age of heart failure in the community is approximately 73 years, being higher than the mean age in the patients admitted to those trials, approximately 60 years.

EFFICACY OF TREATMENT

In extreme examples of heart failure controlled trials are unnecessary. For example, the 3 year survival after heart transplantation is 70% in a population where the 1 year mortality with medical treatment is at least 60%. In patients with pulmonary oedema or with sodium retaining heart failure, diuretics are an essential part of treatment. Even in patients who have had evidence of sodium retention but are subsequently treated with diuretics, continuous treatment with diuretics is necessary rather than treatment with an angiotensin converting enzyme (ACE) inhibitor alone [18].

The key questions recently have been whether other treatment, notably digoxin and ACE inhibitors, add further benefit to patients in terms of symptoms and mortality if those drugs are added to treatment with diuretics [19, 20]. The results for digoxin in terms of efficacy are controversial [21, 22]. A large study is currently underway in the USA organized by the National Institutes of Health in order to investigate the impact of digoxin on mortality. An analysis of observational data in patients 1 year after myocardial infarction raises the possibility that digoxin could be harmful in such patients.

Several recent trials have addressed the question of whether ACE inhibitors added to diuretics reduce mortality [19, 20]. The first study, published in 1987, was the Consensus I study [16]. This showed that in patients with very severe heart failure mortality could be reduced. These patients were overloaded with sodium and water despite a mean dose of frusemide of 200mg. Recently the SOLVD trial [10] has reported and shown not only a reduction in mortality but a reduction in hospitalization. This trial was a large study in two parts, a treatment arm and a prevention arm (Tables I and II). In the prevention arm of the study, patients with an ejection fraction below 35% who were not being treated for heart failure were given either an ACE inhibitor or placebo. In this arm neither total mortality nor cardiovascular mortality was reduced. There was a highly significant reduction in hospitalization, progression to overt heart failure and in myocardial infarction. The results of the SOLVD study have been largely confirmed by reports from the VHeft II study [9] and from a single centre study in Germany [23]. Preliminary reports from the SAVE (survival and ventricular enlargement) study showed similar benefits of ACE inhibitors introduced 3 to 16 days after myocardial infarction in a patient population with an ejection fraction less than 40%. The Consensus II study has reported no difference in mortality if ACE inhibitors are begun intravenously early after infarction. Many other trials with ACE inhibitors in heart failure and after infarction are underway. Current conclusions must be that these drugs should be added to diuretics in patients with established chronic heart failure, and that consideration should be given to using these drugs in patients with left ventricular dysfunction (heart failure without evidence of sodium and water retention), particularly in those with large ventricles. The issue of when these drugs should be initiated after myocardial infarction remains unclear. Comparative studies are needed with nitrates, beta-blockers and aspirin. Overall the conclusions from these studies are that there would be substantial benefit to patients if this policy were followed.

TABLE I. A summary of the clinical implications of the use of an ACE inhibitor for the treatment of overt heart failure or for the prevention of disease events in patients with ventricular enlargement but not on any other form of treatment for heart failure (SOLVD trial – 1000 patients in each arm treated for 3 years)

	Treatment	Prevention
Prevention of heart failure	–	90
Reduced hospitalization	200	65
Prevention of infarct/unstable angina	40	35
Reduced deaths	50	15

TABLE II. Annual mortality in patients with heart failure of different severity in recent trials

		Mortality (%)			
		Placebo	Enalapril	Difference	Change (%)
SOLVD Treatment arm		16	12	4	25
VHeFT I and II		20	9	11	55
Consensus I		52	36	16	31
SOLVD	1 year	16	12	4	25
Treatment arm	2 year	25	19	6	24
	4 year	39	32	7	18

COSTS

In order to undertake a cost versus benefit analysis for the treatment of patients with heart failure, it is necessary to consider efficacy (as above), essential investigations, the cost of those investigations, the time devoted by doctors to the proposed treatments and the number of patients at risk. Only recently have sufficient data become available to allow any form of serious analysis in patients with heart failure. There is also the problematic question of how benefits in terms of the duration of life are assessed by comparison with improvements in the quality of life. That is a human issue where personal judgements may differ. The multiple objectives of the treatment of heart failure are shown in Table III. An attempt [24, 25] has been made to compare the costs of many procedures in cardiology (Table IV).

TABLE III. Objectives of treatment in chronic heart failure

1. Prevention	Myocardial damage	Occurrence Progression Further damage
	Recurrence	Symptoms Fluid accumulation Hospitalization
2. Symptoms	Eliminate oedema and fluid retention Increase exercise capacity Reduce fatigue and breathlessness	
3. Prognosis	Reduce mortality	

TABLE IV. An assessment of costs per quality adjusted life year (QALY) for different procedures in cardiology (derived from Williams [24])

Procedure	Cost per QALY (pounds)
Advice by GPs to stop smoking	180
Pacemaker implantation for AV heart block	700
Valve replacement for aortic stenosis	900
CABG for severe angina with LMD	1040
CABG for severe angina with 3 VD	1270
CABG for moderate angina with LMD	1330
Action by GPs to control hypertension	1700
Action by GPs to lower serum cholesterol	1700
CABG for severe angina with 2 VD	2280
CABG for moderate angina with 3 VD	2400
PTCA for severe angina with 1 VD	2400
CABG for mild angina with LMD	2520
Heart transplantation	8000

CABG: coronary artery bypass grafting; PTCA: percutaneous transluminal coronary angioplasty; LMD: left main coronary artery disease; VD: vessel disease.

Most patients with congestive heart failure will require some simple blood tests including a full blood count, plasma electrolytes and a measure of renal function (plasma urea and creatinine), and possibly thyroid function. A chest X-ray and electrocardiogram are essential. In the view of this writer all patients should have an echocardiogram. Exercise testing and cardiac catherization are necessary in selected patients. Radionuclide ventriculography is not essential because data on the size of the ventricle and the ejection fraction can be obtained from the echocardiogram. The entry criteria for most recent trials exclude patients with a high ejection fraction and often this was measured by a nuclear method. A recent report from America [26] indicated how such tests were used by general practitioners, physicians and cardiologists (Table V). The figures not surprisingly show an increased use of investigations by those who are hospital based physicians. The costs were rather modest.

TABLE V. Investigations in heart failure. Figures are the percentage of patients in whom the investigations were carried out (derived from Fleg et al [26])

Investigation	GP	Physician	Cardiologist	Academic cardiologist
Electrolytes	99	99	99	99
Digoxin level	99	99	91	84
Chest X-ray	97	97	98	98
Electrocardiogram	74	72	89	89
Radionuclide ventriculography	37	52	75	81
Exercise test	57	54	66	67

High costs with young, specialists and urban setting.
NYHA II costs of procedures ranged from $240 to $864 per annum.

The case for the echocardiogram is not established by formal investigation. In our own studies [6, 15] only one-third of patients with heart failure had been investigated with an echocardiogram despite a high percentage, more than 80%, having had a chest X-ray and electrocardiogram. The echocardiogram can often confirm the diagnosis of coronary artery disease or cardiomyopathy, allows a measurement of the ejection fraction, provides an assessment of myocardial contractility, detects left ventricular hypertrophy, detects incoordinate contraction, confirms the absence of any abnormality of the valves and is a reasonable screening test for rare diseases of the heart.

IMPLICATIONS
The data from the recent trials suggest that the treatment of heart failure is particularly efficacious in terms of both reduction of mortality [9, 10, 16, 17] and an improvement in the quality of life [20]. The investigations are cheap. The condition is common and readily detectable. These are important criteria if a major new initiative is proposed in the approach to the treatment of a disease entity. Comparisons can be made with other forms of treatment (Figure 1). The lives saved per ten thousand persons treated are plotted against time in years. It is notable that all the major trials in heart failure demonstrate a considerable number of lives saved in a relatively short period of time. This compares favourably with thrombolytic therapy and cardiovascular surgery

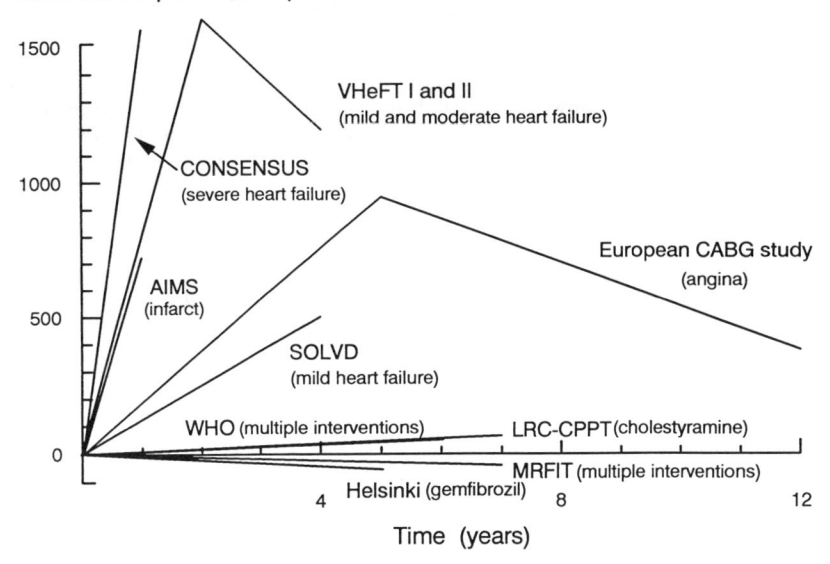

Figure 1. Lives saved per ten thousand patients treated over time. The greatest benefit appears to be from the treatment of heart failure and the use of thrombolytics in the treatment of myocardial infarction.

and is vastly superior to interventions aimed at the prevention of coronary heart disease. The total number of lives saved in the country (the impact on the total community) can be obtained by multiplying the number of lives saved by the prevalence of the disease entity. Since heart failure is extraordinarily common such a calculation is likely to increase the apparent benefit in relation to other treatment.

The conclusion from this brief review of some of the key results in the management of heart failure is simple. Whereas in the last twenty years much emphasis has been placed on the detection and treatment of hypertension and coronary heart disease, more emphasis and resources should now be allocated to the detection and treatment of congestive heart failure. This medical problem has not been ignored, but insufficient emphasis and resources have been given to heart failure in comparison to other common medical conditions.

REFERENCES

1. Poole-Wilson PA. Chronic heart failure: cause, pathophysiology, prognosis, clinical manifestations, investigations. In Julian DG, Camm AJ, Fox KF et al, eds. *Diseases of the Heart*. London: Baillière-Tindall. 1989: 24–36
2. Poole-Wilson PA. Heart failure. *Med Int 1985; 2*: 866–871
3. Harris P. Congestive cardiac failure: central role of the arterial blood pressure. *Br Heart J 1987; 58*: 190–203
4. Poole-Wilson PA. Future perspectives in the management of congestive heart failure.

4. *Am J Cardiol* 1990; 66: 462–467
5. Smith WM. Epidemiology of congestive heart failure. *Am J Cardiol* 1985; 55: 3A–8A
6. Parameshwar J, Poole-Wilson PA, Sutton GC. Heart failure in a district hospital. *J Roy Coll Phys London* 1992; 26: 139–142
7. Kannel WB, Savage D, Castelli WP. Cardiac failure in the Framingham Study: twenty-year follow up. In Braunwald E, Mock MB, Watson JT, eds. *Congestive Heart Failure. Current Research and Clinical Applications.* New York: Grune and Stratton. 1982: 15–30
8. Remes J, Miettinen H, Reunanen A, Pyorala K. Validity of clinical diagnosis of heart failure in primary health care. *Eur Heart J* 1991; 12: 315–321
9. Cohn JN, Johnson G, Ziesche S et al. A comparison of enalapril with hydralazine-isosorbide dinitrate in the treatment of chronic congestive heart failure. *N Engl J Med* 1991; 325: 302–310
10. The SOLVD Investigators. Effect of enalapril on survival in patients with reduced left ventricular ejection fractions and congestive heart failure. *N Engl J Med* 1991; 325: 293–302
11. Eriksson H, Svardsudd K, Larsson B et al. Risk factors for heart failure in the general population: the study of men born in 1913. *Eur Heart J* 1989; 10: 647–656
12. Kannel WB, Belanger JA. Epidemiology of heart failure. *Am Heart J* 1991; 121: 951–956
13. Yusuf S, Thom T, Abbott RD. Changes in hypertension treatment and in congestive heart failure mortality in the United States. *Hypertension* 1989; 13 (suppl 1): 74–79
14. Teerlink JR, Goldhaber SZ, Pfeffer MA. An overview of contemporary aetiologies of congestive heart failure. *Am Heart J* 1991; 121: 1852–1853
15. Parameshwar J, Shackell MM, Richardson A et al. Prevalence of heart failure in north-west London – a general practice survey. *J Gen Practice* 1992; in press
16. The CONSENSUS Trial Study Group. Effects of enalapril on mortality in severe congestive heart failure. Results of the Cooperative North Scandinavian Enalapril Survival Study (CONSENSUS). The CONSENSUS Trial Study Group. *N Engl J Med* 1987; 316: 1429–1435
17. Cohn JN, Archibald DG, Ziesche S et al. Effect of vasodilator therapy on mortality in chronic congestive heart failure. Results of a Veterans Administration Cooperative Study. *N Engl J Med* 1986; 314: 1547–1552
18. Richardson A, Bayliss J, Scriven AJ et al. Double-blind comparison of captopril alone against frusemide plus amiloride in mild heart failure. *Lancet* 1987; ii: 709–711
19. Poole-Wilson PA, Lindsay D. Advances in the treatment of chronic heart failure. Two steps forward, one step back. *Br Med J* 1992; 304: 1069–1070
20. Lindsay DC, Poole-Wilson PA. Angiotensin-converting enzyme inhibitors or vasodilators as therapy in chronic heart failure: a review of the trials. *J Cardiovasc Pharmacol* 1992; 19 (suppl 4): S45–S55
21. Poole-Wilson PA, Robinson K. Digoxin – a redundant drug in the treatment of congestive heart failure. *Cardiovasc Drugs Ther* 1989; 2: 733–741
22. Jaeschke R, Oxman AD, Guyatt GH. To what extent do congestive heart failure patients in sinus rhythm benefit from digoxin therapy? A systematic overview and meta-analysis. *Am J Med* 1990; 88: 279–286
23. Kleber FX, Niemoller L, Doering W. Impact of converting enzyme inhibition on progression of chronic heart failure: results of the Munich Mild Heart Failure Trial. *Br Heart J* 1992; 67: 289–296.
24. Williams A. The cost-effectiveness approach to the treatment of angina. In Patterson D, ed. *Quality of Life: Assessment and Application.* Lancaster: MTP Press. 1987.
25. Williams A. The economics of coronary artery bypass grafting. *Br Med J* 1985; 291: 325–329
26. Fleg JL, Hinton PC, Lakatta EG et al. Physician utilization of laboratory procedures to monitor outpatients with congestive heart failure. *Arch Intern Med* 1989; 149: 393–396

LIPID CLINICS – DO WE NEED THEM?

Glyn R Evans
Dudley Road Hospital, Birmingham

INTRODUCTION

Cardiovascular disease is the major cause of death in North America and Western Europe. The majority of these deaths are due to myocardial or cerebral infarction, atherosclerosis being the principal cause [1].

The development of the atherosclerotic plaque is a highly complex event involving at the very least the interaction of lipoproteins, leucocytes, platelets, macrophages and fibroblasts [2–5]. Atherosclerosis is a fatal disease for which there is no known cure [6].

Although clinically atherosclerosis is a disease of the middle-aged and elderly, pathologically it is not. Atherosclerosis is a progressive process starting with the development of the fatty streak which matures throughout life to the thrombosed, calcified, ulcerated advanced plaque [7]. Post mortem studies on American servicemen killed in both Korea [8] and Vietnam [9] have shown atherosclerotic lesions in men in their late teens and early twenties. Indeed, the earliest lesions develop within the first decade [10]. The inevitable consequence of this is that any attempt to interfere with the natural history of the condition has to be directed not only to those with clinical heart disease, but more importantly to those without.

Coronary heart disease (CHD) has a major impact on our society. It accounts for 150,000 deaths annually in England and Wales [11] which is approximately one in every three deaths. It is primarily a disease of the elderly. The incidence of death from CHD increases with age [11] with 80% of deaths occurring in individuals over 65 years of age. One in five coronary deaths occurs in people of working age, leading to the annual loss of 240,000 man-years of working life [11].

CHD is also a major cause of morbidity. The British Regional Heart Study [11] found that one in four middle-aged men had clinical or electrocardiographic evidence of CHD; 350,000 new cases present annually to general practitioners. This also has economic consequences. CHD accounts for 10% of days off work, costs hundreds of millions of pounds in sickness benefit payments and billions of pounds in lost production [11].

Treatment of CHD is also expensive. The combined costs of primary care, in- and outpatient hospital care, and drugs was £389 million in 1985 for England and Wales [11]. It is likely that this figure is an underestimate. The daily cost of care on a high dependency area such as a coronary care unit is higher than the cost of an 'average' hospital bed, partly because of the higher staff:patient ratio. These figures do not include either Scotland or Northern Ireland where the prevalence of CHD is higher than in the remainder of the UK [11].

The aim of coronary prevention programmes is not the total abolition of death from CHD. Such a goal is, with current knowledge, not possible. The aim of the programme is to reduce the rate of progression of atherosclerosis so that the transition from silent atherosclerosis to clinical coronary heart disease occurs later in life. The goal is the abolition of premature cardiac death.

RISK FACTORS FOR CORONARY HEART DISEASE
CHD is a disease of multifactorial aetiology. The aetiological factors can be considered in three groups [12]. There are factors such as cigarette smoking, obesity and physical inactivity which are totally avoidable. Age, male sex and family history are immutable. Other factors, such as lipid disorders, hypertension and diabetes are open to manipulation. Is treatment of hypercholesterolaemia beneficial?

TREATMENT OF HYPERCHOLESTEROLAEMIA
Hypercholesterolaemia is causally related to the development of atherosclerosis and the risk of CHD [13]. Will reducing an elevated serum cholesterol lead to a reduction in the risk of coronary heart disease?

This question has been addressed by several intervention trials of varying design. Some trials have been of methods of primary prevention, others secondary prevention. Some have considered cholesterol reduction in isolation, others the simultaneous modification of several risk factors. Some have used cholesterol lowering diets, others drugs.

Overview analyses have evaluated the effects of cholesterol lowering in clinical trials, showing that for every 1% cholesterol reduction a 2% reduction is achieved in the risk of CHD [14–16]. Trials have shown reduction in fatal and non-fatal myocardial infarction in groups treated with cholesterol lowering drugs [17–20].

Following an initial case report and early uncontrolled investigations, we now have controlled clinical trials which provide angiographic evidence that cholesterol lowering drugs not only delay the progression of CHD, but can also lead to its regression. These include the National Heart, Lung, and Blood Institute type II study (NHLBI type II), the Cholesterol Lowering Atherosclerosis Study (CLAS), and the Familial Atherosclerosis Treatment Study (FATS) [6].

NHLBI type II involved 116 patients classified as Fredrickson type II who were managed with diet and cholestyramine for 5 years. In those who had 50% or greater stenosis at baseline, lesion progression in those treated with cholestyramine was 12% compared with 33% in controls. CLAS involved 162 patients who had already undergone bypass grafting. They were assigned to either placebo or combination treatment with colestipol and niacin. The treated group had fewer lesions which progressed, fewer new lesions and less adverse changes in the grafts. A 16.2% regression rate in the treated group compared with 2.4% in the controls was also noted [6].

FATS compared two intensive strategies, colestipol with either niacin or lovastatin, with a more conventional approach in men at high risk as a result of established coronary atherosclerosis. Substantial changes in both high density lipoprotein (HDL) and low density lipoprotein (LDL) were seen in both treatment groups with only a slight change in the conventional therapy group. Progression was seen in 46% of the conventional therapy group as compared with 25% in the colestipol-niacin group and 21% in the colestipol-lovastatin group. Regression was more frequently observed in the treatment groups (colestipol-niacin 39%, colestipol-lovastatin 32%) compared with conventional therapy (11%). Clinical events (death, myocardial infarction, revascularization for worsening symptoms) were seen less often in the treatment groups [6].

Overview analysis of randomized trials of cholesterol lowering do suggest that intervention leads to a slight increase in total mortality [14]. It also shows that cholesterol reduction is associated with a weak downward trend in total mortality. It is thought that treatment has a small adverse effect when cholesterol is not reduced, but that this effect is offset by cholesterol lowering. An 8-9% fall in cholesterol is needed before reduction of total mortality is seen [14]. Reductions of at least twice this amount can be expected with 3-hydroxy-3-methylglutaryl coenzyme A (HMG CoA) reductase inhibition [21]. It is also possible that the risks are drug specific. The Coronary Primary Prevention Trial showed no significant adverse medical effects with the long-term use of bile acid binding resins [19].

STRATEGIES FOR CHOLESTEROL REDUCTION
There are two basic approaches to the reduction of cholesterol levels in the community: the population strategy and the high risk or individual strategy.

The population strategy recognizes that many people have more than one risk factor and that these factors interact. Additionally, most CHD results from exposure of a large proportion of the population to moderately elevated levels of risk factors. The strategy seeks to improve the health-oriented behaviour of the community by an education programme leading to an improved diet, smoking cessation, and more exercise. If successful this will reduce the number of people at high risk requiring individual care. It has the major advantage of reducing the risk of those in the middle of the cholesterol distribution [22].

Those with the most severe hypercholesterolaemia are the ones most at risk. They often have an underlying genetic hyperlipidaemia and will only have a partial response to diet. The moderate changes in health habits comprising the population strategy will be inadequate. These people would be helped by the high risk strategy. This involves the identification of those at high risk by some form of screening, either selective screening, opportunistic screening or general screening and offering them more intensive treatment. The disadvantage with this approach is that the benefits would be confined to a relatively small number of individuals.

These strategies are complementary, and what is needed is a population-based approach with public education combined with screening to identify those in the high risk group. The Standing Medical Advisory Committee to the Secretary of State for Health has reported that the most cost-effective approach is an opportunistic screening programme in which coronary risk factors are identified, with priority for cholesterol testing being given to individuals at high overall coronary risk [22].

CONSEQUENCES OF CHOLESTEROL REDUCTION

A cholesterol reduction programme will have economic consequences. On the individual level, the adoption of a healthier diet should save money [22]. On the larger scale, there will be the cost of the education programme and the screening programme, and also the costs of counselling and treatment of those with hypercholesterolaemia.

The impact of prevention is on age-specific coronary risk. Rose and Shipley [23] have shown that a reduction in the number of coronary deaths in one age group will be associated with an increase at a later age. Reducing the probability of a fatal heart attack at each successive age will result in people living longer. Because of this they will incur additional years of exposure to the risk of cardiac death. The risk of CHD rises very steeply with age so that these additional years may add to the life-time probability of dying from CHD. Hence what is achieved by coronary prevention is the postponement of cardiovascular death, with a longer life and more symptom-free years.

Controlling cardiac risk factors is likely to have other effects. Reducing smoking is likely to reduce the number of deaths from bronchial carcinoma and some other malignancies as well as deaths from respiratory disease. Treatment of hypertension might reduce the number of deaths due to stroke. These reductions would be at the expense of increasing the numbers of coronary deaths [22].

THE WORK OF THE LIPID CLINIC

Expending resources on identifying individuals with hypercholesterolaemia is pointless unless resources to treat them are also allocated. A lipid clinic is a suitable setting in which treatment can be provided.

A lipid clinic is concerned with more than just lipids. It is primarily a coronary prevention clinic. Its role is to diagnose and where necessary provide treatment for all lipid abnormalities and also to identify and where possible provide treatment for non-lipid cardiac risk factors.

In order to achieve these goals the clinic must:

1 accurately diagnose and effectively treat primary hyperlipidaemia;
2 identify secondary hyperlipidaemia; and
3 diagnose and treat concurrent cardiac risk factors.

The clinic must also make effective local arrangements for selective screening of individuals likely to have positive findings. Such groups might include those with the following characteristics [24]:

positive family history of CHD;
family history of hyperlipidaemia;
presence of xanthomas;
xanthelasma or corneal arcus in person <40 years old;
obesity;
diabetes mellitus;
hypertension;
smoking;
gout.

It is possible for a lipid clinic to achieve these goals. An audit of a lipid clinic in a district general hospital [25] found it was possible to help 20% of smokers to stop and others to cut down. Weight reduction was achieved, particularly in those weighing between 120 and 150% of ideal body weight. There was an average reduction of 12% in cholesterol level and 33% in triglyceride level. Target reductions in lipid levels were achieved in 42% of those with hypercholesterolaemia and 46% of those with hypertriglyceridaemia. A subsequent audit of the same clinic demonstrated a fall in blood cholesterol level averaging 17% in the first 3 months after intensive dietary advice [26]. The cost of the clinic averaged £470 per patient per year [25]. It cost £35 annually for a patient on diet alone, compared with £601 for a patient on drugs [26]. The high drug bill was a reflection of the frequent use of bile-acid binding resins. The patent on these drugs is due to expire soon, which might reduce the cost. The newest class of drugs, the HMG CoA reductase inhibitors, are potentially even more expensive, but they seem to be more effective. In practice, they can be expected to produce a 20–30% reduction in serum cholesterol and so the cost may well be offset by the reduction in coronary heart disease [22].

ALTERNATIVES TO THE LIPID CLINIC?
In theory, others could do the work of the lipid clinic. Although there are a large number of lipid disorders, most are uncommon. The majority of patients attending the clinic will have hypercholesterolaemia with a normal or slightly elevated triglyceride level. For the most part, management of hypercholesterolaemia is fairly structured. A goal cholesterol level is set, dietary treatment is prescribed. If the response to diet is unsatisfactory, drugs are added in a step-wise manner until the target is achieved or side-effects supervene. It is possible to devise a treatment algorithm so that a non-specialist could manage hypercholesterolaemia [13], and this might be useful in areas lacking local specialist advice.

However, given the importance of diet in management of lipid disorders, the lipid clinic with attached dietician does have the edge over non-specialist clinics or general practice in terms of providing dietary support, which is the most cost-effective part of management [26]. There is also ready access to cardiological advice. It is also important to bear in mind that there are a large number of people with hyperlipidaemia in the community and relatively few doctors trained in its management. Perhaps the need for a lipid clinic is best illustrated by the demands for its services with the increasing number of referrals as more cases are diagnosed.

The problem of hyperlipidaemia can only be adequately tackled by a coordinated partnership between primary care and hospital clinic. GPs should undertake the task of identifying those with hyperlipidaemia, offering basic dietary advice and follow-up. This will be adequate for the majority of patients. Refractory cases should be referred to the hospital clinic for consideration of drug therapy. The lipid clinic should also be the source for lipid advice. The lipid specialist should also develop educational programmes and regularly audit the service to ensure maximum efficiency.

CONCLUSION

The Western world is experiencing a major epidemic of premature CHD. The age-specific death rate from CHD can be reduced by changes in lifestyle combined, where necessary, with the use of drugs to lower serum cholesterol levels. This would lead to a postponement of coronary death and increased symptom-free survival at the cost of ultimately increasing the number of deaths from CHD in old age.

REFERENCES

1. *Report of the Working Group of Arteriosclerosis of the National Heart, Lung, and Blood Institute (1981)* Vol 2. Washington DC: Government Printing Office (DHEW publication no. (NIH) 82-2035
2. Bevilacqua MP, Pober JS, Wheeler ME et al. Interleukin I acts on cultured human vascular endothelium to increase the adhesion of polymorphonuclear leukocytes, monocytes and related leukocyte cell lines. *J Clin Invest 1985; 76*: 2000-2011
3. Mitchinson MJ, Ball RY. Macrophages and atherogenesis. *Lancet 1987; ii*: 8551:146-148
4. Steinberg D. Lipoproteins and atherosclerosis: a look back and a look ahead. *Arteriosclerosis 1983; 3*: 283-301
5. Ross R. The pathogenesis of atherosclerosis – an update. *N Engl J Med 1986; 314(8)*: 488-500
6. Superko HR. Drug therapy and the prevention of atherosclerosis in humans. *Am J Cardiol 1989; 64*: 31G-37G
7. McGill HC Jr. Persistent problems in the pathogenesis of atherosclerosis. *Arteriosclerosis 1984; 4*: 443-451
8. Enos W, Holmes R, Beyer J. Coronary disease among United States soldiers killed in action in Korea. *JAMA 1953; 152*: 1090-1092
9. McNamara JJ, Molot MA, Stemple JF. Coronary artery disease in combat casualties in Vietnam. *JAMA 1971; 216*: 1185-1187
10. Newman WP III, Freedman DS, Voors AW. Relation of serum lipoprotein levels and systolic blood pressure to early atherosclerosis: the Bogalusa Heart Study. *N Engl J Med 1986; 314*: 138-144
11. Wells N. *Coronary Heart Disease – the Need for Action*. Office of Health Economics. 1987
12. Bierman EL. Atherosclerosis and other forms of arteriosclerosis. In Petersdorf RG, Adams RD, Braunwald E et al, eds. *Harrison's Principles of Internal Medicine*, 10th edn. New York: McGraw-Hill. 1983: 1465-1475
13. National Cholesterol Education Program Expert Panel. Report of the National Cholesterol Education Program Expert Panel on Detection, Evaluation, and Treatment of High Blood Cholesterol in Adults. *Arch Intern Med 1988; 148*: 36-69
14. Homle I. An analysis of randomized trials evaluating the effect of cholesterol reduction on total mortality and coronary heart disease incidence. *Circulation 1990; 82(6)*: 1916-1924
15. Lipids Research Clinics Program. The Lipid Research Clinics Coronary Primary Pre-

vention Trial results: II. The relationship of reduction in incidence of coronary heart disease to cholesterol lowering. *JAMA 1984; 251*: 365-374

16 Peto R, Yusuf S, Collins R. Cholesterol lowering trial results in their epidemiological context (abstract). *Circulation 1985; 72 (suppl III)*: III-451

17 Oliver MF, Heady JA, Morris JN, Cooper J. A Co-operative trial in the primary prevention of ischaemic heart disease using clofibrate. Report from the Committee of Principal Investigators. *Br Heart J 1978; 40*: 1069-1118

18 The Coronary Drug Project Research Group. Clofibrate and niacin in coronary heart disease. *JAMA 1975; 231*: 360-381

19 Lipid Research Clinics Program. The lipid research clinics coronary primary prevention trial results: I Reduction in incidence of coronary heart disease. *JAMA 1984; 251*: 351-364

20 Frick MH, Elo O, Haapa K et al. Helsinki heart study: primary-prevention trial with gemfibrozil in middle-aged men with dyslipidemia. *N Engl J Med 1987; 317*: 1237-1245

21 Goldman L, Weinstein MC, Goldman PA, Williams LW. Cost-effectiveness of HMG-CoA reductase inhibition for primary and secondary prevention of coronary heart disease. *JAMA 1991; 265(9)*: 1145-1151

22 Reckless JPD. The economics of cholesterol lowering. In Betteridge DJ, ed. *Baillière's Clinical Endocrinology and Metabolism 1990; 4(4)*: 947-972

23 Rose, G, Shipley M. Effects of coronary risk reduction on causes of death. In Lewis B, Assmann G, eds. *The Social and Economic Contexts of Coronary Prevention*. London: Current Medical Literature. 1990: 24-29

24 European Atherosclerosis Society. Strategies for the prevention of coronary heart disease. A policy statement of the European Anterosclerosis Society Naples, June 18, 1986. In Assmann G, ed. *Lipid Metabolism Disorders and Coronary Heart Disease. Primary Prevention, Diagnosis and Therapy Guidelines for General Practice*. Munchen: MMV-Medizin-Verlag. 1989: 13-34

25 Evans GR, Taylor G, Taylor KG. The work of a lipid clinic: an audit of performance. *Q J Med 1990; 74(275)*: 239-245

26 Le Cornu K. Audit of dietary input into a hospital lipid clinic. *J Hum Nutrition and Dietetics 1991; 4*: 121-126

LIFE-THREATENING ARRHYTHMIAS IN THE DISTRICT GENERAL HOSPITAL – WHAT CAN WE AFFORD?

Ronald WF Campbell
Freeman Hospital, Newcastle upon Tyne

INTRODUCTION
District general hospitals (DGHs) cater for local health needs. They must cope with all types of emergencies and, depending upon circumstances and facilities, must determine whether investigation and management can be completed in the DGH or whether referral to a specialist centre is necessary.

Life-threatening cardiac arrhythmias take many forms but all have acute presentations and most need speedy, accurate initial management. Facilities to support antiarrhythmic life-saving interventions are mandatory in DGHs; e.g. basic pacing and defibrillation, but whether more complex, sophisticated and expensive techniques are available is controversial. Many are appropriate only for a specialist centre but as awareness of arrhythmias gathers pace in the UK, some of these techniques fall within a desirable and affordable category for DGHs.

WHAT ARE LIFE-THREATENING ARRYTHMIAS?
The field of arrhythmology is bedevilled by poor definitions. 'Life-threatening' is one such term; it is imprecise; it involves dimensions other than electrophysiology; and it means different things to different people. Its emotional appeal has helped retain the term in professional usage even to the extent that it is a licensed indication for the use of some antiarrhythmic drugs. Ventricular fibrillation is life-threatening but only a minority of ventricular tachycardia threatens life. Almost all complete heart block is life-threatening but second degree atrioventricular (AV) block is not. Atrial fibrillation is unpleasant but not lethal except in the context of short refractory period accessory pathways. In essence, life-threatening arrhythmias are those that cause important haemodynamic upset – they are either very fast or very slow. Immediate life saving for these arrhythmias is their conversion to a stable 'normal rate' rhythm. This is usually straightforward; the major clinical challenge is to prevent their recurrence. District general hospitals should have facilities for the termination of haemodynamically important arrhythmias

but the optimal DGH role in long-term prophylactic antiarrhythmic strategies is more controversial.

MANDATORY ANTIARRHYTHMIC FACILITIES IN THE DISTRICT GENERAL HOSPITAL

The following are the minimum requirements in a DGH for the purpose of saving life threatened by an arrhythmia:

Equipment and drugs

1 An ECG monitor.
2 A 12-lead ECG machine. A 3-channel ECG machine is essential if supraventricular tachycardia (SVT) is to be distinguished from ventricular tachycardia (VT).
3 A synchronized defibrillator. More salvageable lives will be saved with a defibrillator than with almost any other piece of medical equipment yet defibrillators are not given high priority for upgrading and often too few are distributed about the hospital.
4 A pacemaker generator.
5 A supply of sterile pacing catheters. An emergency pacing pack should be readily available.
6 Access to fluoroscopy.
7 Antiarrhythmic drugs – adenosine (or verapamil), lignocaine.

Training and support

1 Basic arrhythmia knowledge.
2 Expertise in the use of the equipment.
3 Maintenance, safety and technical support facilities for the equipment.

Medical staff, particularly those in front line duty, must possess basic arrhythmia knowledge and be able to accurately and reliably diagnose the major lethal arrhythmias (ventricular fibrillation (VF), VT, torsade de pointes, complete heart block). There is little evidence that such diagnostic expertise exists [1, 2]. Ventricular tachycardia is poorly recognized (even by trained cardiologists) and, further, its misdiagnosis as 'SVT with aberration' has led to disaster with inappropriate verapamil administration [3, 4]. Medical, nursing and technical staff must be familiar with life-saving equipment. Newly appointed staff must be shown how to operate defibrillators and be versed in their *safe* use. Finally, equipment and supplies must be serviced regularly. This is particularly relevant for rechargeable defibrillators and for emergency drug carts.

PROGRAMMED ELECTRICAL STIMULATION

No discussion of arrhythmia management can avoid consideration of the role of programmed electrical stimulation. Introduced in 1969, this procedure has added greatly to knowledge of cardiac arrhythmias and is the keystone of specialized arrhythmia investigation. Performed under local anaesthetic, one or more multipole electrode catheters are introduced via peripheral veins to specific intracardiac locations. Electrograms from these sites are recorded and pacing stimuli can be delivered. The ability to deliver critically timed pacing impulses is programmed stimulation. With such stimulation, conduction capability and refractory periods of cardiac tissue can be measured. More important, critically timed stimuli will initiate and terminate a wide range of clinically important arrhythmias including VT. Moreover, when VT can be reliably induced, suppressive drug therapy can be identified: after its administration VT will no longer be inducible [5]. Electrophysiological testing may similarly be of great value in assessing survivors of acute myocardial infarction [6-8] and for evaluating resuscitated survivors of out-of-hospital cardiac arrest [9]. Thus, programmed electrical stimulation is a powerful clinical tool. Perhaps *all* patients with symptomatic VT should have this investigation but, in reality, few do in the UK. Programmed stimulation requires moderately sophisticated equipment and a reasonable level of electrophysiological knowledge. Multicatheter programmed stimulation is expensive to set up and is time consuming to perform; it has little place in DGH management. Single catheter programmed stimulation, however, is affordable and, particularly in the context of VT, has an important management contribution. It *could* reasonably be offered in a DGH.

ARRHYTHMIA MANAGEMENT IN THE DGH

Arrhythmia management appropriate for the DGH can be decided on several criteria; but quality is not one. DGH arrhythmia management should not represent 'second best'. What is offered should be modern optimal therapy. The DGH limitation should be only in the extent to which procedures and managements are pursued. Expertise, procedural time, equipment and case load are the important factors.

Expertise

It is reprehensible that medical training in the UK has paid scant attention to arrhythmia diagnosis and management. Cardiac arrhythmias are responsible for a majority of sudden, unexpected deaths in the UK. Arrhythmias are also responsible for substantial morbidity. Most arrhythmias are treatable and a wide range of prophylactic and curative strategies are available. Sadly for the majority of afflicted patients, suboptimal management is offered. Most large cities in the USA have more clinical arrhythmologists than exist in the whole of the UK. This situation must change. Cardiology is a complex medical subspecialty with demanding training needs. Expertise in arrhythmia management is relevant for *all* those with cardiological responsibilities – the more so for the DGH cardiologist who must be a 'jack of all trades'. Expertise in the present context means knowledge and familiarity rather than technical competence in a practical technique. The DGH cardiologist should be able to distinguish the following arrhythmias: VF, torsade de pointes, polymorphic VT, monomorphic VT, para/intra AV nodal re-entry tachycardia, reciprocating tachycardias using accessory pathways, true atrial tachycardia, atrial flutter and atrial fibrillation. He/she should also know the practical management strategies, natural history and aetiological associations of each.

Procedural time
Much can be accomplished in arrhythmia diagnosis and management by knowledgeable assessment of the surface ECG allied to a good clinical history but intracardiac electrode catheter placement is the keystone of more advanced arrhythmia assessment. Once considered the domain of specialist electrophysiological centres, invasive electrophysiological studies can be economic, simple and supported to a high standard in a DGH. Their acceptability in this setting, however, relates to the time they demand. A procedural time of more than one hour might be a point at which support in a DGH becomes difficult. Nonetheless, a considerable number of important antiarrhythmic managements fall within this time frame.

The need for critically timed extra stimuli
Programmed electrical stimulation involves the delivery of sequences of critically timed extra stimuli during normal rhythms, during tachycardias and during 'drive' pacing. The delivery of such impulses requires a sophisticated cardiac stimulator. User-friendly commercial systems have not been available but that situation is changing. Nonetheless, the need for signal timing and the ability to deliver several programmed extra stimuli may take arrhythmia investigation to a level of sophistication that would not be reasonable to expect in all DGHs. Simple pacing (with high rate option) is of some value but in most circumstances is suboptimal.

Number of catheters
Electrophysiological diagnosis and management complexity increases exponentially with the number of catheters (and with the number of recording poles per catheter). Insertion and placement of multiple catheters takes time, and can be tedious (especially when cardiac movement frequently displaces catheters from critical positions such as the His bundle). Multiple catheters can place great demands on equipment – each recording site needs a conditioning amplifier and display and printout facilities. Multi-catheter procedures can be performed in DGHs but in general they are more appropriate for a specialist centre.

Load
Experience and constant practical application of skills is important in offering service quality. There are a remarkable range of cardiac arrhythmias – many are uncommon and their management may reasonably be considered the province of a specialist centre. Nonetheless, for life-threatening arrhythmias, management must be available in a DGH and must be of a high standard even if encountered only rarely.

THE DGH ROLE
Table I details a range of procedures in arrhythmia diagnosis and management

and lists procedural time, the need or otherwise for critically timed extra stimuli, catheter needs and, finally, suggests whether a typical DGH is likely to deal with that problem on more than four occasions per year.

TABLE I. Procedures in arrhythmia management and diagnosis

Procedure	Procedure > 1 hour	Critically timed extra stimuli needed	Multiple catheters needed	DGH need > 4/year
Paced termination of VT	No	Not necessarily	No	Yes
Assessment of accessory pathway risk	No	No	No	Yes
Drug assessment of VT therapy	No	Yes	No	Yes
Evaluation of ICDs	No	Yes	No	Yes
Drug assessment of accessory pathways	No	Yes	No	Yes
Post-MI assessment	No	Yes	No	Yes
Assessment of resuscitated out-of-hospital cardiac arrest	No	Yes	No	Yes
Work-up of syncopal patient	Yes	Yes	Yes	Yes
Mapping of VT origin	Yes	Yes	Yes	No
Accessory pathway mapping	Yes	Yes	Yes	No
Radio-frequency ablation of arrhythmia	Yes	Yes	Yes	Yes
VT and WPW surgical procedures	Yes	Yes	Yes	No

Abbreviations: ICDs = implantable cardioverter defibrillators; MI = myocardial infarction; VT = ventricular tachycardia; WPW = Wolff–Parkinson–White syndrome.

WHAT IS APPROPRIATE IN DGH MANAGEMENT OF LIFE-THREATENING ARRHYTHMIAS?

Pace termination of ventricular tachycardia and assessment of accessory pathway risk demand little and are important procedures in arrhythmia management and prognostication. Assessment of drug therapy for VT and accessory pathway arrhythmias, evaluation of implantable cardioverter defibrillators, assessment of sudden death and VT risk post-infarction and assessment of resuscitated victims of out-of-hospital cardiac arrest are also very cost-effective procedures which reasonably could be offered at a DGH. They require a programmable cardiac stimulator but this can be justified by the frequency with which it would be used and by the importance of the results.

The electrophysiological work-up of a syncopal patient, mapping of ventricular tachycardia and accessory pathways, radio-frequency ablation and antiarrhythmic surgical procedures are complex and time consuming. They demand expensive equipment and high levels of technical and clinical expertise. These procedures should be available in specialist centres. It is long overdue that such centres be established in the UK to offer regional support for what are highly effective life-saving managements often offering a cure rather than mere palliation of cardiovascular disease. Such centres would encourage and support DGH provision of arrhythmia management.

ACKNOWLEDGEMENT

Academic Cardiology is supported by the British Heart Foundation.

REFERENCES

1. Dancy M, Camm AJ, Ward D. Misdiagnosis of chronic recurrent ventricular tachycardia. *Lancet 1985; ii*: 320–323
2. Griffith MJ, De Belder M, Micklewright J et al. Multivariate analysis to simplify the differential diagnosis of broad complex tachycardia. *Br Heart J 1991; 66*: 166–174
3. Buxton AE, Marchlinski FE, Doherty JU et al. Hazards of intravenous verapamil for sustained ventricular tachycardia. *Am J Cardiol 1987; 59*: 1107–1110
4. Rankin AC, Rae AP, Cobbe SM. Misuse of intravenous varapamil in patients with ventricular tachycardia. *Lancet 1987; ii*: 472–474
5. Waller TJ, Kay HR, Spielman SR et al. Reduction in sudden death and total mortality by antiarrhythmic therapy evaluated by electrophysiologic drug testing: criteria of efficacy in patients with sustained ventricular tachyarrhythmia. *J Am Coll Cardiol 1987; 10*: 83–89
6. Richards DA, Byth K, Ross DL, Uther JB. What is the best predictor of spontaneous ventricular tachycardia and sudden death after myocardial infarction? *Circulation 1991; 83*: 756–763
7. Cripps T, Bennett ED, Camm AJ, Ward DE. Inducibility of sustained monomorphic ventricular tachycardia as a prognostic indicator in survivors of recent myocardial infarction: a prospective evaluation in relation to other prognostic variables. *J Am Coll Cardiol 1989; 14*: 289–296
8. Uther JB, Richards DAB, Denniss AR, Ross DL. The prognostic significance of programmed ventricular stimulation after myocardial infarction: a review. *Circulation 1987; 75 (Suppl 3)*: 161–165
9. Skale BT, Miles WM, Heger JJ et al. Survivors of cardiac arrest: prevention of recurrence by drug therapy as predicted by electrophysiologic testing or ECG monitoring. *Am J Cardiol 1986; 57*: 113–119

NEW TESTS IN IMMUNOLOGY FOR THE CLINICIAN

HF Sewell, AM Farrell
University Hospital, Queen's Medical Centre, Nottingham

INTRODUCTION
The multidisciplinary nature of immunology has ensured its continued enrichment by the advances in biomedical science. Outstanding examples in the recent past are the development of hybridoma technology producing monoclonal antibodies and recombinant DNA techniques resulting in the cloning and expression of individual genes and their products. The science of immunology as applied in medicine also continues to gain from astute clinicopathological observations and the mixture of these advances has resulted in the generation of a plethora of immunological tests. The clinician when considering patient management needs to evaluate these tests. The evaluation must consider whether the tests are essential to patient management or may be useful or are merely interesting but still constitute clinical research. Additionally clinicians need to be cognizant of the quality assurance and the costs of such new tests.

In this selective review emphasis is placed on relatively new tests which are considered to be important in the clinician's armamentarium. The two areas selected are: (1) newer autoantibody tests and (2) immunophenotyping of lymphocytes.

AUTOANTIBODY TESTS
The relevance and quality assurance of many autoantibody tests in clinical management is well established [1].

In the past 5 years two new and now relatively well-defined autoantibody tests have emerged which have been shown to be essential within the clinical arena. These antibodies are: (a) antineutrophil cytoplasmic antibodies (ANCAs) and (b) antiphospholipid antibodies (APAs).

Essential requirements of clinically useful autoantibody tests are their sensitivity and specificity. Sensitivity defines the proportion of individuals with a disease in whom a test for that disease is positive using a stated method. Tests of high sensitivity can, if negative, be used to exclude a disease. Specificity defines the proportion of individuals without the disease in whom the test is negative. The test should be negative in healthy persons as well as individuals with diseases of differing aetiology but similar clinical presentation. Tests of high specificity can be used as positive confirmation of a disease. The two tests to be defined have high sensitivity and specificity within a clinical context.

Antineutrophil cytoplasmic antibodies

These autoantibodies have specificity for various enzymes found within the cytoplasmic granules of myeloid cells. They are commonly detected by an indirect immunofluorescent (IIF) assay using a substrate preparation of human granulocytes/polymorphonuclear leucocytes. The quantity of antibody can be documented by the serial dilution of the patient's serum. Two distinct patterns of positive ANCAs are noted which have been well characterized by various internationally agreed workshops. The patterns are:

1 Cytoplasmic pattern termed C-ANCA.
2 A perinuclear pattern termed P-ANCA.

Recent biochemical and molecular biological techniques have resulted in the isolation and protein sequencing of the myeloid antigens which appear to be the predominant targets associated with the immunofluorescent pattern. A serum proteinase enzyme termed proteinase-3 (PR3) correlates with the C-ANCA pattern whilst the P-ANCA pattern correlates predominantly with the antigen myeloperoxidase (MPO). Using the purified antigens as substrates in sensitive enzyme-linked immunosorbent assay (ELISA) and radio-immunoassay (RIA) systems, the two way correlations for both patterns of antigens with the IIF assay have been above 85% [2].

Clinical usefulness of ANCA

ANCA has proved to be valuable in the diagnosis and assessment of disease activity in patients with pauci immune (systemic) necrotizing vasculitides involving many tissues. ANCA tests are very useful in the diagnosis of Wegener's granulomatosis (WG), microscopic polyarteritis and idiopathic necrotizing and crescentic glomerulonephritis [3]. ANCA tests have high sensitivity (85-98%) and specificity (95-100%) for diagnosing active generalized Wegener's granulomatosis [4]. ANCA levels correlate with disease activity [5] and are predictive of disease relapse [6]. P-ANCA positivity has been shown typically in other vasculitides, e.g. Churg-Strauss syndrome, polyarteritis nodosa, polyangiitis and debatably Henoch-Schönlein purpura [7]. Many (Wegener's and microscopic polyarteritis) sera possess ANCA of both patterns confirmed by using the specific ELISA and radio-immunoassays. It is clear that neither pattern correlates reliably with any single pattern of predominant organ involvement (e.g. renal, respiratory) in the ANCA-related diseases [8].

ANCA may represent more than a marker of vasculitis and may play a role in pathogenesis [3]. Recent experience has revealed atypical forms of C-ANCA, e.g. in HIV infection [9], and of P-ANCA in inflammatory bowel disease [10]. Most often these atypical antibodies do not have specificity for the defined antigens proteinase-3 and myeloperoxidase using the ELISA and

RIA systems. The inference is that clinical laboratories offering these tests should perform or have access to the ELISA/RIA systems using defined antigens.

Concluding remarks

Management of the often complex vasculitides has hitherto depended on clinical features and histopathological identification of typical necrotizing vasculitis and/or granulomata which may require biopsy of tissues as diverse as nasal mucosa, renal tissue or lung. Testing for ANCA provides a rapid assay requiring 5–10ml of clotted blood, a result being obtainable within 1–2 hours with the IIF assay, leading to rapid diagnosis and institution of therapy. ANCA is also useful in monitoring disease activity and in differentiating intercurrent infection from disease relapse, both of which may present with neutrophilia and raised ESR and C-reactive protein. Intercurrent infections will not be associated with a raised ANCA.

ANCA testing is rapid and of little cost. It is essential in cases of unexplained vasculitis and/or of rapidly progressive glomerulonephritis. Serial quantitation of ANCA is also useful in monitoring disease activity.

Antiphospholipid antibodies (APAs)

These autoantibodies are directed predominantly against negatively charged phospholipids, e.g. cardiolipin, phosphatidic acid, phosphatidyl serine, which are common components of many cell membranes. The term APA is often used to cover detection of autoantigens reacting in the anticardiolipin antibody (ACA) test, and in anticoagulant assays. The ACA test is based upon a sensitive ELISA or RIA system. Antiphospholipid antibodies have been classically associated with systemic lupus erythematosus (SLE) [11]. Historically in vitro tests have documented factors in SLE sera that prolong clotting as defined by tests such as the activated partial thromboplastin time and the kaolin clotting time, i.e. the so-called lupus anticoagulant (LAC) test.

Some lupus sera are known to cause a false positive test for syphilis, i.e. a positive Wassermann (WR) with a negative confirmatory test and these false positive WRs are now known to be due to anticardiolipin antibodies.

From a large series of detailed studies [11–13] it has become apparent in SLE patients having at least four of the revised American Rheumatism Association (ARA) criteria [14] that the presence of antiphospholipid antibodies correlates with the risk of thrombotic events, recurrent foetal loss, and thrombocytopenia. Additionally patients with non-classical SLE, e.g. with negative antinuclear antibodies (ANAs) or negative double-stranded DNA autoantibodies and possessing fewer than three ARA criteria, have also been documented to have antiphospholipid antibodies which also correlate with the above defined complications [15]. This has led to the suggestion of an entity termed the antiphospholipid syndrome. More recently a number of patients have been defined who possess antiphospholipid antibodies but who do not satisfy the current criteria for the diagnosis of classical or non-classical SLE. These individuals are referred to as having a 'primary antiphospholipid syndrome' [16, 17] and present with the complications of thrombosis (i.e. arterial and/or venous) together with recurrent foetal loss and thrombocytopenia.

The anticardiolipin antibody assays measuring separately IgM and IgG specificities and the LAC assay are not recognizing the same antigenic epitopes on the target phospholipid antigens [18]. In many sera both specificities are coincident but in some sera there is clear separation, one being positive whilst the other is negative. For patient management the clinician should request both tests, i.e. the anticardiolipin antibody assay and the LAC test.

Experimental data indicate that antiphospholipid antibodies may have a direct pathological role. For instance, mice injected with purified antiphospholipid antibodies or with monoclonal antibodies with APA specificity develop recurrent foetal loss [19].

Clinical usefulness of APA testing
APA tests should be requested in patients with classical and non-classical SLE who have a history of thrombosis (venous or arterial, e.g. deep vein thrombosis, pulmonary embolism, myocardial infarction, premature stroke, etc.). The antibody should also be sought in SLE patients who are planning a pregnancy or who are pregnant or who give a history of foetal loss. SLE patients with unexplained thrombocytopenia should also be tested.

On the basis of current evidence it would be wise to test for antiphospholipid antibodies in young patients (non-SLE) presenting with a history of unexpected or recurrent thrombosis or with idiopathic thrombocytopenia or with a history of recurrent foetal loss. A few studies have indicated that up to 10% of these patients may possess antiphospholipid antibodies. The clinical relevance of APA detected in some patient groups (e.g. isolated myocardial infarction) is uncertain and requires more detailed studies. Treatment decisions based on detection of antiphospholipid antibodies are varied and difficult. Options considered include low dose aspirin 75mg/day, steroids, azathioprine, subcutaneous heparin, intravenous immunoglobulin and, in the presence of a previous thrombotic episode, standard anticoagulation. The best treatment modalities are not clear but many are the focus of current ongoing clinical trials.

Concluding remarks
APA testing is essential in classical and non-classical SLE patients presenting with the index complications of thrombosis, foetal loss and/or thrombocytopenia. The test may be useful in young non-SLE patients with unexpected or recurrent thrombosis, or indeed with a history of recurrent foetal loss and/or thrombocytopenia. Both ACA and LAC assays should be requested.

IMMUNOPHENOTYPING OF LYMPHOCYTES
Lymphocytes which confer the properties of specificity, diversity and memory to the specific immune response display a vast array of molecules associated with their membrane, cytoplasm and nucleus. Many of the lymphocyte molecules (antigens) have been partially characterized and importantly there is a large series of monoclonal antibodies which define these antigens. These

antigens have been designated CD (cluster of differentiation) numbers which are recognized by complementary monoclonal antibodies. Table I lists some well known CDs and their association with normal T- and B-lymphocyte development. The availability of this wide range of monoclonal antibodies has made possible the widespread use of *immunophenotyping* of lymphocytes in clinical management. Immunophenotyping is the technique of using labelled antibodies to document the expressed characteristics (defined as CD antigens) of individual lymphocytes which depends on their genotype and how the genes are expressed. Diseases resulting in altered lymphocyte phenotype are readily and efficiently analysed giving vital diagnostic and prognostic information. The concurrent development of flow cytometry technology resulting in bench-top user-friendly relatively inexpensive machines has given access to automated immunophenotyping for district general hospital laboratories. Flow cytometry is a system of sensing cells as they move in a liquid stream through a laser beam. When cells (e.g. lymphocytes reacted with fluorescent monoclonal antibodies to CD antigens) pass the sensing area the laser light is scattered and colour discriminated fluorescence is measured. Cells are thus analysed on the basis of their size and cytosolic content (physical parameters causing scattering of the laser light) and whether they are carrying various CD antigens reacting with fluorescently labelled monoclonals. The quantity and intensity of fluorescence are recorded by a computer system and displayed on visual units of the flow cytometer machine. The machines can analyse in excess of 10,000 cells within seconds thus giving rapid, accurate and precise multiparametric analysis of lymphocyte phenotype. Cells from blood, cerebrospinal fluid (CSF) and other body fluids as well as single cell suspensions derived from tissue biopsies can all be used for flow cytometric immunophenotyping. With respect to clinical medicine, immunophenotyping is particularly useful in the following areas where lymphocytes become the target of or reflect disease processes:

1 Leukaemia/lymphoma immunophenotyping and investigation of idiopathic lymphadenopathy/lymphocytosis
2 Evaluation and monitoring of immunodeficiency disorders

Leukaemia/lymphoma immunophenotyping and investigation of idiopathic lymphadenopathy/lymphocytosis

The ontogeny of T- and B-lymphocytes (associated with defined CD antigenic profiles) is well documented using a series of monoclonal antibodies as shown in Table I. Well-known examples of CD antigens are CD4 and CD8 characterizing respectively T-helper and T-cyctotoxic/suppressor cells. The knowledge of the detailed antigenic profile of normal lymphocytes (Table I) is exploited in defining neoplastic acute and chronic lymphoid proliferations (leukaemias and non-Hodgkin's lymphomas) whereby the neoplastic cells express qualitative, quantitative or aberrant deviations from the normal lymphocyte antigenic profile [20, 21]. The initial assessment of newly diagnosed leukaemia and lymphoma patients is assisted by immunophenotyping. The classification of these diseases according to the

TABLE I. CD antigen profile of T- and B-cells

	T-cell maturation				
	Thymus			Blood and other sites Peripheral T-cells	
Immature thymocyte	Common thymocyte	Mature thymocyte	$T_{H/I}$		$T_{C/S}$
CD2	CD1	CD2	CD2		CD2
*CD3	CD2	CD3	CD3		CD3
CD5	CD3	CD4 or D8	CD4	or	CD8
CD7	CD5	CD5	CD5		CD5
CD38	CD7	CD7	CD7		CD7
*Tdt	CD4	Tdt±			
	+				
	CD8				
	*Tdt				

⟶ Maturation

	B-cell maturation					
B-cell precursors						
I	II	III	IV	Pre B-cell	B-cell	Plasma cell
HLA-DR	HLA-DR	HLA-DR	HLA-DR	HLA-DR	HLA-DR	HLA-DR(±)
Tdt	CD19	CD19	CD19	CD19	CD19	Cyto Ig
	Tdt	CD10	CD10	CD10	CD20	
	CD24	Tdt	CD20	CD20	Sm Ig	
		CD24	Tdt	Cyto μ	CD24	
			CD24	Tdt ±		
				CD24		

⟶ Maturation

* Indicates intracellular antigen; Tdt = terminal deoxynucleotidyl transferase; $T_{H/I}$ = T-helper/inducer cells; $T_{C/S}$ = T-cytotoxic/suppressor cells; Cyto μ/Ig = cytoplasmic IgM(μ) heavy chain/immunoglobulin; Sm Ig = cell surface membrane immunoglobulin; HLA-DR = human leucocyte antigen-DR.

expression of CD markers as shown in Table II has led to the definition of sub-groups with different prognoses. Additionally, immunophenotyping is also useful in guiding and monitoring response to therapy. Some markers on neoplastic lymphoid cells can be used as tumour specific antigens, e.g. a clone of neoplastic B-cells often expresses a single immunoglobulin light chain (kappa or lambda) on its surface membrane (Sm Ig). This is in marked contrast to an equal mixture of kappa (κ) and lambda (λ) positive clones represented within the multiclones present in normal or 'reactive' lymphocyte populations in vivo. This simple marker of immunophenotyping light chains present on the cell can give a rapid answer when investigating whether *an idiopathic lymphadenopathy or lymphocytosis is neoplastic (one light only) or reactive (mixture of κ and λ positives) in origin.* This is particularly useful when it is realized that the majority of neoplastic lymphoid proliferations are of

TABLE II. CD antigen profile of neoplastic lymphoid proliferations

Type of leukaemia/lymphoma	Immunophenotypic profile
Acute lymphoblastic leukaemia (ALL)	Usual antigenic profile
Non-T ALL (B-lineage): Null cell ALL (~10%)	HLA-DR, Tdt, variable (±) CD19, CD24
Common ALL (~70%)	HLA-DR, CD19, CD10, Tdt, CD24
Pre-B ALL (~15–20%)	HLA-DR, CD19, CD10, Tdt, CD24, Cyto μ
B-ALL (<1% of ALL)	HLA-DR, CD19, Sm Ig
T-ALL (~15–20% ALL): Early thymocyte / Common thymocyte / Mature thymocyte	Profile of normal counterparts + Important features of aberrant expression of CDs
Chronic lymphoid leukaemia (CLL)	
B-CLL	Weak Sm Ig: (M+D), *kappa or lambda ±CD5, CD19, HLA-DR, CD24 (CD22)
T-CLL (~2% CLL)	CD2, CD3, CD5, CD7, CD4 or CD8
B-PLL (~80% PLL)	Strong Sm Ig, ±CD5, CD19, DR, CD24, CD22
T-PLL	As T-CLL
HCL	Strong Sm Ig, CD11, CD19, CD25++, HLA-DR, CD5 (±)
Non-Hodgkin's lymphoma (NHL)	
T-NHL	
Lymphoblastic	CD7, CD5, CD38, CD1, CD2, CD4, CD8 (surface CD3/TCR neg) (similar phenotype to T-ALL)
Peripheral T-cell lymphoma	CD2, CD3/TCR, CD5, CD7, CD4 or CD8 – may need genotyping – aberrant expression most useful
B-NHL	
FCC lymphoma	HLA-DR, CD19, CD20, CD21, Sm Ig, CD10(±) – aberrant expression useful – rarely genotyping
SLL	CD5, CD19, HLA-DR, Sm Ig, CD24, CD20 (similar phenotype to B-CLL)
Immunoblastic	HLA-DR, CD20, Sm Ig, CD19±

* Indicates detection of a single light chain associated with a neoplastic clone.
FCC = follicle centre cell; SLL = small lymphocytic lymphoma; PLL = prolymphocytic leukaemia; HCL = hairy cell leukaemia.
Genotyping – using molecular DNA probes to genetic elements of the T- and B-cell antigen receptors to examine gene rearrangements which can identify neoplastic clones.

B-cell lineage. More recently monoclonal antibodies to the V region of the human T-lymphocyte antigen-binding receptor (with some similarity to B-cell Sm Ig (cell surface membrane immunoglobulin)) have proved useful in defining neoplastic and oligoclonal T-cell proliferations [22].

Evaluation and monitoring of immunodeficiency disorders

The final diagnosis of many primary and secondary immune deficiency [23] disorders requires the evaluation of lymphocytes. Immunophenotyping is one aspect of this evaluation. It is now accepted that immunophenotypic monitoring of the absolute CD4 T-lymphocyte count is valuable in the management of HIV seropositive individuals and populations. The level of CD4 T-cells which are the target of HIV – the virus uses a CD4 molecule as its specific receptor for infecting and dysregulating lymphocytes – gives useful prognostic information and influences therapeutic decisions regarding antimicrobial prophylaxis and primary anti-HIV therapy [24].

Concluding remark
Clinicians should liaise and consult directly with their clinical pathologist colleagues when considering the use of immunophenotyping.

REFERENCES

1. Gooi HC, Chapel H. *Clinical Immunology: A Practice Approach.* Oxford University Press. 1990: 255 pp
2. Falk RJ, Becker M, Terell R, Jennette JC. *Antigen specificity of P-ANCA and of C-ANCA [Abstract].* The 3rd International Workshop on ANCA. Washington DC, 1990: 2–3
3. Kallenberg CG, Cohen Tervaert JW, van der Woude FJ et al. Autoimmunity to lysosomal enzymes: new clues to vasculitis and glomerulonephritis? *Immunol Today 1991; 12:* 61–64
4. van der Woude FJ, Rasmussen N, Lobatto S et al. Autoantibodies against neutrophils and monocytes: tool for diagnosis and marker of disease activity in Wegener's granulomatosis. *Lancet 1985; ii*: 425–429
5. Egner W, Chapel HM. Titration of antibodies against neutrophil cytoplasmic antigens is useful in monitoring disease activity in systemic vasculitides. *Clin Exp Immunol 1990; 82*: 244–249
6. Cohen Tervaert JW, Huitema MG, Hené RJ et al. Prevention of relapses in Wegener's granulomatosis by treatment based on anti-neutrophil cytoplasmic antibody titre. *Lancet 1990; 336:* 709–711
7. Gueirard P, Delpech A, Gilbert D et al. Anti-myeloperoxidase antibodies: immunological characteristics and clinical associations. *J Autoimmun 1991; 4*: 517–527
8. Falk RJ, Jeanette JC. Wegener's granulomatosis, systemic vasculitis, and antineutrophil cytoplasmic autoantibodies. *Ann Rev Med 1991; 42*: 459–469
9. Koderisch J, Andrassy K, Rasmussen N et al. 'False-positive' anti-neutrophil cytoplasmic antibodies in HIV infection [Letter]. *Lancet 1990; 335*: 1227–1228
10. Saxon A, Shanahan F, Landers C et al. A distinct subset of auto-antineutrophil cytoplasmic antibodies is associated with inflammatory bowel disease. *J Allergy Clin Immunol 1990; 86*: 202–210
11. Harris EN, Gharavi AE, Boey ML et al. Anticardiolipin antibodies: detection by radioimmunoassay and association with thrombosis in systemic lupus erythematosus. *Lancet 1983; ii*: 1211–1214
12. Love PE, Santoro SA. Antiphospholipid antibodies: anticardiolipin and the lupus anticoagulant in systemic lupus erythematosus (SLE) and in non-SLE disorders. Prevalence and clinical significance. *Ann Intern Med 1990; 112*: 682–698

13 Petri M, Rheinschmidt M, Whiting-O'Keefe Q et al. The frequency of lupus anticoagulant in systemic lupus erythematosus: a study of sixty consecutive patients by activated partial thromboplastin time, Russell viper venom time, and anticardiolipin antibody level. *Ann Intern Med 1987; 106:* 524-531

14 Tan EM, Cohen AS, Fries JT et al. The 1982 revised criteria for the classification of systemic lupus erythematosus. *Arthritis Rheum 1982; 25*: 1271-1277

15 Asherson RA, Khamashta MA, Gil A et al. Cerebrovascular disease and antiphospholipid antibodies in systemic lupus erythematosus, Lupus-like disease, and the primary antiphospholipid syndrome. *Am J Med 1989; 86*: 391-399

16 Asherson RA, Khamashta MA, Ordi-Ros J et al. The 'primary' antiphospholipid syndrome: major clinical and serological features. *Medicine (Baltimore) 1989; 68*: 366-374

17 Alarcón-Segovia D, Sanchez-Guerrero J. Primary antiphospholipid syndrome. *J Rheumatol 1989; 16*: 482-488

18 Derksen RHWM, Hasselaar P, Blokzijl L et al. Coagulation screen is more specific than the anticardiolipin antibody ELISA in defining a thrombotic subset of lupus patients. *Ann Rheum Dis 1988; 47*: 364-371

19 Blank M, Cohen J, Toder V, Shoenfeld Y. Induction of anti-phospholipid syndrome in naive mice with mouse lupus monoclonal and human polyclonal anti-cardiolipin antibodies. *Proc Natl Acad Sci 1991; 88*: 3069-3073

20 Chan LC, Pegram SM, Greave MF. Contribution of immunophenotype to the classification and differential diagnosis of acute leukaemics. *Lancet 1985; i*: 475-479

21 Sewell HF, Milton JI, MacKenzie R et al. Immunophenotyping of leukaemias by flow cytometry and APAAP: a two-year comparative analysis in hospital practice. *Disease Markers 1988; 6*: 221-229

22 Clark DM, Hall PA, Boylston AW, Carrel S. Antibodies to T cell antigen receptor beta chain families detect monoclonal T cell proliferation. *Lancet 1986; ii*: 835-837

23 Buckley RH. Immunodeficiency disorders. *JAMA 1987; 258*: 2841-2851

24 Phillips AN, Lee CA, Elford J et al. Serial CD4 lymphocyte counts and development of AIDS. *Lancet 1991; 337*: 389-392

THE THERAPY OF PRIMARY IMMUNODEFICIENCY

Mansel Haeney
Hope Hospital, Salford

INTRODUCTION
The study of primary immunodeficiency has been of enormous benefit to the fundamental understanding of how the immune system works and in stimulating the applied science of immunology, e.g. in bone marrow transplantation. Advances in management have led to progressive increases in survival of patients with primary immunodeficiency disease. Children with severe combined immunodeficiency or chronic granulomatous disease are now surviving into adolescence and early adulthood, while recognition of newer forms of antibody deficiency has uncovered patients with previously unexplained bacterial infections. Consequently, increasing numbers of patients with primary immunodeficiencies are being managed by general physicians.

PRINCIPLES OF MANAGEMENT
Early diagnosis is essential if treatment is to be started early enough to influence outcome. In severe combined immunodeficiency, for instance, bone marrow transplantation is the only cure: without it, children die before they are 1 year old [1]. Even in antibody deficiency, early diagnosis helps to prevent infections and reduce the incidence of complications [2].

Infections should be treated early with full doses of antimicrobial agents. Where possible, narrow spectrum drugs should be used. Prophylactic antibiotics are not generally recommended; they increase the hazard of infection with fungi or resistant organisms.

Blood transfusions should never be given to patients with proven or suspected defects of cellular immunity unless blood has been irradiated to destroy lymphocytes capable of causing graft-versus-host disease [1, 3]. Lymphocytes also remain viable in washed red blood cells, unprocessed plasma, and platelet preparations [3].

Immunodeficient patients have developed adverse reactions following immunization with living attenuated organisms [3]. Thus 'live' vaccines should be avoided in patients with suspected or proven immune defects.

Killed bacterial vaccines are generally harmless. In patients on immunoglobulin therapy, the passive immunity provided considerably reduces the risk of endemic infection.

ANTIBODY DEFICIENCY

Excluding selective IgA deficiency, where the prevalence is about 1 in 600 [4], the prevalence of hypogammaglobulinaemia in the UK is about 1 in 25,000 [5]. However, wide regional variations occur [6], ranging from 3.4 to 16 per million males (Figure 1) and 3.2 to 12.5 per million females. Primary antibody deficiency can be overlooked for years. One survey [7] found a delay in

Prevalence of CVI in the United Kingdom*, 1990 (♂)

- Scotland 7.3
- Northern Ireland 10.3
- Northern 10.7
- Yorkshire 8.5
- North Western 13.9
- Mersey 3.4
- Trent 10.4
- Wales 10.8
- West Midlands 11.3
- East Anglian 16
- Oxford 13.5
- N.W. Thames 11.7
- N.E. Thames 4.4
- South Western 10.2
- Wessex 11.9
- S.W. Thames 11.8
- S.E. Thames 10.2

□ Greater Than
▨ Less Than
National Prevalence Rate of 10/Million

* Health Regions

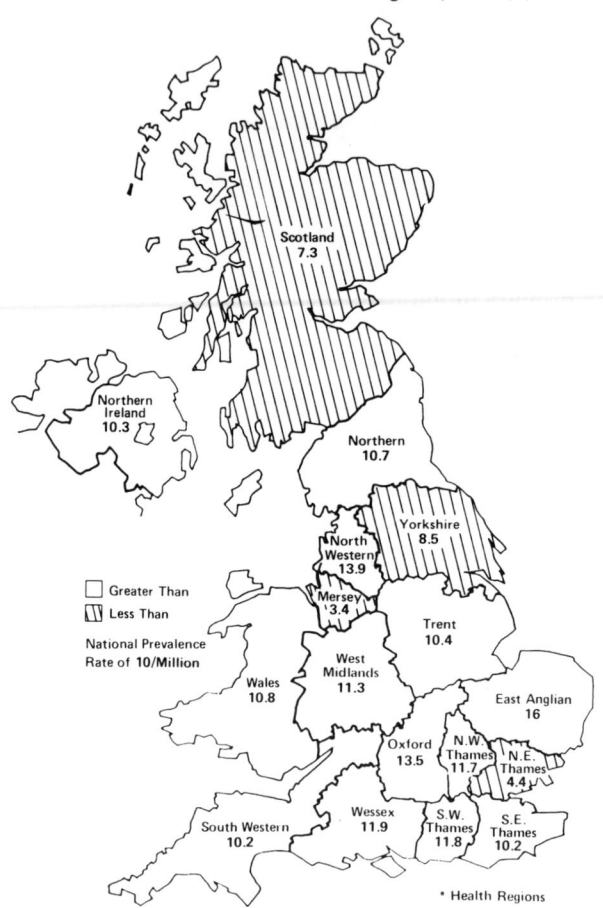

Figure 1. Prevalence of common variable immunodeficiency in males in different health regions of the UK, 1990. (No. per million population.) Reproduced from Gooi [6] by kind permission of the author and Royal Society of Medicine Services.

diagnosis in half of all children with antibody deficiency and virtually all adults. The delay ranged from 2 to 27 years in adults (median 5.5 years) and from 1 to 4 years in children (median 2.5 years) and entailed considerable morbidity. The diagnosis was rarely considered in adults or when patients were referred to organ-based specialties [7, 8]. Sometimes, the diagnosis was considered but inappropriate tests were done or abnormal results were overlooked [7].

Immunoglobulin replacement therapy
Immunoglobulin replacement therapy is mandatory for patients with defective antibody production. If treatment is started early, and given frequently enough, the cycle of recurrent infection and progressive lung damage can be slowed or stopped [9].

Intramuscular immunoglobulin
Intramuscular immunoglobulin is prepared from out-dated, pooled blood-bank plasma. The manufacturing procedure is virucidal to known viruses transmitted via blood or blood products, e.g. human immunodeficiency virus [10]. Most of the material is IgG and its antibody activity reflects that of the donor pool.

Unfortunately, there are drawbacks to the use of intramuscular immunoglobulins: the most serious problem is that 20% of patients will develop a systemic reaction although these are usually isolated episodes. The reaction occurs within minutes and resembles a classic anaphylactic attack; it is probably caused by aggregates of IgG which activate complement and trigger mast cell degranulation. Consequently, this preparation must never be injected intravenously. Local side-effects include pain, nerve damage and sterile abscess formation. Absorption of intramuscular immunoglobulin is variable and, coupled with the limitation on the volume injected, means that serum IgG levels rarely exceed 2–3g/l on this form of therapy. For the management of most patients, intravenous immunoglobulin therapy is the treatment of choice.

Intravenous immunoglobulin
Intravenous immunoglobulin (IVIG) is produced according to WHO criteria: each lot should be derived from plasma pooled from over 1000 donors; it should contain over 90% intact IgG, with the IgG subclasses corresponding to normal plasma, and be as free as possible of aggregates; its IgG molecules should maintain all their biological activities, such as opsonization capacity and the ability to fix complement; and the preparations should be free from kinins, plasmin, prekallikrein activator and from infectious agents [11].

IVIG preparations have several advantages over intramuscular immunoglobulin: larger doses can be given, so higher serum IgG levels are reached; infusions are less painful and less frequent; and adverse reactions are rare [12–14].

There is the potential for self-administration of IVIG at home in a way similar to factor VIII therapy in haemophilia. Home IVIG therapy began in the

USA and has been taken up in other countries including the UK. Home therapy is safe provided patients receive formal instruction at a recognized centre, which is a medico-legal requirement in the UK [15]. It is also cost-effective [12].

The efficacy of IVIG in reducing the frequency and severity of infections is dose-dependent [16]: given at a dose of 0.2–0.4g IgG/kg body weight every 3–4 weeks, trough serum IgG levels of 5–6g/l are obtained, although it may take 3–6 months to reach this steady state. It is important that the dose of IVIG is tailored to each patient's need.

A remaining concern about IVIG is the risk of transmissible disease, notably hepatitis C. All donor plasma is screened for hepatitis B surface antigen, human immunodeficiency virus and elevated levels of alanine aminotransferase, and soon will be screened for antibodies to hepatitis C. Nevertheless, there have been several outbreaks of non-A, non-B hepatitis involving different IVIG preparations [17]; some were associated with licensed products that had previously been safe, suggesting that the manufacturing processes were on the margin of safety as regards elimination of hepatitis C. It is important, therefore, that any change of therapy should be made on clinical and not on economic grounds. Plasma infusions have no place in the long-term treatment of antibody deficiency.

Subcutaneous immunoglobulin
Recently, it has been shown that intramuscular immunoglobulin can be given safely by rapid subcutaneous infusion [18]. The technique can be taught to patients for home treatment and trough levels of IgG obtained are similar to those with IVIG [18].

IgG subclass deficiency and immunoglobulin therapy

Recurrent bacterial infections occur in patients deficient in one or more of the four subclasses of IgG [19–21]. Individuals with IgG2 subclass deficiency are vulnerable to pneumococcal infection, presenting as septicaemia, meningitis, pneumonia or peritonitis. There is an association between deficiency of IgA and IgG2 (and IgG4) [21]. There is considerable debate as to which of the other claimed associations of IgG subclass deficiencies are true clinical entities [19–21]: these include respiratory tract infections, allergic disease, mouth ulcers and epilepsy. However, some patients with absent or deficient subclasses remain healthy [22]. It is an impaired antibody response, not a deficiency of an IgG subclass protein, that is associated with an increased risk of infection and a beneficial response to IVIG. An association between a clinical syndrome and a low level of an IgG subclass does not necessarily imply a causal link. A causal linkage will depend on the demonstration of several postulates (Table I). Many patients with selective impairment of antibody production to thymus-independent antigens have normal serum IgG subclasses [21]. In some of these cases, the antibody response can be corrected using protein-polysaccharide conjugate vaccines.

TABLE I. Suggested modified Koch postulates for determining causal link between IgG subclass deficiencies and associated clinicopathological changes

1. Deficiency must be consistently associated with given pathological condition
2. Clinical problem should be resolved by correcting defect or replacement
3. It should be possible to explain clinical association according to the known or experimentally determined physiological properties of the relevant IgG isotype
4. Induction of similar deficiencies in animal experimental models should result in analogous pathological changes

Reproduced from Jefferis and Kumararatne [21] by kind permission of the authors and *Clinical and Experimental Immunology*.

Other forms of therapy

Common variable immunodeficiency (CVI) represents a collection of defects, patients having either primary B-cell abnormalities, or B-cell dysfunction due to inadequate T-cell or macrophage function. Some patients have B-cells capable of responding to exogenous T-cell-derived differentiation signals, suggesting that, given an appropriate stimulus, these B-cells could be made to function more or less normally. One possibility is a state of relative interleukin-2 (IL-2) deficiency. This has led to in vitro studies on the use of recombinant IL-2 conjugated to polyethylene glycol (PEG-IL-2) to enhance T-cell, and potentially B-cell function in patients with CVI. PEG-IL-2 has a longer half-life than IL-2 with no apparent alteration in biological function. Preliminary experiments [23] show that B-lymphocytes from CVI patients respond to IL-2 in culture by secreting immunoglobulin, albeit at a lower level than B-cells from normal donors. In vivo studies of PEG-IL-2 in CVI patients are in progress.

SEVERE COMBINED IMMUNODEFICIENCY

Most defects involving cell-mediated immunity present within the first 6 months of life. Severe combined immunodeficiency (SCID) is the most serious form and occurs in 1 in 60,000 births. Infants with SCID grow and develop normally for a few weeks only but then fail to thrive, frequently with a clinical triad of intractable diarrhoea, pneumonia, and mucocutaneous candidiasis [1]. Because SCID is fatal within a year unless treated [1], this diagnosis must be excluded as early as possible, remembering that the differential diagnosis includes infection with human immunodeficiency virus.

Bone marrow transplantation

The first successful allogeneic bone marrow transplants (BMT) were performed in children with severe SCID. The only therapy that has been reproducibly successful for all forms of SCID is the transplantation of normal donor lymphoid stem cells, so allowing engraftment by donor T-lymphocytes. Ideally, donor and recipient should be identical at the major histocompatibility

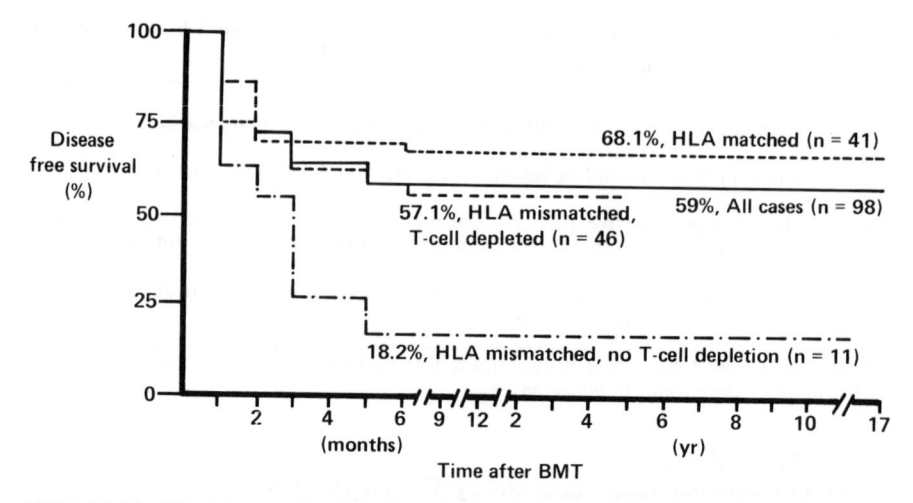

Figure 2. Probability of survival for patients with severe combined immunodeficiency following bone marrow transplantation. Reproduced from Fischer et al [25] by kind permission of the authors and *The Lancet*.

(MHC) Class I and II loci but two-thirds of patients with SCID do not have a compatible donor. Consequently, BMT for SCID may be achieved either using HLA-matched bone marrow or HLA-mismatched marrow which has been depleted of mature T-lymphocytes, separated physically by soybean agglutination and E rosetting or killed using monoclonal antibodies and complement [24].

In Europe, between 1968 and 1985, HLA-matched BMT achieved 68% disease-free survival [25] (Figure 2), similar to that reported elsewhere in the world [24]. Reanalysis of the European data up to February 1989 shows that 183 patients out of 314 with primary immune deficiencies or inborn errors of metabolism have been transplanted because of severe combined immunodeficiency [26]. The probability of survival for recipients of HLA identical BMT was 75.9%, reaching 96.9% for those treated since 1983. Recipients of T-cell-depleted, HLA non-identical BMT had a lower probability of survival of 52.2%. Four factors significantly influence the outcome of HLA non-identical BMT [26]: the presence of lung infection prior to BMT (relative risk (RR) 9.3), absence of protection (RR 11.07), female to male transplantation (RR 3.4) and absence of conditioning regimen (RR 3.3). A favourable combination of the three modifiable factors increased survival probability to 76% [26].

Graft-versus-host disease (GVHD), when it occurs, appears 8–20 days after a transplant and is characterized by fever, an erythematous, maculopapular skin rash, bloody diarrhoea, hepatosplenomegaly and pancytopenia [3, 27], and is frequently fatal. Low-grade GVHD, reflected in hepatomegaly, jaundice and skin rash, can persist for many months and become chronic and severely debilitating [3, 27]. Children restored immunologically have died occasionally of pre-existing pulmonary infections with *Pneumocystis carinii* or other organisms and prophylactic treatment with cotrimoxazole has proved useful in preventing these complications.

Liver transplantation
Transplantation of liver from foetuses of 9 to 11 weeks' gestation has reconstituted T- and B-cell function in some patients with SCID. The delay in reconstitution is very long (6 to 18 months) and the survival rate only 15% [3]. In the absence of an HLA identical bone marrow donor, haploidentical bone marrow transplantation is a better alternative than foetal liver transplantation.

Enzyme replacement
Frozen, irradiated red blood cells [28] or polyethylene-glycol modified adenosine deaminase (ADA) [29] provide partial replacement of enzymes in infants with the ADA form of SCID or purine nucleoside phosphorylase deficiency. Bone marrow transplantation is, however, the treatment of choice, the oldest survivors now approaching 20 years.

Gene therapy
Adenosine deaminase (ADA) deficiency is the cause of about 25% of cases of SCID [1, 3]. It causes accumulation of deoxyadenosine in tissue and body fluids which can be phosphorylated to form toxic dATP: this occurs readily in T-cells, leading to a combined immunodeficiency. The gene for ADA has been isolated on chromosome 20 and cDNA cloned. ADA deficiency is the first disease for which somatic gene therapy has been attempted.

To transfer the ADA gene to patient cells, a modified Moloney retrovirus vector called SAX has been prepared [30]. SAX contains a bacterial gene for neomycin resistance as a selectable marker and the human ADA gene driven by a promotor from simian virus 40 (SV40) [30]. Basic experiments showed that SAX-infected mouse T-cells produced a high level of human ADA, lasting over 4 months in vivo, and that gene transfer could correct the metabolic abnormalities in SCID patients in vitro [30]. This evidence provided the platform for the first attempts at gene therapy for patients with ADA-SCID. Treatment involves repeated apheresis to collect peripheral T-cells from patients, culture with anti-CD3 antibody and IL-2 to induce T-cell expansion, gene transfer by SAX and reinfusion of up to 2×10^{10} cells into the patient (Figure 3). Two patients with ADA-SCID have been treated so far [31]. Both have shown immunological improvement with an increase in ADA activity in T-cells from 1% to 35% of normal levels. Although the number of CD4+ T-cells remains subnormal, positive delayed type hypersensitivity skin tests and lymphocyte proliferative responses to antigens have been demonstrated [31].

CHRONIC GRANULOMATOUS DISEASE
Chronic granulomatous disease (CGD) is a group of congenital phagocytic disorders characterized by recurrent pyogenic infections with catalase-positive bacteria and fungi [32]. CGD results from a defect in one of the four com-

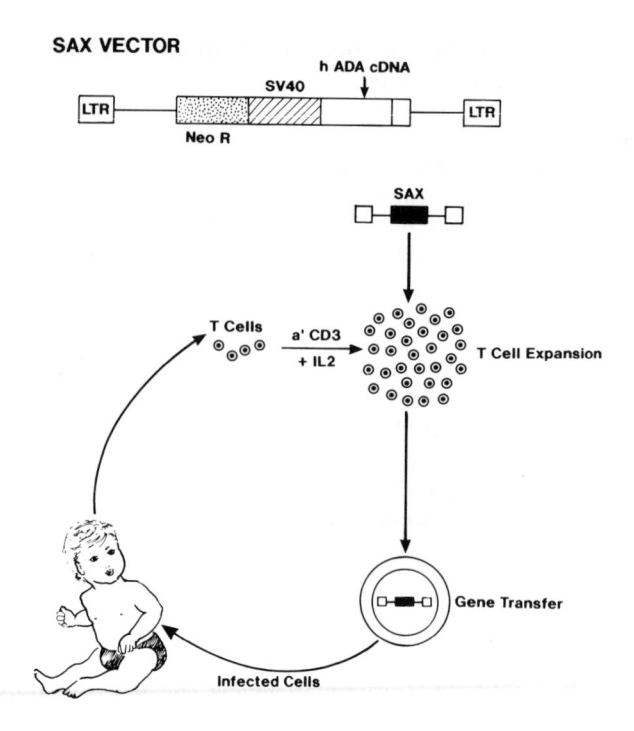

Figure 3. Schematic representation of somatic gene therapy for the treatment of ADA deficient SCID using the SAX vector.

ponents of the NADPH-oxidase system (two cytosol factors (p47-phox and p67-phox), and cytochrome b heavy and light chains (gp91-phox and p22-phox)). The phagocytic cells of CGD patients are unable to generate reactive oxygen metabolites and kill ingested microorganisms properly. The most common abnormality is the X-linked form, in which there is a defective gene for the 91 kD chain of cytochrome b-558 [32].

General measures
Until recently, the management of CGD had been largely supportive. Prolonged use of antibiotics and aggressive surgery for deep-seated infections remain central to patient management. Antibiotic prophylaxis with cotrimoxazole seems to improve the clinical course, and prolongs the interval between infections from about one every 9 months to about one every 4 years [33], although controlled prospective trials have not been performed. Despite these approaches, many patients still get terrible infections and die.

Interferon therapy
Treatment with recombinant human interferon-γ (IFN-γ) induces a marked increase in phagocyte bactericidal activity in CGD patients although only some show increased superoxide production, implying that IFN-γ acts by

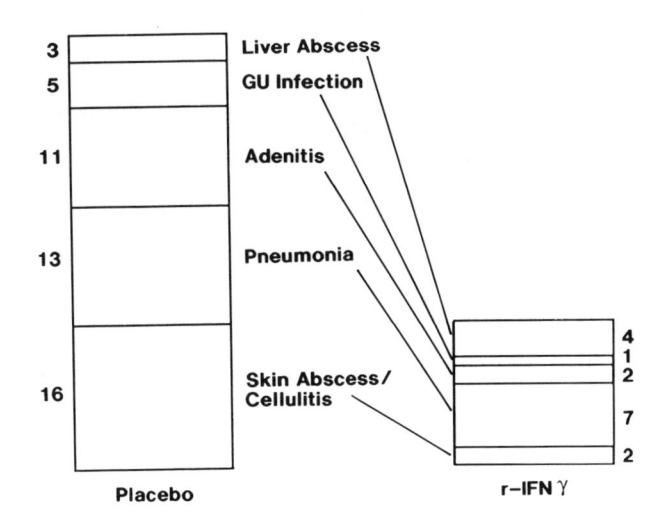

Figure 4. Clinical events requiring hospitalization and intravenous antibiotics in patients with chronic granulomatous disease treated with interferon or placebo. There was a 67% reduction in the relative risk of serious infection in the interferon group (p = 0.0006). Data derived from [35].

multiple mechanisms [34]. An international double-blind study [35] has assessed the clinical efficacy of IFN-γ in CGD. The number of infections that occurred in CGD patients treated with subcutaneous IFN-γ was significantly reduced compared with patients on placebo (Figure 4). Seventy-seven per cent of treated patients were free of serious infection 12 months after randomization compared with only 30% in the placebo group. Thirty of 65 patients in the placebo group experienced at least one serious infection compared with 14 of 63 patients in the IFN-γ group. Several patients had multiple serious infections. IFN-γ was most effective in reducing skin abscesses, pulmonary infections and lymphadenopathy (Figure 4) [35]. These studies suggest that IFN-γ holds promise for long-term prophylactic treatment of CGD but is only palliative. Cure, in the form of somatic gene therapy, has not been achieved but is currently under investigation in several centres.

REFERENCES
1. Rosen FS. Defects in cell-mediated immunity. *Clin Immunol Immunopathol 1986; 41*: 1–7
2. Björkander J, Bake B, Hanson LÅ. Primary hypogammaglobulinaemia: impaired lung function and body growth with delayed diagnosis and inadequate treatment. *Eur J Resp Dis 1984; 65*: 529–536
3. Scientific Group on Immunodeficiency. Primary immunodeficiency diseases. Report of a WHO sponsored meeting. *Immunodef Reviews 1989; 1*: 173–205
4. Hanson LÅ, Björkander J, Oxelius V-A. Selective IgA deficiency. In Chandra RK, ed. *Primary and Secondary Immunodeficiency Disorders.* Churchill Livingstone: Edinburgh. 1983: 62–84

5   Bird AG. Diagnosis of antibody deficiency states. In Levinsky RJ, ed. *IgG Subclass Deficiencies*. London: Royal Society of Medicine Services. 1989: 3-11
6   Gooi HC (for Immunology Travellers' Club, UK). Primary immunodeficiency register – United Kingdom. In Chapel HM, Levinsky RJ, Webster ADB, eds. *Progress in Immune Deficiency III* London: Royal Society of Medicine Services International Congress and Symposium Series No 173. 1991: 103-105
7   Blore J, Haeney MR. Primary antibody deficiency and diagnostic delay. *Br Med J 1989; 298*: 516-517
8   Hansel TT, Haeney MR, Thompson RA. Primary hypogammaglobulinaemia and arthritis. *Br Med J 1987; 295*: 174-175
9   Roifman CM, Lederman HM, Levi S et al. High-dose versus low-dose intravenous immunoglobulin in hypogammaglobulinaemia and chronic lung disease. *Lancet 1987; ii*: 1075-1077
10 Yap PL. Use of intravenous immunoglobulin in infectious disease. *Hosp Update 1990; 16*: 35-42
11 Buckley RH, Schiff RI. The use of intravenous immunoglobulin in immunodeficiency diseases. *N Engl J Med 1991; 325*: 110-117
12 Chapel HM, Brennan V, Delson E. Immunoglobulin replacement therapy by self-infusion at home. *Clin Exp Immunol 1988; 73*: 160-162
13 Schwartz SA. Intravenous immune globulin therapy of immune deficiency disorders. *Clin Immunol Newsletter 1991; 11*: 145-150
14 Ashida E. Use in antibody deficiencies. In: Stiehm ER, moderator. Intravenous immunoglobulins as therapeutic agents. *Ann Intern Med 1987; 107*: 367-382
15 Spickett GP, Misbah SA, Chapel HM. Primary antibody deficiency in adults. *Lancet 1991; 337*: 281-283
16 Gelfand EW, Reid B, Roifman CM. Intravenous immune serum globulin replacement in hypogammaglobulinaemia: a comparison of high- versus low-dose therapy. *Monogr Allergy 1988; 23*: 177-186
17 Editorial. Immunoglobulin therapy. *Lancet 1991; 338*: 157-158
18 Gardulf A, Hammarstrom L, Smith CIE. Home treatment of hypogammaglobulinaemia with subcutaneous gammaglobulin by rapid infusion. *Lancet 1991; 338*: 162-166
19 Morgan G, Levinsky RJ. Clinical significance of IgG subclass deficiency. *Arch Dis Child 1988; 63*: 771-773
20 Kumararatne DS, Bignall A, Joyce HJ, Hazlewood M. Antibody deficiency syndromes. In Gooi HC, Chapel HM, eds. *Clinical Immunology: A Practical Approach*. Oxford: Oxford University Press. 1990: 1-22
21 Jefferis R, Kumararatne DS. Selective IgG subclass deficiency: quantitation and clinical relevance. *Clin Exp Immunol 1990; 81*: 357-367
22 Hanson LA, Soderstrom R, Friman V et al. Update on IgA and IgG subclass deficiency. In Chapel HM, Levinsky RJ, Webster ADB, eds. *Progress in Immune Deficiency III*. London: Royal Society of Medicine Services International Congress and Symposium Series No. 173. 1991: 1-6
23 Cunningham-Rundles C, Mayer L. Potential use of polyethylene glycol-conjugated IL-2 in common variable immunodeficiency. In Chapel HM, Levinsky RJ, Webster ADB, eds. *Progress in Immune Deficiency III*. London: Royal Society of Medicine Services International Congress and Symposium Series No. 173. 191: 61-66
24 Lenarsky C, Parkman R. Bone marrow transplantation for the treatment of immune deficiency states. *Bone Marrow Transplantation 1990; 6*: 361-369
25 Fischer A, Griscelli C, Friedrich W et al. Bone marrow transplantation for immunodeficiencies and osteopetrosis: European survey 1968-1985. *Lancet 1986; ii*: 1080-1084
26 The EBMT/EGID working party on bone marrow transplantation for inborn errors. Bone marrow transplantation for immunodeficiencies and osteopetrosis in Europe. In Chapel HM, Levinsky RJ, Webster ADB, eds. *Progress in Immune Deficiency III*. London: Royal Society of Medicine Services International Congress and Symposium Series No. 173. 1991: 241
27 Ferrara JLM, Deeg HJ. Graft-versus-host disease. *N Engl J Med 1991; 324*: 667-674

28 Hirschhorn R. Inherited enzyme deficiencies and immunodeficiency: adenosine deaminase (ADA) and purine nucleoside phosphorylase (PNP) deficiencies. *Clin Immunol Immunopathol* 1986; *40*: 157-165
29 Hershfield MS, Buckley RH, Greenberg ML. Treatment of adenosine deaminase deficiency with polyethylene-glycol modified adenosine deaminase. *N Engl J Med* 1987; *316*: 589-596
30 Blaese RM. Progress toward gene therapy. *Clin Immunol Immunopathol* 1991; *61*: S47-S55
31 Matsumoto S, Sakiyama Y, Ariga T et al. Progress in primary immunodeficiency. *Immunol Today* 1992; *13*: 4-5
32 Dinaeur MC, Orkin SH. Molecular genetics of chronic granulomatous disease. *Immunodef Reviews* 1988; *1*: 55-69
33 Margolis DH, Melnick DA, Alling DW, Gallin JI. Trimethoprim-sulfamethoxazole prophylaxis in the management of chronic granulomatous disease. *J Infect Dis* 1990; *162*: 723-726
34 Ezekowitz RA, Dinauer MC, Jaffe HS et al. Partial correction of the phagocyte defect in patients with X-linked chronic granulomatous disease by subcutaneous interferon gamma. *N Engl J Med* 1988; *319*: 146-151
35 The International Chronic Granulomatous Disease Cooperative Study Group. A controlled trial of interferon gamma to prevent infection in chronic granulomatous disease. *N Engl J Med* 1991; *324*: 509-516

ANTIBODIES AS KILLERS

PL Amlot
Royal Free Hospital School of Medicine, London

INTRODUCTION
The selective killing of certain cells in the body is a therapeutic goal in cancer, transplantation and autoimmune diseases. The fortuitous and largely undesigned properties of cytotoxic drugs, immunosuppressive agents and corticosteroids fulfil this role but the inherent specificity of antibodies makes them a particularly appropriate vehicle with which to destroy cells selectively. The development of monoclonal antibodies was the technological step required to provide a wide range of antibodies with reliable and reproducible specificity for cell membrane antigens. The membrane antigens which can provide targets for monoclonal antibody (Mab) therapy are cell lineage differentiation antigens, receptors (e.g. growth factors), oncogene products, tumour associated antigens (e.g. carcinoembryonic antigen), tumour specific antigens or viral antigens. The purpose of this paper is to outline how the exquisite specificity of antibodies can be harnessed to provide an effective means of killing cells.

EFFECTOR MECHANISMS

Natural effector functions

Complement mediated cell lysis
Against bacteria and non-nucleated cells, complement is one of the principal lytic effector mechanisms activated by antibodies. However, Mabs are rarely able to induce complement mediated lysis against nucleated cells in homologous systems. This means that although many mouse and rat Mabs are lytic in the presence of rabbit complement, very few are similarly lytic using human complement to kill human cells. Prevention of complement lysis within a species by restriction factors is called homologous inhibition. Examples are: decay accelerating factor (CD55), which inhibits the convertase for the third component of complement (C3); homologous restriction factor (HRF),

which binds to and inhibits the eighth component of complement (C8); and CD59 (gp18), which inhibits the membrane attack complex of complement. All of these restriction factors are widely expressed on human nucleated cell membranes. The only potent complement lytic antibody which has been of value clinically is Campath 1 (CDw52; rat IgM) which binds to most leucocytes and is effective both in vitro and in vivo [1]. Complement lytic mechanisms function efficiently in intravascular and perivascular compartments but are probably of limited value at other tissue sites.

Antibody dependent cellular cytotoxicity (ADCC)
A large number of both mouse and rat Mabs are able to induce ADCC but it is difficult to gauge how effective this is in vivo. Almost all attempts to treat cancer patients with Mabs alone have either had no effect or a very transient effect. Administration of Mabs, up to doses of a gram in some cases, has only had a temporary lowering effect upon the leukaemic cell count in the blood of patients [2–5]. The suppression by OKT3 (CD3) of T-cells in the blood of transplant patients as treatment for rejection is rapidly reversed. Human IgG1, rat IgG2b and mouse IgG2a are the most effective isotypes for mediating ADCC. The use of an IgG2b immunoglobulin switch variant of Campath 1 and its humanized IgG1 form have both produced clinically significant responses in patients with leukaemia/lymphoma [6].

Idiotype network
Among the few truly tumour specific antigens are immunoglobulin and T-cell receptor idiotypes on B- and T-cell lymphomas. Anti-idiotype Mabs raised against lymphoma cells have been used to treat patients from whom the lymphoma cells were obtained. There have been one or two notable successes with this form of treatment [7, 8] but in general it has been as ineffective as other serotherapies using Mabs alone and there has been little evidence to suggest that special idiotype network control mechanisms are activated by these measures in malignant lymphomas.

Other mechanisms
Linking two Mabs together so that one reacts with a target cell and the other binds to an effector cell (T-cell, NK-cell) is a method by which cytotoxic cells can be concentrated at the site of a tumour. The method is effective in vitro but awaits validation by in vivo studies. Mabs which react with receptors (e.g. interleukin-2, transferrin and epidermal growth factor receptors) essential for cell proliferation could also be used to control cells and anti-IL-2 receptor antibodies have been used effectively for this purpose in transplantation but less so in lymphomas [9, 10].

Natural effector mechanisms are attractive as a means of therapy for cancer, transplantation and autoimmune diseases because they avoid the potent drugs and poisons normally used for this purpose. However, it should be remembered that natural effector mechanisms involved in combating infectious disease often lead to symptoms of illness. The use of antibodies such as OKT3 (CD3) or Campath 1 (CDw52) can produce fever, rigors, nausea, anorexia, headache, backache, leucocytosis, fluid retention, capillary leak syndrome, myalgia, rashes, arthralgia, eosinophilia and encephalitis. On the other hand, Mabs which do not induce natural effector mechanisms have been given to many patients, sometimes in large doses, with the minimum of toxicity.

Radioisotopes

Conjugation of a radioisotope to Mabs is the simplest method of increasing their cytotoxic potential. This approach is particularly appealing because the same technique will allow detection and imaging as well as treatment of the tumour. γ-Emission is needed for imaging whereas β-emission is essential for cell damage. The radioisotope most widely used has been ^{131}I which emits both β- and γ-rays and can be used for both therapy and imaging. However, there are advantages in selecting other radioisotopes, some of which are not yet freely available (e.g. ^{67}Cu and ^{210}Bi). In comparison with ^{131}I, yttrium (^{90}Y) is twice as potent in emitting β-irradiation and should therefore prove a more effective therapeutic radioisotope although it is of no value for imaging. An important functional aspect of radioimmunoconjugates is shown in Figure 1. β-Irradiation from a radioimmunoconjugate damages not only the cell to which it is attached but all cells within several cell diameters. The area affected depends on the isotope used. This 'bystander effect' is both desirable and undesirable because irradiation of malignant cells in the immediate vicinity means that it is not essential for the radioimmunoconjugate to bind to every cell in the tumour. On the other hand it also means that damage can occur to normal tissues nearby. Dose limiting toxicity of radioimmunoconjugates is entirely due to bone marrow damage. The maximum tolerated dose for ^{131}I-immunoconjugates (as a single dose) ranges from 50 to 100 mCi/m^2 [11, 12]. The major challenge in the development of radioimmunoconjugates is how effectively they can be concentrated and retained at the tumour site

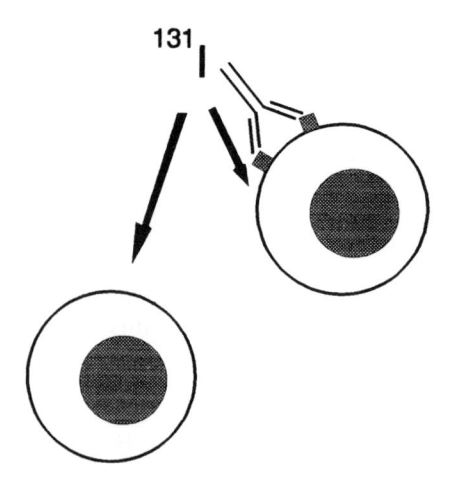

Figure 1. Radioimmunoconjugate, ^{131}Iodine linked to Mab, demonstrating the 'bystander effect'.

compared to the blood and bone marrow. About 10% of the injected dose of isotope will normally accumulate in tumour deposits for 48 hours and thereafter declines at the same rate as radioisotope elsewhere in the body. The bone marrow damage is a considerable disadvantage because it overlaps with the toxicity caused by conventional anticancer therapy (cytotoxic drugs and radiotherapy), which means that both modalities cannot be used together at full dosage.

Toxins and drugs
These studies began initially with cytotoxic drug conjugation to antibodies [13, 14] but this has been replaced by plant toxins which are more potent. Immunotoxins are made largely from ribosomal poisons originating from plants: ricin, abrin, saporin or gelonin. Immunotoxins have also been made with *Pseudomonas* exotoxin A and diphtheria toxin. The mechanism of action is illustrated in Figure 2. Several of the toxins consist of molecules made up of two chains (A and B). The B chain is capable of binding non-specifically to eukaryotic cell surfaces (to galactose side chains in the case of ricin) and facilitates the transfer of the A chain into the cytosol of the cell. This cellular routing is an essential step for cytotoxicity mediated by the A chain [15, 16]. The development of efficient immunotoxins requires the replacement of the non-specific B chain by a Mab to provide specificity and the removal of any chemical reactivity between the A chain and cell membranes (the ricin A chain still has mannose and fucose groups capable of binding mannose and fucose receptors in the liver).

For an immunotoxin to be effective, it must not only enter the cell but also dissociate from the antibody carrying it and enter the cytosol. If it enters lysosomal compartments it is inactivated and becomes totally harmless. These conditions place severe constraints on selecting (a) membrane targets which internalize rapidly on binding to antibody, (b) the linkage between the toxin and the Mab which must not break down in the bloodstream but should dissociate on entering the cell, and (c) an optimal Mab–toxin combination for entry into the cytosolic compartment of the cell so as to be lethal [17]. Attempts have been made to get round the problem of internalization by linking the whole ricin molecule to a Mab and modifying the B chain so as to interfere with its binding to galactose residues on the cell membrane while

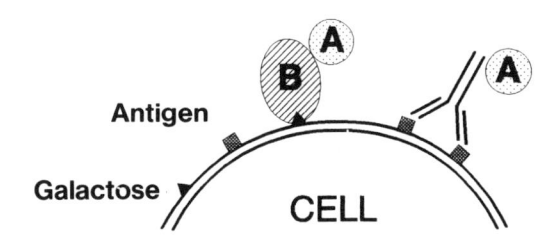

Figure 2. Immunotoxin compared with native ricin as an example of a two chain plant toxin.

still retaining the ability of the B chain to facilitate internalization of the A chain [18].

Dosage and antibody response
The maximum tolerated dose (MTD) for an immunotoxin made with blocked ricin is approximately 10-fold less than immunotoxins made with isolated ricin A chains (Table I), which suggests a considerable residue of non-specific toxicity due to the retention of the B chain despite its 'blocked' form. Antibody responses to both components of the immunotoxin are seen, more frequently in patients with melanoma or other solid tumours than with lymphoma and mostly occurring in the first month of treatment. The antibody response is not reduced by using cyclophosphamide (a potent immunosuppressive) but it can be reduced using cyclosporin A. Treatment with Fab' fragments greatly reduces the antibody response to mouse immunoglobulin but has no effect on the response to ricin (Table I). This indicates that humanization of the Mab is unlikely to prolong the time that immunotoxins can be used clinically since this will be determined when either an anti-mouse or an anti-toxin response occurs.

TABLE I. Maximum tolerated doses (MTD) and antibody responses to immunotoxins

Conjugate	Disease	No	MTD (mg/kg)	Antibodies (%)	
				Mouse	Toxin
CD5-ricin A chain	CLL/TALL	11	3.0	0	9
MEL-ricin A chain	Melanoma	22	4.0	95	95
+cyclophosphamide		20	0.4	100	100
CD22-dgA: FAB'	NHL	15	2.0	7	29
IgG		26	1.0	30	35
CD19-blocked ricin	NHL	25	0.25	56	56
– continuous		43	0.35	58	58
IL-2-diphtheria toxin	NHL	47	2.0	n.a.	60

CLL, chronic lymphocytic leukaemia; TALL, T-cell acute lymphoblastic leukaemia; NHL, non-Hodgkin's lymphoma.

Toxicity
Most clinical experience with immunotoxins has been gained using ricin conjugates but the toxic side-effects are likely to be shared by most of the ribosomal poisons. Unwanted toxicity from immunotoxins is shown in Table II. Very little toxicity was seen in the CD5-RTA study. All patients in the CD5-RTA study had leukaemia and it is likely that the immunotoxin was rapidly absorbed out of the circulation onto the leukaemic cells thus preventing some of the toxicity seen with other ricin containing immunotoxins. The vascular leak syndrome (VLS) and myalgia were the main toxicities seen with ricin A containing immunotoxins. In contrast, the main toxicity with 'blocked ricin' was *hepatic* indicating once again that considerable non-

specific activity was retained by the B chain in this form of immunotoxin. VLS and myalgia were not seen with the diphtheria toxin (DT) nor with radioimmunoconjugates. However, DT causes considerable allergic symptoms and radioimmunoconjugates, as mentioned before, cause haematological toxicity almost exclusively.

TABLE II. Comparison of main toxicities seen with immunotoxins and radioimmunoconjugates

Conjugate	Disease	Principal forms of toxicity seen				
		VLS	Blood	Liver	Myalgia	Allergy
CD5-RTA	CLL/TALL	-	-	-	-	-
MEL-RTA	Melanoma	++	+	-	++	-
CD22-dgA	NHL	++	-	-	++	-
CD19-BR	NHL	+	+	++	+	-
IL-2-DT	NHL	-	-	-	-	++
^{131}I-LYM	NHL	-	++	-	-	-
^{131}I-anti-CEA	Colorectal	-	++	-	-	-

VLS, vascular leak syndrome. Abbreviations of diseases are defined in footnote to Table I. Scale: ++ dose limiting; + significant; and - none or minimal toxicity.
Conjugates are in the same order as in Table I but are given here as abbreviations.

Clinical responses

Promising responses for Phase I studies are seen in lymphomas (NHL) but not in the other solid tumours (Table III). Immunotoxins containing isolated ricin A chain produce clinical responses more frequently than those containing 'blocked ricin'. This is consistent with the evidence elsewhere that the B chain in blocked ricin has considerable non-specific binding activity (especially liver) which may reduce its chances of penetrating to and localizing in tumours. The clinical responses seen in patients with lymphomas are consistent with their greater responsiveness to all forms of therapy. Thus lymphomas respond well with immunotoxins and radioimmunoconjugates whereas other solid tumours fare badly with both these modalities.

Enzyme and prodrug combinations

A different approach to antibody–drug complexes is shown in Figure 3. A Mab coupled to an enzyme is used to digest a non-toxic prodrug into a toxic drug at the site of the tumour. This produces a high concentration of cytotoxic drug locally. The Mab–enzyme complex needs to be injected some time before the prodrug so that it can localize to the tumour optimally and there should be a minimum of Mab–enzyme complex in the blood. Cellular routing is not critical and this approach can optimize the therapeutic index of highly toxic drugs. Enzymes like plant toxins are highly immunogenic and are likely to provoke antibody responses in most patients unless immunosuppressive strategies are used.

TABLE III. Phase I clinical responses to immunotoxins and immunoconjugates

Conjugated to	% of responses		Disease	Reference no.
	CR	PR		
CD5-ricin A	0	0	CLL/TALL	[19]
MEL-ricin A	0	4	Melanoma	[20]
CD22-ricin dgA	5	40	NHL	[21]
CD19-blocked ricin	4	8	NHL	[22]
– continuous	5	12	NHL	
IL-2 diphtheria toxin	6	10	NHL/CTCL	[23]
^{131}Iodine-LYM	13	57	NHL	[11]
^{131}Iodine-anti-CEA	0	6	Colorectal	[12]

CTCL, cutaneous T-cell lymphoma. Abbreviations of other diseases are defined in footnote to Table I.

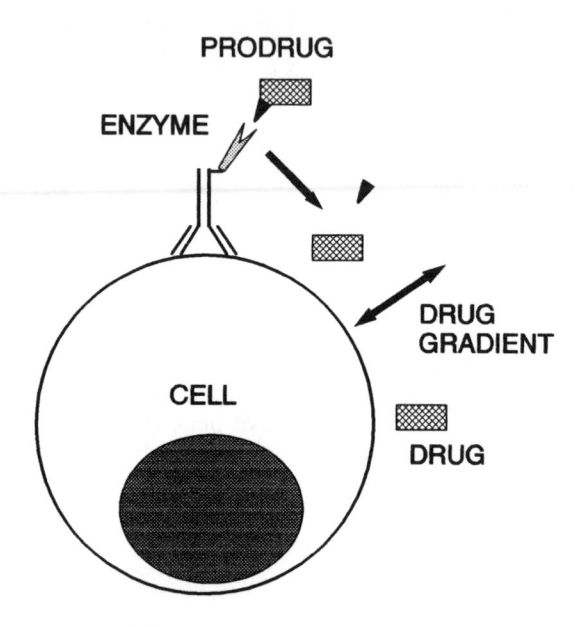

Figure 3. Antibody-directed enzyme prodrug therapy (ADEPT).

SUMMARY: PROS AND CONS

Immunogenicity
It is feasible that immunogenicity can be avoided by chimaerizing or humanizing the murine Mabs. This will benefit both natural effector mechanisms and radioimmunoconjugates but will not be of benefit to immunotoxins or immunoenzymes. Repeated use is possible if immunogenicity is overcome.

Potency
Both radioimmunoconjugates and immunotoxins have been found clinically effective in treating lymphomas. Further refinement of technical aspects may bring about real progress in the treatment of other solid tumours. In general Mabs which induce natural effector mechanisms are unlikely to be sufficiently potent for cancer therapy but have already been effective in transplantation and autoimmune diseases.

Handling
Immunotoxins are stable and retain their cytotoxicity for long periods of time whereas radioimmunoconjugates have to be prepared fresh with each treatment. However, radio-labelling procedures have been made rapid and simple to perform. There is still the problem of disposing of radioactive waste but if predominantly β-emitters like yttrium are used treatment of patients will be greatly simplified. Further impetus for a move to more appropriate isotopes is that de-iodination is an important process leading to dissociation of the ^{131}I from its Mab in vivo.

Selection
Mabs with adequate binding affinity and any target membrane antigen can form suitable systems for radioimmunoconjugates but very stringent conditions are required in the selection of immunotoxins because of the intracellular routing necessary. Any non-specific binding by the toxin moiety will impair the therapeutic effect.

Mode of action
Immunotoxins have a novel mode of action with toxicities which differ from conventional therapies and will allow maximum dosage of each simultaneously. The main side-effects of both radioimmunoconjugates and antibody-directed enzyme prodrug therapy (ADEPT) will be bone marrow toxicity which they share with conventional therapies. ADEPT will be susceptible to multidrug resistance.

REFERENCES
1. Dyer MJS, Hale G, Hayhoe FGJ et al. Effects of CAMPATH-1 antibodies in vivo in patients with lymphoid malignancies: influence of antibody isotype. *Blood 1989; 73*: 1431-1439
2. Houghton A, Scheinberg DA. Monoclonal antibodies in the treatment of hematopoietic malignancies. *S Hematology 1988; 25*: 23
3. Ritz J, Pesando JM, Sallan SE et al. Serotherapy of acute lymphoblastic leukaemia with monoclonal antibody. *Blood 1981; 58*: 141-152
4. Ball ED, Bernier GM, Cornwell III GG et al. Monoclonal antibodies to myeloid differentiation antigen: In vivo studies of three patients with acute myelogenous leukaemia. *Blood 1983; 62*: 1203-1210
5. Dillman RO, Shawler DL, Dillman JB et al. Therapy of chronic lymphocytic leukaemia and cutaneous T-cell lymphoma with T-101 monoclonal antibody. *J Clin Oncol 1984; 2*: 881-891
6. Hale G, Dyer MJS, Clarke MR et al. Remission induction in non-Hodgkin lymphoma with reshaped human monoclonal antibody Campath-1H. *Lancet 1988; ii*: 1394-1398

7 Meeker TC, Lowder J, Maloney DG et al. A clinical trial of anti-idiotype therapy for B-cell malignancy. *Blood 1985; 65*: 1349–1363
8 Hamblin TJ, Cattan AR, Glennie MJ et al. Initial experience in treating human lymphoma with a chimeric univalent derivative of monoclonal anti-idiotype antibody. *Blood 1987; 69*: 790
9 Soulillou J-P, Cantarovich D, Le Mauff B et al. Randomised controlled trial of a monoclonal antibody against the interleukin-2 receptor (33B3.1) as compared with rabbit antithymocyte globulin for prophylaxis against rejection of renal allografts. *N Engl J Med 1990; 322*: 1175–1182
10 Waldmann TA, Goldman CK, Bongiovanni KF et al. Therapy of patients with human T-cell lymphotrophic virus 1 induced adult T-cell leukaemia with anti-Tac, a monoclonal antibody to the receptor for interleukin-2. *Blood 1988; 72*: 1805–1816
11 DeNardo GL, DeNardo SJ, O'Grady LF et al. Fractionated radioimmunotherapy of B-cell malignancies with (131)I-LYM-1. *Cancer Res 1990; 50*: 1014s–1016s
12 Begent RHJ, Ledermann JA, Green AJ et al. Antibody distribution and dosimetry in patients receiving radiolabelled antibody therapy for colorectal cancer. *Br J Cancer 1989; 60*: 406–412
13 Ghose T, Norvell ST, Guclu A et al. Immunochemotherapy of cancer with chlorambucil-carrying antibody. *Br Med J 1972; iii*: 495–499
14 Kanellos J, Pietersz GA, McKenzie IFC. Studies of methotrexate-monoclonal antibody conjugates for immunotherapy. *J Natl Cancer Inst 1985; 75*: 319–329
15 Olsnes S, Sandvig K. How protein toxins enter and kill cells. *Cancer Treat Res 1988; 37*: 39
16 Calafat J, Molthoff C, Janssen H et al. Endocytosis and intracellular routing of an antibody-ricin A chain conjugate. *Cancer Res 1988; 48*: 3822–3827
17 Thorpe PE, Wallace PM, Knowles PP et al. Improved antitumor effects of immunotoxins prepared with deglycosylated ricin A-chain and hindered disulfide linkages. *Cancer Res 1988; 48*: 6396–6403
18 Lambert JM, Goldmacher VS, Collinson AR et al. An immunotoxin prepared with blocked ricin: a natural plant toxin adapted for therapeutic use. *Cancer Res 1991; 51*: 6236–6242
19 Hertler AA, Frankel AE. Immunotoxins: a clinical review of their use in the treatment of malignancies. *J Clin Oncol 1989; 7*: 1932–1942
20 Oratz R, Speyer JL, Wernz JC et al. Antimelanoma monoclonal antibody-ricin A chain immunoconjugate (XMMME-001-RTA) plus cyclophosphamide in the treatment of metastatic malignant melanoma: results of a phase II trial. *J Biol Response Mod 1990; 9*: 345–354
21 Vitetta ES, Stone M, Amlot PL et al. Phase I immunotoxin trial in patients with B-cell lymphoma. *Cancer Res 1991; 51*: 4052–4058
22 Grossbard ML, Freedman AS, Ritz J et al. Serotherapy of B-cell neoplasms with anti-B4-blocked ricin: A Phase I trial of daily bolus infusion. *Blood 1992; 79*: 576–585
23 LeMaistre CF, Von Hoff D, Meneghetti C et al. $DAB_{486}IL-2$ is effective therapy for some patients with IL-2 receptor expressing malignancies. *Proc ASCO 1991; 10*: 280

HEPATITIS C

Geoffrey M Dusheiko
Royal Free Hospital and School of Medicine, London

INTRODUCTION
In 1989, Houghton and co-workers succeeded in isolating nucleic acid clones of the major non-A non-B (NANB) agent by recombinant DNA technology [1–3]. A viral protein (5-1-1) was subsequently expressed in bacteria. Immunoblot analysis was performed on bacterial lysates using serum obtained from chimpanzees which had been experimentally infected with NANB hepatitis, enabling the detection of circulating antibody. A radio-immunoassay was subsequently developed for detection of antibody in patients with chronic NANB hepatitis.

The timely identification of this agent, which has been given the name hepatitis C virus (HCV), and the development of specific serologic tests for the diagnosis of HCV, have rapidly enhanced our understanding of type C hepatitis, and have improved the treatment of this disease.

Preliminary epidemiological assessment suggests most cases of NANB hepatitis in Europe, the Americas, and the Far East are caused by hepatitis C.

VIROLOGY OF HCV
HCV is now believed to be an enveloped virus, approximately 50nm in size, and is known to possess an RNA genome of approximately 9000 nucleotides (Figure 1). The genomic organization suggests some homology to flavi- or pestiviruses, but HCV may be sufficiently unique to be placed in its own genus [4]. Genomic sequences have been published for the prototype strain isolated in the USA (HCV 1), and two strains isolated in Japan (HCV-J and HCV-JH). Partial sequences of other isolates are being reported from other geographic regions [5].

The viral genomic RNA is a single stranded plus sense RNA, with a single long open reading frame. The gene product is a viral polyprotein precursor of 3011 amino acids, which undergoes proteolytic post-translational cleavage to yield structural (core and envelope) and non-structural (proteases, helicases, RNA-dependent RNA polymerase) proteins.

Hepatitis C Virus

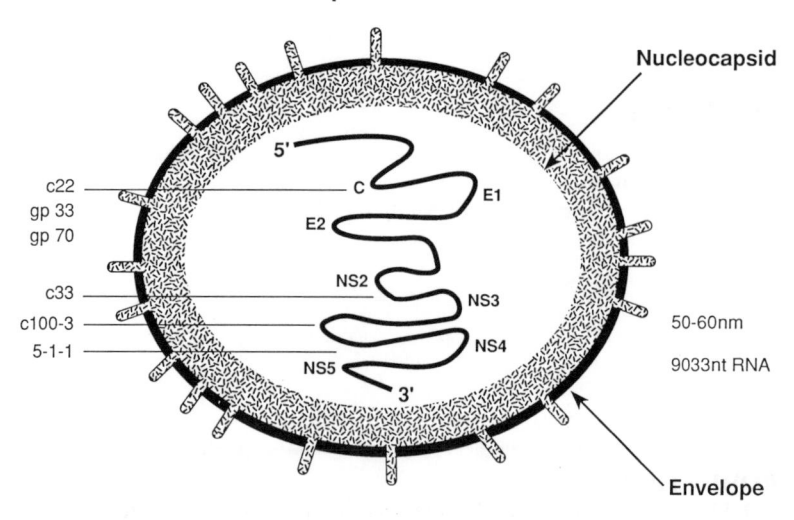

Figure 1. A stylized depiction of the hepatitis C virus, showing the viral particle, nucleocapsid, RNA genome, non-coding 5′ region, coding region, and proteins expressed from the viral genome and used in serological assays for antibody to HCV. C = nucleocapsid protein coding region; E = envelope protein coding region; NS = non-structural region.

The 5′ non-coding region appears to be highly conserved [6, 7]. Two glycosylated proteins, gp 35 and gp 70, may be coded by the E1 and E2 regions of the genome, and could be envelope proteins of the hepatitis C virus [8]. Variable and hypervariable regions within the putative envelope glycoproteins have been described [9, 10]. The first commercially available diagnostic tests were based on antibodies to an expressed protein (c100-3), derived from the NS3/NS4 region. This antigen represents 363 amino acids of viral sequence from the NS4 region (4% of total viral protein), and includes a fusion protein (superoxide dismutase (SOD)) for expression in yeast.

DIAGNOSIS OF HCV

HCV antibodies

There are no tests for antigens of HCV in serum, as the virus circulates in serum at a concentration below the level of detection of antigen by standard immunoassays. Most of the sero-epidemiological and diagnostic studies of hepatitis C were initially based on the prevalence of antibodies to c100-3. More recently, other antigens have been expressed, including a 22 kDa structural protein of HCV, whose coding region has been mapped to the aminoterminal (C, Figure 1) region of the HCV polyprotein, and which is ostensibly a nucleocapsid (core) antigen of HCV [11]. A second series of non-structural antigens, including c33 and c200, have been derived from the NS3 and NS4 regions and expressed in yeast or *Escherichia coli*. Together these antigens are the basis for second generation solid phase enzyme-linked immunoassays for antibodies to HCV, which considerably improve the sensitivity of diagnosis.

The antibodies detected are probably not neutralizing as they are found in chronic carriers. It is suspected, but unproven, that antibodies to the E (envelope) glycoproteins are neutralizing. Assays based on antibodies to synthetic peptides derived from immunodominant regions of both core and non-structural antigens have been developed [12]. IgM antibody tests have also been developed.

Supplemental antibody tests

Initial surveys of antibody to hepatitis C in blood donors indicated a high rate of false positive tests. This has necessitated the development of 'supplemental' assays for confirmation of a positive anti-HCV result. The most widely used supplemental test is the recombinant immunoblot assay (RIBA) in which four HCV antigens are fixed to a nitrocellulose filter, along with control proteins. The four antigens comprise one structural (c22) and three non-structural antigens (c33, c100-3, 5-1-1).

A close correlation has been found between 4-RIBA positive samples and viraemia, which enables discrimination between infective and non-infective donors [13].

HCV RNA testing

Since the antigens of HCV are present in very low titres, direct tests for viraemia in HCV have relied on the detection of HCV RNA in serum. RNA detection necessitates an amplification of the circulating HCV RNA, and thus sensitive assays for HCV RNA have been developed, based on the polymerase chain reaction (PCR). RNA is detected in the majority (60–80%) of anti-HCV positive patients, and is also detectable in a percentage of anti-HCV-negative patients with chronic NANB hepatitis [14].

Sensitivity of the test is improved by using an internal (nested) set of primers, and by using primers derived from the 5' untranslated region of the genome, which is highly conserved [15].

Serological diagnosis: acute hepatitis C

Anti-c100-3 appears in the circulation after a mean interval of 15 weeks from the acute illness and first elevations of the aminotransferase (ALT) [16]. Although roughly one-third of seroconversions take place early in the acute phase of the disease, sometimes as early as 2 weeks [17], seroconversion can be delayed for a year or longer. The average time from transfusion to seroconversion is of the order of 11–12 weeks with the first generation tests, and 7–8 weeks with the second generation tests. Seroconversion occurs much less frequently, and in lower titre, in acute self-limiting infections compared with those that progress to become chronic [18–20]. Thus tests for anti-HCV are of limited benefit in diagnosing acute hepatitis C.

During the early phase of primary HCV infection, serum HCV RNA is the only diagnostic marker of infection, and RNA testing therefore remains the only means of diagnosis in seronegative patients. Serum HCV RNA has been detected within 1 to 3 weeks of transfusion in patients with hepatitis C, and usually lasts less than 4 months in patients with acute self-limited hepatitis C, but may persist for decades in patients with chronic disease [21].

A suitable immunodiagnostic test for resolved infection and immunity is not available, but antibodies to the envelope region are being sought.

Serological diagnosis: chronic hepatitis C

Anti-HCV antibodies persist in the majority of patients with chronic post-transfusion NANB hepatitis; in studies in chimpanzees, anti-HCV (i.e. anti-c100-3) was not neutralizing. The development and maintenance of current diagnostic antibodies to hepatitis C virus therefore appears to reflect concomitant virus replication, and consequently a high potential for infectivity.

A proportion of patients may improve spontaneously, but the number of patients who do so is unclear. These patients lose antibody after follow-up of at least 5 years, and usually develop normal serum aminotranferases [22]. Other patients may have a decline in anti-HCV titre with time [18].

HCV RNA usually persists in patients with abnormal serum aminotransferases and anti-HCV. However, HCV RNA, and hence viraemia, can also be found in patients with normal liver function tests. Preliminary, but unconfirmed, reports have suggested the HCV antigens can be detected in liver biopsy preparations in chronic carriers.

EPIDEMIOLOGY AND TRANSMISSION OF HEPATITIS C

Transmission

Although the precise mode of acquisition of hepatitis C is often uncertain, hepatitis C is known to be transmitted by parenteral, or inapparent parenteral contact routes. The virus circulates in relatively low titres in blood, but transmission by blood transfusion, and blood products including factor VII, factor IX, fibrinogen and cryoglobulin has been unequivocally documented. A number of studies in chimpanzees have documented serial passage of NANB hepatitis (now known to be HCV) using sera derived from blood donors implicated in cases of NANB post-transfusion hepatitis [23]. Similarly, transmission among intravenous drug abusers through shared needles accounts for the high prevalence of infection in this group.

Community-acquired transmission

The majority of cases of NANB hepatitis cannot be accounted for by past blood transfusion, or indeed an identifiable source of parenteral exposure to this virus. The disease is prevalent in many parts of the world where the transmission cannot be explained by blood transfusion or intravenous drug abuse. The precise mechanism of most cases of transmission of community-acquired disease is uncertain, but transmission by close person-to-person contact from carriers of HCV is the most plausible method of explaining transmission in these societies.

Sexual transmission seems certainly possible, albeit a relatively inefficient and infrequent means. Anti-HCV has been found in 11% of sexual partners of anti-HCV positive intravenous drug abusers, and may correlate with the presence of HIV [24]. The overall HCV infection rate is also higher in sexually promiscuous groups.

Transmission by saliva (or saliva containing blood) and by a human bite has been reported [25-27]. Dentists in New York, particularly those practising oral surgery, have a higher prevalence of anti-HCV antibody compared to blood donors [28].

The advent of serological testing has shown that most community-acquired NANB hepatitis is also due to hepatitis C. The rate of seropositivity is higher in patients who progress to chronicity. It would appear that patients with no history of transfusion are just as likely to go on to chronic hepatitis. A substantial proportion of acute community-acquired cases remain unclassified, and studies using PCR to detect HCV RNA remain the only diagnostic test to exclude another virus.

Fulminant hepatitis is more common in sporadic NANB hepatitis, but the aetiology of most cases is not apparently due to hepatitis C virus.

Intrafamilial transmission
The role of intrafamilial transmission requires clarification, but is relatively infrequent. In Japan, up to 8% of family members of an index patient with HCV have been found to be anti-HCV positive, but no specific relative could be linked to HCV positivity, making it difficult to identify the route of infection [29].

Maternal-infant transmission
Mother-to-infant transmission has been observed, but appears to be relatively uncommon. The importance of this route remains controversial. Wejstal et al [30] showed that children born to anti-HCV positive mothers acquired passively transferred antibodies that were present transiently in serum and disappeared within 7 months. A disturbing finding, however, has been the detection of persistent HCV RNA in serum in the absence of anti-HCV in newborn babies delivered by women who were anti-HCV positive, suggesting silent transmission of HCV [31]. It is not clear, however, how important this route is in perpetuating the reservoir of human infection.

Population studies
The prevalence of type C hepatitis in blood donors has now been ascertained in many countries. The positive immunoassay rate ranges from 0.18 to 1.4%; in most Western countries, the prevalence ranges from 0.3 to 0.7%; in Japan and southern Europe, 0.9 to 1.2%. A higher prevalence has been found in southern Italy and eastern Europe than in northern Europe [32]. The prevalence in commercial (paid) donors is higher (10-15%) [33]. A higher prevalence has been found in Africans; for example, in South Africa up to 4.2% of men are anti-HCV positive [34, 35]. False positive results can occur in stored serum from tropical areas. Most anti-HCV positive donors give no history of blood transfusion, but a proportion admit to previous drug use.

Post-transfusion hepatitis C
Prior to the introduction of HCV screening, the incidence of post-transfusion NANB hepatitis ranged from 2 to 19% [36]. Serological testing now indicates that seroconversion to anti-HCV occurs in 85-100% of patients with chronic post-transfusion NANB hepatitis [37]. Retrospective studies have shown a higher prevalence of anti-HCV at onset in those developing chronic disease (83%) than those who recover from post-transfusion hepatitis. Anti-HCV persists for years and even decades in chronic hepatitis C but may decline in titre or disappear with resolution.

Anti-HCV testing should effect at least a further 50% reduction in the incidence of post-transfusion hepatitis. In both Spain and Japan, the incidence has already been reduced from 9.6% and 4.6% to 1.6% and 1.9% respectively [37, 38]. A low incidence of post-transfusion hepatitis C still occurs after transfusion of blood that is negative for anti-HCV [39]. Although the cost effectiveness of screening is unknown, screening is demanded by countries willing and able to pay for health care. Blood banks in the USA voluntarily began testing donations for anti-HCV in 1990, and in the UK in September 1991 [40].

Hepatitis C in high risk populations
A high prevalence of anti-HCV is found in many at-risk groups exposed to blood or blood components, particularly where a single unit containing the virus contaminates the batch. The highest prevalences worldwide are found in haemophiliacs, 50-90% of whom are anti-HCV-positive, depending upon age, the duration of infection, factor VIII requirement, and the source of factor VIII [41]. The high prevalence in haemophiliacs reflects the frequent use of factor VIII, which is derived from thousands of donors. Solvent detergent inactivation and pasteurization have been shown to reduce the risk of transmitting HCV infection [42].

The prevalence of anti-HCV is high in multiply transfused patients with thalassaemia major, but varies geographically according to the source of the blood administered to patients [43]. The prevalence in intravenous drug users is extremely high (70-92%), because of repeated exposure to carriers of HCV through shared, contaminated needles. Several other groups have been shown to be at risk. These include haemodialysed patients, particularly in endemic areas such as the Middle East or Japan [44].

Anti-HCV is apparently also common in transplant patients requiring frequent blood transfusions, including renal, liver and bone marrow transplant recipients [45-47]. Nosocomial or occupational exposure is being evaluated. Health care workers appear to be at comparatively low risk [48, 49].

Prevalence of anti-HCV in chronic liver disease
Serological testing has shown a high prevalence of anti-HCV in patients with chronic active hepatitis (CAH) and/or cirrhosis considered due to NANB hepatitis [18]. The majority (75-95%) of patients with post-transfusion chronic NANB hepatitis in the USA and Europe are positive for anti-HCV. The disease in many persons with chronic NANB hepatitis may or may not be associated with a history of blood transfusion. The prevalence varies

according to the background endemicity of hepatitis C in the population [50]. Test for anti-HCV are now important in establishing a diagnosis of what was formerly considered cryptogenic cirrhosis.

Autoimmune hepatitis
There are conflicting reports regarding the occurrence of hepatitis C antibodies in patients with autoimmune liver disease. Clearly the enzyme-linked immunosorbent assay (ELISA) for anti-HCV is prone to false positive results in patients with high concentrations of immunoglobulins in serum [51]. These false reactive anti-HCV antibodies in patients with anti-smooth muscle antibody may actually disappear with immunosuppressive treatment, as globulin levels decrease [52]. In Japan, 80% of patients with chronic NANB hepatitis have circulating antibodies to a pentadecapeptide (GOR), an epitope of normal hepatocytes; this phenomenon may represent an autoimmune response peculiar to type C hepatitis [53].

Up to 50% of patients with type II autoimmune hepatitis (anti-liver kidney microsomal (LKM), antibody positive) are anti-HCV positive, and anti-HCV and anti-LKM in association may also represent another example of autoimmune disease associated with a virus infection. Anti-HCV positive patients with anti-LKM positive CAH are usually male, older, and have lower titres of anti-LKM than patients without anti-HCV. They are also frequently anti-GOR positive. The target antigen of antibodies to LKM is a portion of the cytochrome P450 II D6 molecule; some sequence homology between HCV and cytochrome P450 may exist [54]. This association has some therapeutic implications, as the autoimmune LKM positive disease is responsive to corticosteroids, and may be aggravated by alpha interferon.

Hepatitis B and HIV
HCV may cause disease concurrently with hepatitis B, particularly in at-risk groups such as haemophiliacs and drug abusers, or where these diseases are endemic in the same environment: the combination may cause aggravated disease [55, 56]; likewise, in drug abusers and haemophiliacs, HIV and HCV may coexist and cause severe, accelerated liver disease.

Alcoholic liver disease
In several countries, a higher prevalence of anti-HCV has been found in patients with alcoholic liver disease. The prevalence of hepatitis C antibodies correlates with the severity of liver injury, and is higher in patients with cirrhosis than in those with only fatty change [57].

Hepatocellular carcinoma (HCC)
Serological analysis of patients with HCC has shown a high prevalence of anti-HCV in these patients. Several case control studies in Europe have suggested that up to 70% of male patients with HCC are anti-HCV positive [58, 59]. The mean interval between the date of transfusion and the diagnosis of cirrhosis and HCC is usually long: 21 and 29 years respectively [60].

Other diseases
Although NANB hepatitis has been thought to be associated with aplastic anaemia, to date there is no conclusive evidence to link HCV infection with aplastic anaemia [61].

Cryoglobulinaemia has been associated with hepatitis C, and up to 54% of patients with mixed cryoglobulinaemia are anti-HCV positive (verified by RIBA). The surprising role of HCV in the pathogenesis of this disease is unknown [62, 63].

CLINICAL FEATURES

Acute hepatitis C
The mean incubation period of hepatitis C is 6–12 weeks. However, with a large inoculum, such as in cases following administration of factor VIII, the incubation period is reduced to 4 weeks or less [17, 64]. The acute course of HCV infection is clinically mild, and the peak serum ALT elevations are less than those encountered in acute hepatitis A or B. Only 25% of cases are icteric. Subclinical disease is common; such patients may first present decades later with sequelae such as cirrhosis or HCC. During the early clinical phase the serum ALT levels may fluctuate, and may become normal or near normal, making the determination of true convalescence difficult. Severe or fulminant hepatitis C is rare, but may occur. The diagnosis of such cases requires confirmation by HCV RNA testing. Arthritis, rashes, glomerulonephritis, vasculitis, neurological syndromes and aplastic anaemia have been reported in association with hepatitis C.

Chronic hepatitis C
The clinical and epidemiological features of transfusion-associated and sporadic NANB hepatitis have been well documented. The disease has a disturbing propensity to progress to chronic hepatitis. Fifty to seventy-five per cent of patients with type C post-transfusion hepatitis continue to have abnormal serum aminotransferase levels after 12 months, and chronic hepatitis histologically [16]. The risk of chronic infection after sporadic hepatitis C is probably similar. Most patients with chronic hepatitis C are asymptomatic, or only mildly symptomatic. In symptomatic patients, fatigue is the most common complaint. Many patients do not give a history of acute hepatitis or jaundice. Physical findings are generally mild and variable, and there may be no abnormalities. With more severe disease, spider angiomata and hepatosplenomegaly may be found. Serum aminotransferases decline from the peak values encountered in the acute phase of the disease, but remain two- to eightfold abnormal. The serum ALT concentrations may fluctuate over time, and may even intermittently be normal. Many patients have a sustained elevation of the serum aminotransferases. A characteristic histological pattern of mild chronic hepatitis with portal lymphoid follicles and varying degrees of lobular activity is found in many patients [65].

The spectrum of chronic disease varies. Most patients appear to have an indolent, only slowly progressive course with little increase in mortality after

20 years. However, cirrhosis develops in approximately 20% of patients with chronic disease within 10 years, albeit that the cirrhosis remains indolent and only slowly progressive for a prolonged period [66, 67]. The disease is not necessarily benign, however, and rapidly progressive cirrhosis can occur. Older age of infection, concomitant alcohol abuse, concurrent HBV or HIV infection or other illness may be important aggravating co-factors. With the development of cirrhosis, weakness, wasting, oedema, and ascites become progressive problems. Older patients may present with complications of cirrhosis, or even HCC.

Several histological studies in asymptomatic anti-HCV positive donors have shown that 45–62% had chronic active hepatitis, and 7–15% had active cirrhosis [68]. Progression to hepatocellular carcinoma is also well documented, and despite the indolent and slowly progressive nature of the disease in many, it is apparent from serological testing for anti-HCV that HCV is a leading cause of morbidity from liver disease in the Western world.

MANAGEMENT

Acute hepatitis C
The management of acute sporadic or transfusion-related hepatitis C is along conventional lines, and is largely non-specific and supportive. The serum aminotransferases should be measured at weekly intervals; during the recovery phase, these levels should be measured periodically (monthly to 3 monthly), as the determination of true convalescence in this illness can be difficult.

Therapeutic trials of alpha interferon have been undertaken. Most have not reduced the rate of chronic disease, but might indicate an amelioration of the severity of the chronic hepatitis lesion. A trial of beta interferon in Japan, given intravenously for 1 to 3 months, did significantly reduce the risk of chronic hepatitis [69]. Until these findings can be reproduced, however, the routine administration of interferon for acute hepatitis C cannot be advised. Liver transplantation is necessary for the treatment of fulminant hepatitis C where indices indicate a high probability of a fatal outcome.

Chronic hepatitis C
Asymptomatic patients detected through blood screening will require a supplemental test to verify their HCV status. Ideally HCV RNA should be measured in all patients to confirm viraemia, but the test is not generally available for routine diagnosis. Serum aminotransferases, bilirubin, alkaline phosphatase, and prothrombin time should be measured. In patients whose lifestyle or geographic origin suggest that they are at risk of other forms of viral hepatitis, HBsAg and HIV infection should also be considered. In equivocal cases, the diagnosis of chronic hepatitis C may still require confirmation, and careful exclusion of all other forms of chronic hepatitis, including alcoholism, inborn errors of metabolism, hepatoxicity, and disease of the biliary tract. Because autoimmune hepatitis is treated differently, it is particularly advisable to exclude this diagnosis by measuring the titres of anti-smooth muscle, and anti-LKM antibodies even in those with a positive anti-HCV test,

and to measure HCV RNA in anti-HCV positive patients in whom interferon therapy is contemplated.

In patients with more than twofold elevations in serum aminotransferases, a liver biopsy to ascertain the degree of inflammatory activity and fibrosis in the liver should be considered. The patient should be monitored for 1 to 3 months to assess the trend in serum aminotransferases.

Individuals with chronic hepatitis C with elevated ALT and chronic hepatitis histologically should be considered for antiviral therapy.

Major restrictions need not be placed on the lifestyle of the patient with compensated hepatitis C. The drinking of excess spirituous liquor is discouraged, as there is evidence that the combination of type C hepatitis and alcohol abuse may be detrimental to the liver. The patient should be counselled and advised not to donate blood. It is not yet clear how efficiently hepatitis C may be transmitted by sexual contact. It can occur, however, in highly viraemic individuals after prolonged contact. It is prudent therefore to test regular sexual partners for anti-HCV.

Alpha interferon

Preliminary therapeutic trials of alpha interferon have indicated that a proportion of patients may respond to treatment with this agent. Larger, placebo-controlled studies have indicated that approximately 50% of patients will have normal serum aminotransferases after treatment courses of alpha-interferon of approximately 3 million units three times a week for 6 months [70, 71]. Serum HCV RNA may become undetectable in patients after 4–8 weeks of alpha-interferon treatment in patients who respond, but an undetectable HCV RNA at the end of treatment does not preclude relapse in patients.

However, after stopping treatment for 6 months, 50% of the responsive patients will promptly relapse. Serum aminotransferases usually increase in patients who are HCV RNA positive at the end of therapy (Figure 2) [72]. Our studies at the Royal Free Hospital indicate that 20% of patients have a prolonged response to therapy and do not develop elevated serum aminotransferases. These patients also become negative for HCV RNA. Other regimens are being evaluated [73]. Initiating therapy with a dose of 15–20 million units per week, and prolonging therapy for a year, may result in lower relapse rates. However, relapses still occur after higher doses, and patients have more side-effects at higher doses.

The cost of 6 months of treatment is at least £1500. Treatment should not be continued beyond 3 months in patients who do not have reducing levels of serum ALT. Responsive patients usually exhibit histological improvement, and may have a decrease in collagen III propeptide concentrations [74].

Many develop flu-like symptoms, some develop severe psychological side-effects, and patients with cirrhosis are at risk of developing significant thrombocytopenia, leucopenia, and therefore infections [75]. Thyroid abnormalities occur in approximately 3% of treated patients.

When can treatment be considered successful? It is reasonable to infer that patients with normal serum ALT for more than a year after stopping

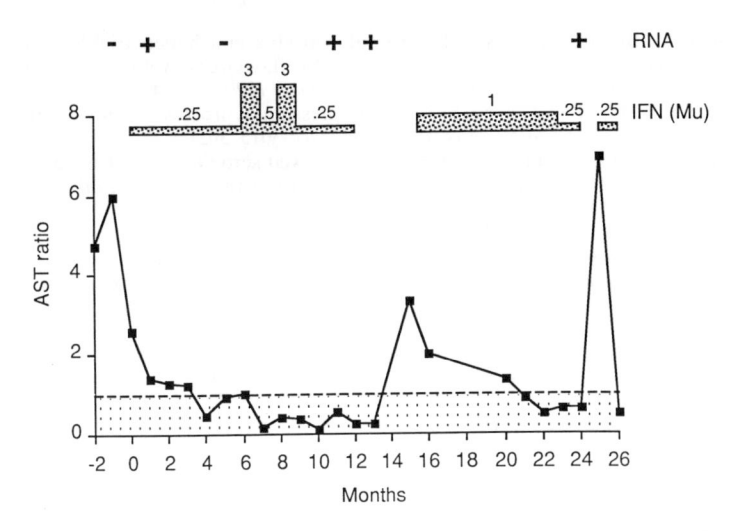

Figure 2. Clinical course in a patient responding to alpha interferon (doses shown) but relapsing when the treatment is stopped. HCV RNA in serum remains positive. AST = aspartate aminotransferase.

interferon treatment, negative HCV RNA in serum for more than a year, with histologically improved disease activity, and a normal serum procollagen III peptide have had a good response.

Ribavirin may be an alternative therapy for chronic hepatitis C [76]. This nucleoside analogue has been shown to suppress HCV, but is weakly efficacious, and doses above 1.2g per day are associated with mild haemolytic anaemia. A multicentre trial of ribavirin for hepatitis C is now in progress.

REFERENCES

1 Kuo G, Choo QL, Alter HJ et al. An assay for circulating antibodies to a major etiologic virus of human non-A, non-B hepatitis. *Science 1989; 244*: 362–364
2 Choo QL, Kuo G, Weiner AJ et al. Isolation of a cDNA clone derived from blood-borne non-A, non-B viral hepatitis genome. *Science 1989; 244*: 359–362
3 Choo QL, Weiner AJ, Overby LR et al. Hepatitis C virus: the major causative agent of viral non-A, non-B hepatitis. *Br Med Bull 1990; 46*: 423–441
4 Takamizawa A, Mori C, Fuke I et al. Structure and organization of the hepatitis C virus genome isolated from human carriers. *J Virol 1991; 65*: 1105–1113
5 Chen P-J, Lin M-H, Tu S-J, Chen D-S. Isolation of a complementary DNA fragment of hepatitis C virus in Taiwan revealed significant sequence variations compared with other isolates. *Hepatology 1991; 14*: 73–78
6 Han JH, Shyamala V, Richman KH et al. Characterization of the terminal regions of hepatitis C viral RNA: identification of conserved sequences in the 5' untranslated region and poly(A) tails at the 3' end. *Proc Natl Acad Sci USA 1991; 88*: 1711–1715
7 Choo QL, Richman KH, Han JH et al. Genetic organization and diversity of the hepatitis C virus. *Proc Natl Acad Sci USA 1991; 88*: 2451–2455
8 Hijikata M, Kato N, Ootsuyama Y et al. Gene mapping of the putative structural region of the hepatitis C virus genome by *in vitro* processing analysis. *Proc Natl Acad Sci USA 1991; 88*: 5547–5551
9 Hijikata M, Kato N, Ootsuyama Y et al. Hypervariable regions in the putative glycoprotein of hepatitis C virus. *Biochem Biophys Res Commun 1991; 175*: 220–228

10   Weiner AJ, Brauer MJ, Rosenblatt J et al. Variable and hypervariable domains are found in the regions of HCV corresponding to the flavivirus envelope and NS1 proteins and the pestivirus envelope glycoproteins. *Virology 1991; 180*: 842–848
11   Harada S, Watanabe Y, Takeuchi K et al. Expression of processed core protein of hepatitis C virus in mammalian cells. *J Virol 1991; 65*: 3015–3021
12   Hosein B, Fang CT, Popovsky MA et al. Improved serodiagnosis of hepatitis C virus infection with synthetic peptide antigen from capsid protein. *Proc Natl Acad Sci USA 1991; 88*: 3647–3651
13   Van der Poel CL, Cuypers HTM, Reesink HW et al. Confirmation of hepatitis C virus infection by new four-antigen recombinant immunoblot assay. *Lancet 1991; 337*: 317–319
14   Kato N, Yokosuka O, Omata M et al. Detection of hepatitis C virus ribonucleic acid in the serum by amplification with polymerase chain reaction. *J Clin Invest 1990; 86*: 1764–1767
15   Cristiano K, Di Bisceglie AM, Hoofnagle JH, Feinstone SM. Hepatitis C viral RNA in serum of patients with chronic non-A, non-B hepatitis: Detection by the polymerase chain reaction using multiple primer sets. *Hepatology 1991; 14*: 51–55
16   Lee S-D, Hwang S-J, Lu R-H et al. Antibodies to hepatitis C virus in prospectively followed patients with posttransfusion hepatitis. *J Infect Dis 1991; 163*: 1354–1357
17   Lim SG, Lee CA, Charman H et al. Hepatitis C antibody assay in a longitudinal study of haemophiliacs. *Br J Haematol 1991; 78*: 398–402
18   Alter HJ, Purcell RH, Shih JW et al. Detection of antibody to hepatitis C virus in prospectively followed transfusion recipients with acute and chronic non-A, non-B hepatitis. *N Engl J Med 1989; 321*: 1494–1500
19   Alter MJ, Sampliner RE. Hepatitis C: and miles to go before we sleep [editorial]. *N Engl J Med 1989; 321*: 1538–1540
20   Nishioka K, Watanabe J, Furuta S et al. Antibody to the hepatitis C virus in acute hepatitis and chronic liver diseases in Japan. *Liver 1991; 11*: 65–70
21   Farci P, Alter HJ, Wong D et al. A long-term study of hepatitis C virus replication in non-A, non-B hepatitis. *N Engl J Med 1991; 325*: 98–104
22   Tanaka E, Kiyosawa K, Sodeyama T et al. Significance of antibody to hepatitis C virus in Japanese patients with viral hepatitis: relationship between anti-HCV antibody and the prognosis of non-A, non-B post-transfusion hepatitis. *J Med Virol 1991; 33*: 117–122
23   Alter HJ, Purcell RH, Holland PV, Popper H. Transmissible agent in non-A, non-B hepatitis. *Lancet 1978; i*: 459–463
24   Tor J, Llibre JM, Carbonell M et al. Sexual transmission of hepatitis C virus and its relation with hepatitis B virus and HIV. *Br Med J 1990; 301*: 1130–1133
25   Abe K, Inchauspe G. Transmission of hepatitis C by saliva. *Lancet 1991; 337*: 248
26   Wang J-T, Wang T-H, Lin J-T et al. Hepatitis C virus RNA in saliva of patients with post-transfusion hepatitis C infection. *Lancet 1991; 337*: 48
27   Dusheiko GM, Smith M, Scheuer PJ. Hepatitis C transmitted by a human bite. *Lancet 1990; 336*: 503–504
28   Klein RS, Freeman K, Taylor PE, Stevens CE. Occupational risk for hepatitis C virus infection among New York City dentists. *Lancet 1991; 338*: 1539–1542
29   Kiyosawa K, Sodeyama T, Tanaka E et al. Intrafamilial transmission of hepatitis C virus in Japan. *J Med Virol 1991; 33*: 114–116
30   Wejstal R, Hermodsson S, Iwarson S, Norkrans G. Mother to infant transmission of hepatitis C virus infection. *J Med Virol 1990; 30*: 178–180
31   Thaler MM, Part C-K, Landers DV et al. Vertical transmission of hepatitis C virus. *Lancet 1991; 338*: 17–18
32   Rassam SW, Dusheiko GM. Epidemiology and transmission of hepatitis C infection. *Eur J Gastroenterol 1991; 3*: 585–591
33   Dawson GJ, Iesniewski RR, Stewart JL et al. Detection of antibodies to hepatitis C virus in US blood donors. *J Clin Microbiol 1991; 29*: 551–556
34   Coursaget P, Bourdil C, Kastally R et al. Prevalence of hepatitis C virus infection in Africa: anti-HCV antibodies in the general population and in patients suffering from cirrhosis or primary liver cancer. *Res Virol 1990; 141*: 449–454
35   Ellis LA, Brown D, Conradie JD et al. Prevalence of hepatitis C in South Africa: Detection

of anti-HCV in recent and stored serum. *J Med Virol 1990; 32*: 249-251
36 Dienstag JL. Non-A, non-B hepatitis. I. Recognition, epidemiology, and clinical features. *Gastroenterology 1983; 85*: 439-462
37 Esteban JI, Gonzalez A, Hernandez JM et al. Evaluation of antibodies to hepatitis C virus in a study of transfusion-associated hepatitis. *N Engl J Med 1990; 323*: 1107-1112
38 Jpn Red Cross Non-A Non-B Hep Res Grp. Effect of screening for hepatitis C virus antibody and hepatitis B virus core antibody on incidence of post-transfusion hepatitis. *Lancet 1991; 338*: 1040-1041
39 Widell A, Sundstrom G, Hansson BG et al. Antibody to hepatitis-C-virus-related proteins in sera from alanine-aminotransferase-screened blood donors and prospectively studied recipients. *Vox Sang 1991; 60*: 28-33
40 Public Health Service inter-agency guidelines for screening donors of blood, plasma, organs, tissues, and semen for evidence of hepatitis B and hepatitis C. *Morb Mort Weekly Rev 1991; 40* RR 4: 1-17
41 Schramm W, Roggendorf M, Rommel F et al. Prevalence of antibodies to hepatitis C virus (HCV) in haemophiliacs. *Blut 1989; 59*: 390-392
42 Pistello M, Ceccherini-Nelli L, Cecconi N et al. Hepatitis C virus seroprevalence in Italian haemophiliacs injected with virus-inactivated concentrates: five year follow-up and correlation with antibodies to other viruses. *J Med Virol 1991; 33*: 43-46
43 Wonke B, Hoffbrand AV, Brown D, Dusheiko G. Antibody to hepatitis C virus in multiply transfused patients with thalassaemia major. *J Clin Pathol 1990; 43*: 638-640
44 Oguchi H, Terashima M, Tokunaga S et al. Prevalence of anti-HCV in patients on long-term hemodialysis. *Nippon Jinzo Gakkai Shi 1990; 32*: 313-317
45 Baur P, Daniel V, Pomer S et al. Hepatitis C-virus (HCV) antibodies in patients after kidney transplantation. *Ann Hematol 1991; 62*: 68-73
46 Poterucha JJ, Rakela J, Ludwig J et al. Hepatitis C antibodies in patients with chronic hepatitis of unknown etiology after orthotopic liver transplantation. *Transplant Proc 1991; 23*: 1495-1497
47 Ponz E, Campistol JM, Barrera JM et al. Hepatitis C virus antibodies in patients on hemodialysis and after kidney transplantation. *Transplant Proc 1991; 23*: 1371-1372
48 Polywka S, Laufs R. Hepatitis C virus antibodies among different groups at risk and patients with suspected non-A, non-B hepatitis. *Infection 1991; 19*: 81-84
49 Hofmann H, Kunz C. Low risk of health care workers for infection with hepatitis C virus. *Infection 1990; 18*: 286-288
50 Pohjanpelto P, Tallgren M, Farkkila M et al. Low prevalence of hepatitis C antibodies in chronic liver disease in Finland. *Scand J Infect Dis 1991; 23*: 139-142
51 McFarlane IG, Smith HM, Johnson PJ et al. Hepatitis C virus antibodies in chronic active hepatitis: pathogenetic factor or false-positive result? *Lancet 1990; 335*: 754-757
52 Schvarcz R, von-Sydow M, Weiland O. Autoimmune chronic active hepatitis: changing reactivity for antibodies to hepatitis C virus after immunosuppressive treatment. *Scand J Gastroenterol 1990; 25*: 1175-1180
53 Mishiro S, Hoshi Y, Takeda K et al. Non-A, non-B hepatitis specific antibodies directed at host-derived epitope: implication for an autoimmune process. *Lancet 1990; 336*: 1400-1403
54 Manns MP, Griffin KJ, Sullivan KF, Johnson EF. LKM-1 autoantibodies recognize a short linear sequence in P450IID6, a cytochrome P-450 mono-oxygenase. *J Clin Invest 1991; 88*: 1370-1378
55 Fong T-L, Di Bisceglie AM, Waggoner JG et al. The significance of antibody to hepatitis C virus in patients with chronic hepatitis B. *Hepatology 1991; 14*: 64-67
56 Fattovich G, Tagger A, Brollo L et al. Hepatitis C virus infection in chronic hepatitis B virus carriers. *J Infect Dis 1991; 163*: 400-402
57 Pares A, Barrera JM, Caballeria J et al. Hepatitis C virus antibodies in chronic alcoholic patients: association with severity of liver injury. *Hepatology 1990; 12*: 1295-1299
58 Tanaka K, Hirohata T, Koga S et al. Hepatitis C and hepatitis B in the etiology of hepatocellular carcinoma in the Japanese population. *Cancer Res 1991; 51*: 2842-2847
59 Bruix J, Barrera JM, Calvet X et al. Prevalence of antibodies to hepatitis C virus in Spanish patients with hepatocellular carcinoma and hepatic cirrhosis. *Lancet 1989; ii*:

60 Kiyosawa K, Sodeyama T, Tanaka E et al. Interrelationship of blood transfusion, non-A, non-B hepatitis and hepatocellular carcinoma: analysis by detection of antibody to hepatitis C virus. *Hepatology 1990; 12*: 671–675
61 Pol S, Driss F, Devergie A et al. Is hepatitis C virus involved in hepatitis-associated aplastic anemia? *Ann Intern Med 1990; 113*: 435–437
62 Ferri C, Greco F, Longombardo G et al. Antibodies to hepatitis C virus in patients with mixed cryoglobulinemia. *Arthritis Rheum 1991; 34*: 1606–1610
63 Durand JM, Lefevre P, Harle JR et al. Cutaneous vasculitis and cryoglobulinaemia type II associated with hepatitis C virus infection. *Lancet 1991; 337*: 499–500
64 Bamber M, Murray A, Arborgh BAM et al. Short incubation non-A, non-B hepatitis transmitted by factor VIII concentrates in patients with congenital coagulation disorders. *Gut 1981; 22*: 854–859
65 Scheuer PJ, Ashrafzadeh P, Sherlock S et al. The pathology of hepatitis C. *Hepatology 1992; 15*: 567–571
66 Patel A, Sherlock S, Dusheiko G et al. Clinical course and histological correlations in post-transfusion hepatitis C: The Royal Free Hospital experience. *Eur J Gastroenterol and Hepatol 1991; 3*: 491–495
67 Mattsson L. Chronic non-A, non-B hepatitis with special reference to the transfusion-associated form. *Scand J Infect Dis Suppl 1989; 59*: 1–55
68 Alberti A, Chemello L, Cavalletto D et al. Antibody to hepatitis C virus and liver disease in volunteer blood donors. *Ann Intern Med 1991; 114*: 1010–1012
69 Omata M, Yokosuka O, Takano S et al. Resolution of acute hepatitis C after therapy with natural beta interferon. *Lancet 1991; 338*: 914–915
70 Davis GL, Balart LA, Schiff ER et al. Treatment of chronic hepatitis C with recombinant interferon alfa. A multicenter randomized, controlled trial. Hepatitis Interventional Therapy Group. *N Engl J Med 1989; 321*: 1501–1506
71 Di-Bisceglie AM, Martin P, Kassianides C et al. Recombinant interferon alfa therapy for chronic hepatitis C. A randomized, double-blind, placebo-controlled trial. *N Engl J Med 1989; 321*: 1506–1510
72 Chayama K, Saitoh S, Arase Y et al. Effect of interferon administration on serum hepatitis C virus RNA in patients with chronic hepatitis C. *Hepatology 1991; 13*: 1040–1043
73 Kakumu S, Arao M, Yoshioka K et al. Recombinant human alpha-interferon therapy for chronic non-A, non-B hepatitis: second report. *Am J Gastroenterol 1990; 85*: 655–659
74 Schvarcz R, Glaumann H, Weiland O et al. Histological outcome in interferon alpha-2b treated patients with chronic posttransfusion non-A, non-B hepatitis. *Liver 1991; 11*: 30–38
75 Renault PF, Hoofnagle JH. Side effects of alpha interferon. *Semin Liver Dis 1989; 9*: 273–277
76 Reichard O, Andersson J, Schvarcz R, Weiland O. Ribavirin treatment for chronic hepatitis C. *Lancet 1991; 337*: 1058–1061

MANAGEMENT OF PORTAL HYPERTENSION WITH BETA-BLOCKERS

Andrew K Burroughs
Royal Free Hospital and School of Medicine, London

In the past 10 years the most important aspect of treating portal hypertension has been the discovery and evaluation of beta-blockers as portal hypotensive agents. Lebrec and his group [1] published a seminal paper in which propranolol was shown to lower portal pressure. Since then there has been an intense research interest in the haemodynamic effects of beta-blockers and other drugs in cirrhotic patients. There have also been numerous randomized clinical trials which have evaluated the use of beta-blockers for both the primary and secondary prevention of variceal bleeding, and bleeding from portal hypertensive gastropathy (congestive gastropathy) which is a common but less severe source of bleeding than varices in cirrhotics [2].

Variceal rupture occurs by explosion and not erosion in the vast majority of cases. The tension on the variceal wall is considered to be the critical factor [3] so that the larger the size of varix the greater the tension (as the latter is a function of the radius), and for similar sized varices, a higher intravariceal pressure will produce a higher tension. Large varices and a higher intravariceal pressure respectively have been found to be independently predictive factors for the risk of first bleeding by the NIEC (North Italian Endoscopic Club) group [4] and Feu et al [5] but in addition both found that red signs on varices (an endoscopic sign) and the severity of liver disease were also independent risk factors. These two factors may affect the integrity of the variceal wall making it thinner. The red signs are thought to be 'varices on varices'. Poor hepatic synthetic function may lead to insufficient or abnormal collagen synthesis. Severity of liver disease also leads to disturbed coagulation, and this may have a role in preventing rapid haemostasis, and sealing of a breach in the variceal wall once it occurs. The author considers that this 'leak and seal' hypothesis may be true, as variations in portal pressure and transmural variation in intravariceal pressure occur many times a day but bleeding is far less frequent. Nevertheless lowering of portal pressure by pharmacological means would reduce variceal wall tension and thus should prevent bleeding.

Portal pressure could be reduced in three ways: diminishing the portal inflow, and/or reducing the intrahepatic vascular resistance, and/or reducing the resistance in the collateral circulation. The drugs that have been evaluated in cirrhotics with portal hypertension, which could be used for long-term administration, are shown in Table I.

TABLE I. Drugs that have been evaluated as portal hypotensive agents and could be used for long-term administration

Non-selective beta-blockers
Cardioselective beta-blockers
Alpha- and beta-blocker (labetalol)
Alpha-antagonists (including clonidine, an alpha-2-antagonist)
Alpha-agonists (methoxamine)
$5HT_2$-antagonists (ritanserin)
Octreotide (subcutaneous)
Nitrate vasodilators
Vasodilators (molsidomine, pentoxifylline)
Diuretics (potassium sparing)

HAEMODYNAMIC CHANGES IN SYSTEMIC AND PORTAL CIRCULATIONS WITH BETA-BLOCKERS

In 1980, Lebrec [1] showed that twice daily oral propranolol (80 to 360mg daily) given to reduce the resting pulse rate by 25% produced a sustained mean decrease in wedge hepatic venous pressure (WHVP) of 25% (4.5mmHg) in alcoholic cirrhotics without jaundice, ascites, or encephalopathy. As WHVP closely reflects portal pressure in alcoholic cirrhosis, in which the site of resistance is sinusoidal and post-sinusoidal [6], this suggested that portal pressure was reduced. There was also a mean decrease in cardiac output of 31% and in hepatic blood flow of 24%. These haemodynamic changes could be maintained at 3 and 9 months with prolonged administration [7] so that tachyphylaxis did not occur. However, there was no correlation between the decrease in hepatic venous pressure gradient (HVPG) and cardiac output, so that the latter could not be the sole explanation for the fall in WHVP.

Hillon et al [8] later showed that for a similar decrease in cardiac output, there was a significantly more marked decrease in HVPG following oral propranolol (40mg) than following oral atenolol (100mg). This suggested that extracardiac mechanisms (beta-2-receptor blockade) were also responsible for the reduction in HVPG following propranolol. This is in part due to unopposed alpha-adrenergic activity in the splanchnic bed causing vasoconstriction, during beta-2-receptor blockade [9]. In man [10] an experimental beta-2-blocker (ICI 118551) caused a 12% drop in WHVP without changing cardiac output, proving that this was part of the mechanism of portal pressure reduction by beta-blockers.

In the early reports propranolol was always found to reduce the HVPG, but the extent was very variable and in some the reduction was so modest that it was within the coefficient of variation of the hepatic venous pressure measurements. The patients studied were nearly all categorized as modified Child's grade A or B, i.e. with good or moderate liver function. However, later reports [11-13] found that acute administration of oral propranolol, even with adequate plasma concentrations, did not reduce the HVPG in some decompensated cirrhotics [12], or had a less-marked effect. In one study [13] one-third of patients showed no HVPG change with 40mg of oral propranolol, and only 43% of a group of these non-responders showed a fall in HVPG with incremental doses of propranolol. The percentage reduction in resting heart rate only correlated with plasma propranolol concentrations and not with HVPG reduction. Even if severity of liver disease was taken into account, neither percentage reduction in resting heart rate nor plasma propranolol concentrations correlated with percentage reduction in HVPG. Other workers have also found that pulse rate reduction was not related to severity of liver disease nor to propranolol concentration [14]. This suggests that a 25% reduction in resting pulse rate is not a reliable index of HVPG reduction and should not be used as such.

The variable effect of propranolol on HVPG reduction and its possible relationship to a reduction in the frequency of variceal bleeding (the therapeutic response) are further complicated by considering other haemodynamic indices. Valla et al [15] found that the reduction in WHVP in alcoholic cirrhotics was not paralleled by a similar reduction in portal pressure reduction when this was measured directly. Other authors [16, 17] have found no fall in portal pressure with direct measurement. The discrepancies between WHVP and direct portal pressure measurement in alcoholic cirrhotics following propranolol administration may be due to an increase in portal collateral resistance and/or intrahepatic vascular resistance that offsets a reduction in portal pressure due to a decrease in portal outflow. Using Doppler ultrasound, Ohnishi et al [16] have shown reduction in portal flow that is greater than the fall in portal pressure.

It is now clear that there are non-responders to propranolol in terms of portal pressure. Bendtsen et al [18] defined non-responders as those exhibiting less than 10% reduction in portal pressure 90 minutes following an oral dose of 80mg propranolol. They compared the haemodynamic indices between responders and non-responders. All patients had evidence of adequate beta-blockade with plasma levels above 50ng/ml, and a fall in cardiac output. The non-responders had a lower baseline cardiac index, and a higher systemic vascular resistance, i.e. their circulations were less hyperdynamic. There was no relationship between the effect of propranolol and the height of portal pressure, severity of liver disease, or presence of ascites.

Propranolol reduces intravariceal pressure, compared to placebo [19]. It is established, therefore, that pressure at the site of variceal rupture can be reduced. Unfortunately, this study was not designed to assess any correlation between variceal pressure reduction and WHVP reduction, as it may be that if collateral resistance is usually increased by propranolol, then intravariceal pressure would fall, and portal pressure would not. This could provide an explanation for the smaller or non-existent decrease in portal pressure.

Azygous blood flow is an indirect measure of collateral blood flow in cirrhotics that includes blood flowing through oesophageal varices [11, 20, 21]. In all studies, azygous blood flow has been reduced in virtually every patient given propranolol. The percentage reduction in azygous blood flow averages 32%, much greater than the average HVPG reduction. This reduction in azygous blood flow appears to be a specific effect of beta-2-blockade in the splanchnic bed because it is not blocked by alpha-adrenergic blockade; that is, it is not caused by unopposed alpha-adrenergic vasoconstriction [22]. The magnitude of the decrease in azygous blood flow following administration of propranolol was not related to the degree of hepatic decompensation in one study [20]. However, in another study intravenous propranolol reduced azygous blood flow less markedly in decompensated cirrhotics [23]. Despite these differences, azygous blood flow appears to be a good index to assess a haemodynamic response to propranolol. However, as for pressure measurements [17], no direct correlation has been found between azygous blood flow and the risk of variceal haemorrhage [21]. In a long-term study versus placebo, azygous blood flow was found to be persistently reduced whereas hepatic venous pressure reduction was no different at 1 year [24].

At present, therefore, there is no reliable baseline haemodynamic index to assess the probability of a therapeutic response to propranolol, viz. the reduction in frequency of variceal bleeding [25, 26]. There is only one preliminary report which has analysed the factors which might predict an absolute reduction of HPVG to 12mmHg or less in a group of cirrhotics, some of whom had bled [27]: 18 of 150 (12%) reduced their HVPG to this extent. The only variables which were independently predictive of this HPVG reduction were a lower baseline HVPG (mean 14.7mmHg versus 20mmHg) and a higher mean arterial pressure (mean 97mmHg versus 88mmHg). A marked acute response to propranolol (>20% reduction from baseline HPVG), which was found in 36 (24%) patients, was predicted by the absence of previous episodes of bleeding (36% *vs* 8% of those who had previously bled) and the absence of ascites (32% *vs* 15% with ascites). When neither previous bleeding nor ascites was present, then 42% of these patients had a marked response. This is the first study which has attempted to look at predictive factors for a haemodynamic response to propranolol. Unfortunately, the correlation with the therapeutic response was not made. However, recently there has been evidence of such an index predicting bleeding in *response* to propranolol. In the Barcelona, Boston and New Haven primary propranolol prophylaxis trial [28], bleeding did not occur in patients whose HVPG fell to 12mmHg or less [29]. In addition a haemodynamic index which might predict re-bleeding from varices has been suggested by Sacerdoti et al [30]. Patients who had a percentage reduction of HVPG of greater than 12% at 1 month following nadolol administration did not re-bleed. The value of these haemodynamic indices needs to be evaluated prospectively, and new clinical trials should be designed to achieve target pressures in as many patients as possible either by increasing the dosage of propranolol or adding other drugs, to reduce portal pressure further.

NITROVASODILATORS AND COMBINATIONS WITH BETA-BLOCKERS

Nitroglycerin, isosorbide mononitrate and dinitrate are vasodilators which act via nitric oxide in vascular smooth muscle cells [31]. Several groups have found that these vasodilators decrease WHVP, portal pressure or intravariceal pressure [32, 33], but as for propranolol, other groups have not detected any pressure reduction [34]. There is a theoretical possibility that WHVP is reduced by vasodilators whereas portal pressure is not, as WHVP is dependent on hepatic arterial blood flow and arterial pressure, as well as portal blood flow and intrahepatic portal resistance. In normal man, low doses of vasodilators decrease venous return by inducing venous pooling, whilst the arterial pressure remains unchanged. The decreased venous return induces constriction in the splanchnic arteriolar bed secondary to reduction in cardiac filling pressure. In turn, this causes unloading of the cardiopulmonary baroreceptors [35]. However, in cirrhotic patients the same low dose of vasodilators has no splanchnic haemodynamic effects [36].

In high doses vasodilators lower arterial pressure as well as reducing venous return. This activates arterial baroreceptors causing constriction of splanchnic arterioles. In cirrhotics this could reduce both portal inflow and pressure. This has been little studied, but it is known that arterial baroreflexes are abnormal in cirrhotics [37]. Rector et al [34] suggest that the response to vasodilators is dependent on the pulmonary wedge pressure (PWP). In those patients whose PWP was <12mmHg there was a reduction in WHVP. However, those with a PWP >12mmHg had an increase in WHVP. Presumably in the latter group there was not a secondary decrease in PWP sufficient to cause cardiopulmonary baroreceptor unloading to trigger splanchnic arteriolar vasoconstriction. Finally vasodilators may act by reducing intrahepatic or collateral vascular resistance, which has been demonstrated in man [38].

Thus, as single agents, nitrate vasodilators are not optimal portal hypotensive agents in cirrhotics. In high doses they induce arterial hypotension, and may decrease systemic oxygen consumption and increase plasma lactate concentrations, if the reduction in blood pressure is of the order of 20% or more [36]. This would suggest tissue hypoxia. Tolerance to vasodilators could be a problem and one study has shown an anti-aggregatory platelet effect. Moreover, there is some evidence that isosorbide 5 mononitrate (ISMN) may impair renal function [39].

However, the combination of nitrate vasodilators with other drugs could theoretically enhance portal pressure reduction. In a short-term haemodynamic study [40], the addition of ISMN to propranolol caused a further reduction in mean HVPG: 21.5mmHg ± 3.9 to 18.6mmHg ± 4.2 with propranolol and to 15.7mmHg ± 3.1mmHg following the addition of ISMN without a further decrease in azygous venous blood flow. However, mean arterial pressure fell by 22% and hepatic blood flow by 15.5%. In the long-term part of the study ISMN also caused a further reduction in HVPG in comparison to propranolol alone, with only a 12% reduction in mean arterial blood pressure.

Although free hepatic venous pressure (FHVP) increased in this study, the additional fall in HVPG was entirely due to a further decrease in WHVP. A further interesting observation was that the propranolol 'non-responders' became 'responders' following the addition of ISMN, and this sub-group of patients was the one which had the greatest pharmacological response. The same group [41] have furthered their evaluation by comparing the effects of oral propranolol alone and the combination of propranolol and isosorbide mononitrate in a randomized controlled trial over 3 months. The HPVG decreased by more than 20% of the baseline values in only 10% of propranolol treated patients, but in 50% of the combined therapy group. The ISMN did not further reduce hepatic blood flow or intrinsic clearance of indocyanine green, compared to propranolol alone.

ISMN has no first pass effect (unlike isosorbide dinitrate), making dosage easier to determine in cirrhotic patients, and appears to maintain its effect over time, i.e. tolerance was not induced.

MOLSIDOMINE

This vasodilator does not induce tolerance and has little effect on arterial pressure in normal man. However, it is metabolized to its active form in the liver. Three groups have now published data on this. In the first Vinel et al [42] the mean WHVP (−11%) and portohepatic venous gradient (−15%) were reduced by molsidomine as was arterial pressure (−13.5%) and hepatic blood flow (−17.4%). Free hepatic venous pressure was not affected and neither was the intrinsic hepatic clearance of indocyanine green. Interestingly heart rate did not change suggesting that baroreceptor constricting reflexes were not involved. Therefore, the action of molsidomine may be that of a direct portal vasodilator. However, three of 13 (24%) patients did not respond. In a German study 28% had no reduction in the HVPG [43].

In the third study (Del Arbol et al [44]) similar reductions in WHVP and HPVG were found with 2mg or 4mg orally and these effects could also be shown at 2 hours − 13% of patients did not respond (1 in 8) in terms of HVPG reduction. Mean azygous blood flow did not change, despite reduction in cardiac output and liver blood flow suggesting a reduction in resistance in the collateral vessels. Thus the action of molsidomine may be due to both portal-collateral and hepatic vasodilation, as well as reduced portal inflow secondary to reflex arteriolar vasoconstrictor in splanchnic organs. However, hepatic blood flow and intrinsic clearance of indocyanine green were also significantly reduced, in contrast to the first study [42], but to a similar extent as propranolol combined with 40mg ISMN. However, care should be taken in long-term studies, particularly, as hepatic metabolism is crucial to the action of molsidomine. Its active metabolite has a greatly prolonged half-life in cirrhotic patients [45].

DIURETICS

In 1985 it was reported that long-term spironolactone reduced WHVP [46]. This observation passed unnoticed for some time as did the original reports of the 1960s.

Volume contraction might theoretically induce a reduction in portal inflow due to reflex vasoconstrictor secondary to baroreceptor reflexes. Okumara et al [47] evaluated the haemodynamic effects of a 4 week oral administration of of 100mg spironolactone (n=15) or 40mg frusemide (n=10) in cirrhotics with ascites. They showed a mean reduction of HVPG of 22% and of WHVP of 16% in the spironolactone group but none in the frusemide group. The circulating volume did not fall in the frusemide group but did fall in the spironolactone group, but there was no correlation with HVPG reduction. However, there was a negative correlation with the post-treatment aldosterone concentrations. In neither group was there a change in the estimated hepatic blood flow. However, the cardiac output and mean arterial pressure fell in both groups, without change in heart rate. The systemic vascular resistance did not change in the spironolactone group but fell in the frusemide group. It is not clear if these differences between spironolactone and frusemide are real, as theoretically volume contraction should occur with both diuretics, following chronic administration. It is not known if similar effects could be induced in cirrhotic patients without ascites but who have increased plasma volumes, nor is it known whether the combination with beta-blockers might enhance the portal pressure reduction.

RANDOMIZED CLINICAL TRIALS OF BETA-BLOCKERS

Prevention of the first gastrointestinal haemorrhage

The risk of first gastrointestinal bleeding in cirrhotics with varices is approximately 30% during their lifetime [48]. The mortality due to bleeding is very high, approximately 50%, and this has led to therapeutic trials. However, these deaths due to bleeding represent only a third of deaths in cirrhotics with varices, and affect only 15% of such patients. Consequently to prove an overall reduction in mortality, by the prevention of first bleeding alone, would require a very large number of patients [48].

There are nine trials which have included 996 patients, seven with propranolol and two with nadolol (Table II). The author was involved in a comprehensive meta-analysis [49] and updates [50; D'Amico 1992, unpublished] which showed that the incidence of first bleeding is significantly reduced by propranolol compared to no treatment. There was no statistical heterogeneity, i.e. the variation in treatment effect is consistent with 'normal' variability. The pooled odds ratio of bleeding patients taking beta-blockers is almost half that of placebo: 0.54 (95% confidence interval, 0.39–0.74), p<0.001, with only one trial [51] showing an increased risk of bleeding with propranolol. Using the method proposed by Jaeschnke et al [52] the number of patients who need to be treated to prevent one adverse bleeding event is 10 (95% confidence interval, 8–18). The mortality rate is also reduced but not significantly so, 0.75 (95% confidence interval, 0.57–1.06) [50; D'Amico 1992, unpublished].

Using individual patient data, rather than trial outcomes, a meta-analysis of four of the trials comprising 589 patients [53] has shown that after 2 years (taking age and severity of cirrhosis into account as these affected mortality) the survival rate was not significantly increased but was slightly better in the

TABLE II. Randomized trials of beta-blockers for the primary prevention of variceal bleeding

Trial (author)*	Sample size	Mean or median follow-up (months)	Bleeding rate (%)		Death rate (%)	
			Controls	Beta-blocker	Controls	Beta-blocker
Pascal	230	16	27	17	36	21
IMPP	174	28	35	21	31	44
Ideo*	79	23	22	3	18	10
Lebrec* [67]	106	12	19	13	19	19
Conn [28]	102	34	22	4	22	16
Strauss	36	16	25	20	44	35
Andreani† [68]	84	ca 20	32	5	41	30
PROVA† [69]	140	15	18	18	22	15
Colman [51]	48	24	8	34	28	26

* Nadolol.
† Also had a prophylactic sclerotherapy group.
References to trials are in Pagliaro et al [49].

beta-blocker group (p=0.09). However, prevention of fatal bleeding by beta-blockers was highly significant (p=0.004), a saving of eight lives amongst 100 patients followed for 2 years each. This was also true for the prevention of bleeding per se: a mean of 78% patients were free of bleeding in the propranolol group versus 65% in the control group (p=0.002). These differences remained after adjustment for the cause and severity of cirrhosis, ascites and size of varices. The former two factors were associated with bleeding and death in both the beta-blocker and control groups. The advantage of analysing individual patient data (the first such meta-analysis in hepatology or gastroenterology) is that censored data and prognostic data can all be taken into account. Secondly data can be combined after the same period of follow-up. Comparison between proportional hazard models and adjusted log rank tests can be made for several sub-groups of particular interest, e.g. alcoholics versus non-alcoholics, ascitic versus non-ascitic, and nadolol versus propranolol as was done in this meta-analysis. However, none of these analyses affected the overall difference between treatment groups.

This evaluation suggests that screening for moderate and large varices in cirrhotics should become part of routine clinical practice, and that if these types of varices are found, beta-blockers should be given to reduce the incidence of bleeding and death from bleeding. The 10 patients who need to take treatment to prevent one adverse event is a similar number to the 14 needed to be treated to prevent one stroke or death by using aspirin in patients with transient ischaemic attacks [54]. Although mortality is not reduced by beta-blockers the reduction in bleeding is a very useful clinical goal, and is sufficient to justify the use of propranolol, which is cheap and has few side-effects. It is important to note that in a recent trial of aspirin or warfarin for the prevention of stroke and embolism the trial was stopped when there was evidence of a reduction in these complications but not in death [55].

Prevention of bleeding from portal hypertensive gastropathy
In the first propranolol trial, patients who had gastric mucosal bleeding were also included, and propranolol was shown to protect from re-bleeding from this source but the numbers were too small to establish statistical significance. Portal hypertensive gastropathy is now a recognized entity, also known as congestive gastropathy. It may lead to chronic anaemia as well as upper gastrointestinal bleeding [2]. In animal models the mucosa has a microvasculopathy which results in reduced oxygenation of the surface gastric mucosa and is more susceptible to injurious agents [56]. Whatever the triggering agent for occult or frank blood loss, propranolol has been shown to prevent both acute and chronic bleeding in a single blind randomized study [57]. Thus the actuarial percentages of patients free of re-bleeding from portal hypertensive gastropathy at 12 months were 65% versus 38% ($p<0.05$) and at 30 months 52% versus 7% ($p<0.05$). There were also fewer episodes of acute re-bleeding (mean episodes/patient/month: 0.01 vs 0.12).

Prevention of re-bleeding from varices: beta-blockers compared to no treatment
Once bleeding from varices has occurred the risk of re-bleeding is 70% or more. The risk of re-bleeding is partly related to the severity of liver disease, but no haemodynamic index has been shown to be correlated with re-bleeding.

There are 12 trials comprising 637 patients (Table III). The same meta-analyses [49, 50] show that the risk of re-bleeding is significantly reduced by beta-blockers. The pooled odds ratio is 0.4 (95% confidence intervals, 0.3–0.5), $p<0.001$, with no statistical heterogeneity. However, there is no significant effect on mortality, the pooled relative risk being 0.7 (95% confidence intervals, 0.5–1.04). However, the difference in mortality is far less than in the primary

TABLE III. Randomized trials of beta-blockers for the prevention of re-bleeding from varices

Trial	Sample size	Mean or median follow-up (months)	Bleeding rate (%)		Death rate (%)	
			Controls	Beta-blocker	Controls	Beta-blocker
Lebrec [67]	74	29	64	16	22	8
Burroughs [70]	48	21	59	54	23	15
Villeneuve [71]	79	23	81	76	38	45
Queuniet [72]	99	25	65	57	21	24
Gatta [73]	24	14	67	25	25	8
Colombo* [74]	62	12	47	25	23	12
Colombo [74]	62	12	47	31	23	10
Sheen [75]	36	12	56	28	11	0
Garden [76]	81	16	77	47	44	37
Cerebelaud [77]	84	16	66	34	–	–
Von Kobe [78]	54	–	46	38	32	23
Colman [51]	100	–	50	35	4	4

* Atenolol.

prevention trials whether examined individually or collectively. Clinical factors which might predict the therapeutic response for re-bleeding with propranolol are not fully established, but non-compliance, presence of a hepatocellular carcinoma, alcoholism and non-reduction of resting heart rate have been suggested by Lebrec's group [58]. Some haemodynamic criteria may be shown to be useful in the future [30] but their measurement remains invasive and not practical. A future solution to this problem may be the correlation of intravariceal pressure reduction measured endoscopically with the incidence of re-bleeding. However, there is no simple 'splanchnic sphygmomanometer', as for systemic hypertension.

Prevention of re-bleeding from varices: beta-blockers compared to sclerotherapy
There are eight trials comprising 644 patients (Table IV). The same meta-analysis [49] showed that the two therapies are equivalent, with a pooled odds ratio of 1 (95% confidence intervals, 0.7–1.7) for mortality, and 0.7 (95% confidence intervals, 0.5–1.1) for re-bleeding. Thus, on this basis beta-blockers would be the treatment of first choice for the prevention of re-bleeding, barring contraindications, as they are less expensive and invasive than long-term sclerotherapy, and they do not increment endoscopy work load. However, many groups still use long-term sclerotherapy despite this evidence. In the future combination drug therapy should make the pharmacological approach more effective.

TABLE IV. Randomized trials of beta-blockers versus sclerotherapy for the prevention of variceal bleeding

Trial	Sample size	Mean or median follow-up (months)	Bleeding rate (%)		Death rate (%)	
			Beta-blockers	Sclero-therapy	Beta-blockers	Sclero-therapy
Alexandrino	65	29	74	55	32	29
Fleig	105	26	48	31	32	36
Dollet	51	36	44	64	32	29
Westaby [87]	108	24	52	42	77	64
Teres	72	11	49	21	31	21
Liu [80]	118	?	75	35	41	53
Rossi [81]	53	19	48	50	26	23
Martin [82]	76	36	53	55	23	31

References to trials are in Pagliaro et al [49].

Prevention of re-bleeding from varices: addition of beta-blockers to sclerotherapy versus sclerotherapy alone, or versus beta-blockers alone
There are seven trials of the combination of sclerotherapy and beta-blockers versus sclerotherapy alone comprising 347 patients (Table V). There is no advantage in combining beta-blockers with long-term sclerotherapy: pooled odds ratio 0.7, (95% confidence intervals, 0.45–1.2). Theoretically the drug

might prevent re-bleeding before variceal obliteration. Only one group (Jensen et al [59, 60]) shows re-bleeding is significantly decreased both before and after eradication and only one other trial shows a significant advantage of adding a beta-blocker (Vinel et al [61]). Mortality is unchanged: pooled odds ratio 0.95 (95% confidence intervals, 0.5–1.75).

TABLE V. Randomized trials of beta-blocker combined with sclerotherapy versus sclerotherapy alone

Trial	Sample size	Mean or median follow-up (months)	Bleeding rate (%)		Death rate (%)	
			Beta-blocker and sclerotherapy	Sclerotherapy	Beta-blocker and sclerotherapy	Sclerotherapy
Westaby [79]	53	6	27	30	35	26
Vickers [83]	69	24	51	44	37	26
Vinel [61]	65	12	21	38	12	19
Jensen [59, 60]	31	–	20	75	7	6
Gerunda [84]	60	6	20	17	–	–
Lundell [85]	41	–	12e	11e	5	26
Bertoni [86]	28	–	7	29	7	21

e = episodes.

There are two trials of sclerotherapy and beta-blockers versus beta-blockers alone [62, 63]. Both show a significant advantage of adding sclerotherapy to beta-blockers in terms of re-bleeding: beta-blockers alone re-bleeding 65% – combination 45% (O'Connor et al [62]); beta-blockers alone re-bleeding 60% – combination 39% (Ink et al [63]). There was no improvement in mortality. The results of these nine trials do not justify a routine use of the combination of beta-blockers and sclerotherapy.

COMPLICATIONS OF BETA-BLOCKERS: EFFECTS ON KIDNEY AND LIVER FUNCTION AND HEPATIC ENCEPHALOPATHY

There are no reports of fatal complications of beta-blockers in cirrhotic patients. Withdrawal due to the expected side-effects (e.g. heart failure, asthma) is infrequent. A recent review reports effects on kidney, liver and brain function in cirrhotic patients [64]. Occasionally hepatic encephalopathy may be precipitated by propranolol but the effect is reversible.

THE FUTURE OF LONG-TERM MEDICAL THERAPY FOR THE MANAGEMENT OF PORTAL HYPERTENSION

The future management of portal hypertension will increasingly be based on medical therapy. Drug combinations will be used as in systemic hypertension. It may even be possible to prevent the development, or the extension, of the collateral circulation and thus the development of varices. This has already been shown in animal models of schistosomal portal hypertension

[65] and portal vein stenosed rats [66], using propranolol. Anti-fibrotic drugs may achieve the same result. However, the current problem is the lack of a 'splanchnic sphygmomanometer' which could be used to monitor therapy precisely. In addition there is no reliable haemodynamic index which can be measured prior to therapy, which will reliably predict the therapeutic efficacy. However, gradient changes in hepatic venous pressure measurement following propranolol administration may predict the therapeutic response, but this requires invasive measurement. As yet an easily measured clinical or haemodynamic variable that correlates with one or more cardinal splanchnic haemodynamic indices does not exist. Future studies will be directed at simple ways of establishing individual patient response to portal hypotensive agents in relation to target haemodynamic effects.

SUMMARY

Propranolol is the drug of choice for long-term prevention of re-bleeding and prevention of the first variceal bleed. For primary prophylaxis it significantly reduces the rate of bleeding; there is a trend towards reducing mortality. It should be used in cirrhotic patients with large varices. For secondary prophylaxis, propranolol significantly reduces re-bleeding but does not improve survival. The reduction in re-bleeding is similar to long-term sclerotherapy when compared in randomized studies. There is no value in adding beta-blockers to sclerotherapy compared to sclerotherapy alone. Beta-blockers can be used as the first line therapy to prevent variceal re-bleeding. They also have been shown to reduce the frequency of re-bleeding from congestive gastropathy.

Many patients do not have a portal pressure reduction with propranolol. The addition of isosorbide mononitrate converts many 'non-responders' to responders. Current clinical tests are evaluating if therapeutic efficacy is improved by these drug combinations.

REFERENCES

1 Lebrec D, Novel O, Corbic M et al. Propranolol – a medical treatment for portal hypertension. *Lancet 1980; ii*: 180–182
2 D'Amico G, Montalbano L, Traina M et al. Natural history of congestive gastropathy in cirrhosis. *Gastroenterology 1990; 99*: 1558–1564
3 Polio J, Groszmann RJ. Haemodynamic factors involved in the development and rupture of esophageal varices. A pathophysiological approach to treatment. *Semin Liv Dis 1986; 6*: 318–328
4 North Italian Endoscopic Club (NIEC) for the Study and Treatment of Oesophageal Varices. Prediction of the first variceal haemorrhage in patients with cirrhosis of the liver and oesophageal varices: a prospective study. *N Engl J Med 1988; 319*: 983–989
5 Feu F, Bordas JM, Garcia-Pagan JC, Bosch J, Rodes J. Endoscopic measurement of variceal pressure in patients with cirrhosis. Correlation with the NIEC index and with the risk of first haemorrhage. *J Hepatol 1991; 11 (suppl 2)*: S22 (abstract)
6 Boyer TD, Triger DR, Horisawa M et al. Direct transhepatic measurement of portal vein pressure using a thin needle. Comparison with wedged hepatic vein pressure. *Gastroenterology 1977; 72*: 584–589
7 Lebrec D, Hillon P, Munoz C et al. The effect of propranolol on portal hypertension in patients with cirrhosis. A haemodynamic study. *Hepatology 1982; 2*: 523–527
8 Hillon P, Lebrex D, Munoz C et al. Comparison of the effects of a cardioselective and a non-selective beta-blocker on portal hypertension in patients with cirrhosis. *Hepatology 1982; 2*: 528–531

9   Price HL, Cooperman LH, Warden JC. Control of the splanchnic circulation in man. Role of beta-adrenergic receptors. *Circ Res 1967; 21*: 333-340
10 Bihari D, Westaby D, Gimson AES et al. Reductions in portal pressure by selective beta 2 adrenoceptor blockade in patients with cirrhosis and portal hypertension. *Br J Clin Pharmacol 1984; 17*: 753-757
11 Bosch J, Mastai R, Kravetz D et al. Effects of propranolol on azygous venous blood flow and hepatic and systemic haemodynamics in cirrhosis. *Hepatology 1984; 4*: 1200-1205
12 Colman JC, Jennings GL, McLean AJ et al. Propranolol in decompensated alcoholic cirrhosis [letter]. *Lancet 1982; ii*: 1040-1041
13 Garcia-Tsao G, Grace ND, Groszmann RJ et al. Short-term effects of propranolol on portal venous pressure. *Hepatology 1986; 6*: 101-106
14 Caujolle B, Ballet F, Poupon R. Relationship among beta-adrenergic blockade, propranolol concentration and liver function in patients with cirrhosis. *Scand J Gastroenterol 1988; 23*: 925-930
15 Valla D, Bercoff E, Menu Y et al. Discrepancy between wedged hepatic venous pressure and portal venous pressure after acute propranolol administration in patients with alcoholic cirrhosis. *Gastroenterology 1984; 86*: 1400-1403
16 Ohnishi K, Nakayama T, Saito M et al. Effects of propranolol on portal haemodynamics in patients with chronic liver disease. *Am J Gastroenterol 1985; 80*: 132-135
17 Rector WG. Propranolol for portal hypertension. Evaluation of therapeutic response by direct measurement of portal vein pressure. *Arch Intern Med 1985; 145*: 648-650
18 Bendtsen F, Henriksen JH, Sorensen TIA. Propranolol and haemodynamic response in cirrhosis. *J Hepatol 1991; 13*: 144-148
19 Feu F, Bordas JM, Garcia-Pagan J, Bosch J, Rodes J. Double blind investigation of the effects of propranolol and placebo on the pressure of oesophageal varices in patients with portal hypertension. *Hepatology 1991; 13*: 917-922
20 Cales P, Braillon A, Hiron MI et al. Superior portosystemic collateral circulation estimated by azygous blood flow in patients with cirrhosis. *Hepatology 1984; 1*: 37-46
21 Bosch J, Mastai R, Kravetz D et al. Measurements of azygous venous blood flow in the evaluation of portal hypertension in patients with cirrhosis. Clinical and haemodynamic correlations in 100 patients. *J Hepatol 1985; 1*: 125-139
22 Mastai R, Bosch J, Navasa M. Reduction in azygous blood flow is an intrinsic effect of beta adrenergic blockade in patients with cirrhosis [abstract]. *Hepatology 1985; 2 (suppl)*: S282 (abstract)
23 Braillon A, Cales P, Valla D et al. Influence of the degree of liver failure on systemic and splanchnic haemodynamics and on the response to propranolol in patients with cirrhosis. *Gut 1986; 27*: 1204-1209
24 Bendtsen F, Henriksen JH, Sorensen TIA. Long-term effects of oral propranolol on splanchnic and systemic haemodynamics in patients with cirrhosis and oesophageal varices. *Scand J Gastroenterol 1991; 26*: 933-939
25 Valla D, Jiron I, Poynard T et al. Failure of haemodynamic measurements to prevent recurrent gastro-intestinal bleeding in cirrhotic patients receiving propranolol. *J Hepatol 1987; 5*: 144-148
26 Vorobioff J, Picabea E, Villavicencio R et al. Acute and chronic haemodynamic effect of propranolol in unselected cirrhotic patients. *Hepatology 1987; 7*: 648-653
27 Pereira O, Garcia-Pagan J, Feu F et al. Factors influencing the portal pressure response to propranolol administration in patients with cirrhosis. *Hepatology 1991; 14*: 133A (abstract)
28 Conn HO, Grace ND, Bosch J et al. Propranolol in the prevention of the first haemorrhage from esophagogastric varices: A multicentre randomized clinical trial. *Hepatology 1991; 13*: 902-912
29 Groszmann RJ, Bosch J, Grace ND et al. Haemodynamic events in a prospective randomized trial of propranolol versus placebo in the prevention of a first variceal haemorrhage. *Gastroenterology 1990; 99*: 1401-1407
30 Sacerdoti D, Merkel C, Gatta A. Importance of the 1 month-effect of nadolol on portal pressure in predicting failure of prevention of re-bleeding in cirrhosis. *J Hepatol 1991;*

12: 124-125 (correspondence)
31 Waldman SA, Murad F. Cyclic GMP synthesis and function. *Pharmacol Rev 1987; 39*: 163-196
32 Moreau R, Lebrec D. Leader. Nitrovasodilators and portal hypertension. *J Hepatol 1990; 10*: 263-267
33 Iwao T, Toyonaga A, Sumino M et al. Hemodynamic study during transdermal application of nitroglycerin tape in patients with cirrhosis. *Hepatology 1991; 13*: 124-128
34 Rector WG, Hossack KF, Ready JB. Nitroglycerin for portal hypertension. A controlled comparison of the haemodynamic effects of graded doses. *J Hepatol 1990; 10*: 375-380
35 Hirsch AT, Levenson DJ, Cutler SS et al. Regional vascular responses to prolonged lower body negative pressure in normal subjects. *Am J Physiol 1989; 257*: H219-H225
36 Moreau R, Roulot D, Braillon A et al. Low dose of nitroglycerin failed to improve splanchnic haemodynamics in patients with cirrhosis: evidence for an impaired cardiopulmonary baroreflex function. *Hepatology 1989; 10*: 93-97
37 Koshy A, Moreau R, Cerini R et al. Effects of oxygen inhalation on tissue oxygenation in patients with cirrhosis. Evidence for an impaired arterial baroreflex control. *J Hepatol 1989; 9*: 240-245
38 Navasa M, Bosch J, Chesta J, Rodes J. Isosorbide 5 mononitrate reduces hepatic vascular resistance and portal pressure in patients with cirrhosis. *Gastroenterology 1988; 96*: 1110-1118
39 Salmeron JM, Del Arbol L, Gines A et al. Isosorbide 5-mononitrate increases plasma renin activity and aldosterone and impairs renal function in cirrhosis with ascites. *J Hepatol 1991; 13 (suppl 2)*: S67 (abstract)
40 Garcia-Pagan JC, Navasa M, Bosch J et al. Enhancement of portal pressure reduction by the association of isosorbide 5 mononitrate to propranolol administration in patients with cirrhosis. *Hepatology 1990; 11*: 230-238
41 Garcia-Pagan JC, Feu F, Bosch J, Rodes J. Propranolol compared with propranolol plus isosorbide mononitrate for portal hypertension in cirrhosis. A randomised controlled study. *Ann Intern Med 1991; 114*: 869-873
42 Vinel JP, Monnin J-L, Combis J-M et al. Haemodynamic evaluation of molsidomine: a vasodilator with antianginal properties in patients with alcoholic cirrhosis. *Hepatology 1990; 11*: 239-242
43 Huppe D, Jager D, Tromm A et al. Einflub von molsidomin aut die portale und kardiale haemodynamik bei Leberzirrhose. *Dtsch Med Wschr 1991; 116*: 841-845
44 Del Arbol L, Garcia-Pagan J, Feu F et al. Effects of molsidomine, a long acting venous dilator on portal hypertension. *J Hepatol 1991; 13*: 179-186
45 Spreux-Varoquaus O, Doll J, Dutot C et al. Pharmacokinetics of molsidomine and its active metabolite, linsidomine in patients with liver cirrhosis. *Br J Clin Pharmacol 1991; 32*: 399-401
46 Klein CP. Spironolactone in der Behandlung der portalen hypertonie bei Leberzirrhoses. *Dtsch Med Wschr 1985; 110*: 1774-1776
47 Okumara H, Aramaki T, Katsuta Y et al. Reduction in hepatic venous pressure gradient as a consequence of volume contraction due to chronic administration of spironolactone in patients with cirrhosis and no ascites. *Am J Gastroenterol 1991; 86*: 46-52
48 Burroughs AK, D'Heygere F, McIntyre N. Pitfalls in studies of prophylactic therapy for variceal bleeding in cirrhotics. *Hepatology 1986; 6*: 1407-1413
49 Pagliaro L, Burroughs AK, Sorensen T et al. Therapeutic controversies and randomised controlled trials (RCT's): prevention of bleeding and re-bleeding in cirrhosis. *Gastroenterol Int 1989; 2*: 71-84
50 Pagliaro L, Burroughs AK, Sorensen TIA et al. Beta-blockers for preventing variceal bleeding. *Lancet 1990; 336*: 1001-1002 (correspondence)
51 Colman J, Jones P, Finch C, Dudley F. Propranolol in the prevention of variceal haemorrhage in alcoholic cirrhotic patients. *Hepatology 1990; 12*: 851 (abstract)
52 Jaeschke R, Oxman A, Guyatt G et al. To what extent do congestive heart failure patients in sinus rhythm benefit from digoxin therapy? A systemic overview and meta-analysis. *Am J Med 1990; 88*: 279-286
53 Poynard T, Cales P, Pasta L et al. Beta-adrenergic antagonist drugs in the prevention of

gastro-intestinal bleeding in patients with cirrhosis and esophageal varices. *N Engl J Med 1991; 324*: 1532-1538
54 Laupacis A, Sackett DL, Roberts R. An assessment of clinically useful measures of the consequences of treatment. *N Engl J Med 1988; 318*: 1728-1733
55 Stroke Prevention in Atrial Fibrillation Study Group. Preliminary report of the stroke prevention in atrial fibrillation study. *N Engl J Med 1990; 322*: 863-868
56 Sarfeh IJ, Tarnawski A. Increased susceptibility of the portal hypertensive gastric mucosa to damage. *J Clin Gastroenterol 1991; 13 (suppl)*: S18-S21
57 Perez-Ayuso R, Pique J, Bosch J et al. Propranolol in prevention of recurrent bleeding from severe portal hypertensive gastropathy in cirrhosis. *Lancet 1991; 337*: 1431-1434
58 Poynard T, Lebrec D, Hillon P et al. Propranolol for the prevention of recurrent gastro-intestinal bleeding in patients with cirrhosis: a prospective study of factors associated with re-bleeding. *Hepatology 1987; 7*: 447-451
59 Jensen LS, Krarup N. Propranolol may prevent recurrence of oesophageal varices after obliteration by endoscopic sclerotherapy. *Scand J Gastroenterol 1990; 25*: 352-356
60 Jensen LS, Krarup N. Propranolol in prevention of re-bleeding from esophageal varices during the course of endoscopic sclerotherapy. *Scand J Gastroenterol 1989; 24*: 339-345
61 Vinel JP, Lamouliliette H, Cales P et al. Propranolol reduced the re-bleeding rate during injection sclerotherapy: results of a randomized study. *Gastroenterology 1990; 98*: A644 (abstract)
62 O'Connor KW, Lehman G, Yune H et al. Comparison of three non-surgical treatments for bleeding esophageal varices. *Gastroenterology 1989; 96*: 899-906
63 Ink O, Martin T, Poynard T et al. Does chronic sclerotherapy improve the efficacy of long term propranolol for prevention of recurrent bleeding in patients with severe cirrhosis? A prospective multicenter randomized trial. *J Hepatol 1991; 13 (suppl 2)*: S37 (abstract)
64 Burroughs AK, McCormick PA. Long-term pharmacologic therapy of portal hypertension. *Surg Clin North Am 1990; 70*: 319-339
65 Sarin SK, Groszmann RJ, Mosca PG et al. Propranolol ameliorates the development of portal-systemic shunting in a chronic murine schistosomiasis model of portal hypertension. *J Clin Invest 1991; 878*: 1032-1036
66 Lin H-C, Soubrane O, Cailmail S, Lebrec D. Early chronic administration of propranolol reduced the severity of portal hypertension and portal-systemic shunts in conscious portal vein stenosed rats. *J Hepatol 1991; 13*: 213-219
67 Lebrec D, Poynard T, Bernuau J et al. A randomised controlled study of propranolol for prevention of recurrent gastrointestinal bleeding in patients with cirrhosis. A final report. *Hepatology 1984; 4*: 355-358
68 Andreani T, Poupon R, Balkau B et al. Preventive therapy of first gastrointestinal bleeding in patients with cirrhosis: results of a controlled trial comparing propranolol, endoscopic sclerotherapy and placebo. *Hepatology 1990; 12*: 1413-1419
69 The PROVA Study Group. Prophylaxis of first haemorrhage from esophageal varices by sclerotherapy, propranolol or both in cirrhotic patients, a randomized multicentre trial. *Hepatology 1991; 14*: 1016-1024
70 Burroughs AK, Mezzanotte G, Phillips A et al. Cirrhotics with variceal haemorrhage: The importance of the time interval between admission and the start of analysis for survival and re-bleeding rates. *Hepatology 1989; 9*: 801-807
71 Villeneuve J-P, Pomier-Layrargue G, Infante-Rivard C et al. Propranolol for the prevention of recurrent variceal haemorrhage. A controlled trial. *Hepatology 1986; 6*: 1239-1243
72 Queuniet AM, Czeznichow P, Lerebours E et al. Etude contrôlée du propranolol dans la prévention des récidives hémorragiques chez les patients cirrhotique. *Gastroenterol Clin Biol 1987; 11*: 41-47
73 Gatta A, Merkel C, Sarcedot D et al. Nadolol for prevention of variceal re-bleeding in cirrhosis. A controlled clinical trial. *Digestion 1987; 37*: 22-28
74 Colombo M, De Franchis R, Tommasini M et al. Beta-blockade prevents recurrent gastrointestinal bleeding in well compensated patients with alcoholic cirrhosis: A multicentre randomized controlled trial. *Hepatology 1989; 9*: 433-438
75 Sheen IS, Chen TY, Liaw YF. Randomized controlled study of propranolol for prevention of recurrent esophageal varices bleeding in patients with cirrhosis. *Liver 1989; 9*: 1-5

76 Garden OJ, Mills PR, Birnie GG et al. Propranolol in the prevention of recurrent variceal haemorrhage in cirrhotic patients: a controlled trial. *Gastroenterology 1990; 98*: 1985-1990
77 Cerbelaud P, Lavignolle A, Perrin D et al: Propranolol et prévention des récidives par rupture de varice oesophagienne du cirrhotique [abstract]. *Gastroenterol Clin Biol 1989; 18*: A10
78 Von Kobe E, Schentke K-U. Unsichere Rezidiv prophylaxe von osophagusvarizen Blutungen durch Propranolol bei Leber xirrhotikern - eine propektive kontrollierte Studie. *Klin Med 1987; 42*: 507-510
79 Westaby D, Melia E, Hegarty J et al. Use of propranolol to reduce the re-bleeding rate during injection sclerotherapy prior to variceal obliteration. *Hepatology 1986; 6*: 673-675
80 Liu JD, Yeng YS, Chen PH et al. Endoscopic injection sclerotherapy and propranolol in the prevention of recurrent variceal bleeding. *World Congress of Gastroenterology, Sydney 1990*: FP118 (abstract)
81 Rossi V, Cales P, Burtin P et al. Prevention of recurrent variceal bleeding in alcoholic cirrhotic patients: prospective controlled trial of propranolol and sclerotherapy. *J Hepatol 1991; 12*: 283-289
82 Martin T, Taupignon A, Lavignolle A et al. Prevention des récidives hémorragiques chez des malades, atteints de cirrhose. Résultats d'une étude contrôlée comparant propranolol et sclérose endoscopique. *Gastroenterol Clin Biol 1991; 15*: 833-837
83 Vickers C, Rodes J, Hillenbrand P et al. Prospective controlled trial of propranolol and sclerotherapy for prevention of re-bleeding from esophageal varices. *Gut 1987; 28*: A1359 (abstract)
84 Gerunda GE, Neri D, Cangrandi F et al. Nadolol does not reduce early re-bleeding in cirrhotics undergoing endoscopic variceal sclerotherapy: a multicenter randomized controlled trial. *Hepatology 1990; 12*: 988 (abstract)
85 Lundell L, Leth R, Lind T et al. Evaluation of propranolol for prevention of recurrent bleeding for esophageal varices between schlerotherapy sessions. *Acta Chir Scand 1990; 156*: 711-715
86 Bertoni G, Fornaciari G, Beltrami M et al. Nadolol for prevention of variceal re-bleeding during the course of endoscopic injection sclerotherapy: a randomised pilot study. *J Clin Gastroenterol 1990; 12*: 364-365 (letter)
87 Westaby D, Polson RJ, Gimson AE et al. A controlled trial of oral propranolol compared with injection sclerotherapy for the long term management of variceal bleeding. *Hepatology 1990; 11*: 353-359

LAPAROSCOPIC CHOLECYSTECTOMY

David L Carr-Locke, David C. Brooks
Brigham and Women's Hospital, Boston, USA

HISTORY OF LAPAROSCOPY

The marriage of laparoscopy and cholecystectomy represents the culmination of two diverse techniques which have only recently come together to offer an innovative approach to a common surgical disease. Remarkably, the lines of enquiry in both these procedures span the better part of the twentieth century. Although laparoscopy appears to be a relatively modern technique it has its roots in the early years of this century. Kelling is reported to have performed the first coelioscopy in the early 1900s using a cystoscope to examine the abdomen of a dog. Following this, Jacobeus, using similar instruments, performed laparoscopy to diagnose tuberculous peritonitis in man in 1910. The technique of laparoscopy subsequently received little reported attention until 1936 when Bosch developed a sterilization technique using high-frequency current to coagulate the Fallopian tubes [1]. This was followed in 1941 by Power and Barnes's introduction of tubal fulguration as an alternative method. As early as 1946, gynaecologists expanded their techniques to include limited ovarian biopsies as well as pelvic adhesiolysis. These modalities were limited by the amount of heat produced by the light source and there was concern for injury to adjacent gastrointestinal organs. In general, however, laparoscopy remained primarily a diagnostic tool until the early 1970s when the introduction of the 'cold light' and safe monitors of intra-abdominal pressure made routine laparoscopy a reliable, safe and effective technique. The single most important impetus for the development of operative laparoscopy was the desire for an effective, safe and speedy method of permanent sterilization. Since then, millions of women have undergone tubal ligation with a remarkably low complication rate. Thus, although the technique of laparoscopy was originally developed by a surgeon, it has remained almost entirely in the hands of gynaecologists until now.

TREATMENT OF CHOLELITHIASIS

The history of gallbladder surgery began with Karl Langenbuch who performed the first cholecystectomy in Berlin in 1882. As the operation has been performed over the last century, it has become the 'gold standard' against which all other forms of therapy for gallbladder disease must be measured. The evolution of this procedure paralleled the development of safe and reliable surgery over the last 100 years and, with developments in anaesthesia, blood transfusion, antimicrobial therapy and intensive care, so intra-abdominal surgery became safer and more successful [2].

In recent years reported mortality has been well under 1% in selected patients operated upon electively without significant co-morbidity. Moreover, the accompanying morbidity has also been extremely low. The major complication directly related to the procedure is retained or overlooked choledocholithiasis which occurs in approximately 7–10% of cases [3].

Despite the noteworthy advances which have been made in biliary tract surgery over the last 100 years, recent attention has been focused on non-surgical approaches to the treatment of symptomatic cholelithiasis. The last two decades have witnessed the introduction of oral bile salt dissolution therapy, extracorporeal shock wave lithotripsy and, most recently, contact dissolution of stones, all of which techniques are non-operative and which threatened to remove gallbladder disease from the surgical arena [4, 5]. These non-surgical approaches had an obvious allure. They did not require a major incision and nor did they require a 4 to 6 week recuperation period which was associated with conventional cholecystectomy. The surgeon viewed these as relative negatives, limited in their impact and, in the long run, unlikely to represent a significant problem for the patient. After the usual recovery period the patient was back to work, functioning at a normal energy level, and completely cured of the disease. Most importantly, this last fact differentiated surgery from other forms of therapy.

The absence of the gallbladder almost completely guarantees that stones will not re-develop, if one accepts that the majority of bile duct stones seen postoperatively are not primary, and this more than compensates for any short-term drawbacks the operative procedure may entail. In contrast, non-operative forms of therapy which retain the intact gallbladder are accompanied by an inevitable recurrence rate which may range from 10 to 15%, in the case of shock wave lithotripsy, to nearly 50% over 5 years, in the case of oral dissolution therapy.

A further factor which favours surgical removal of the gallbladder is cost-benefit. Recent advances in management have allowed surgeons to admit patients on the day of surgery and to reliably discharge them within 2 to 3 days of the operation. This has had a major impact on costs, which nevertheless remain remarkably high. The hospital and surgican charges associated with gallbladder disease are estimated to be approximately $5,000,000,000 per year in the USA alone, and this figure is exclusive of time lost from work. Strict financial accounting of alternative forms of therapy is difficult to calculate but when costs of retreatment are included many experts acknowledge that lithotripsy and oral dissolution therapy may be more expensive.

PATIENT SELECTION

Finally, in the selection of patients for treatment, surgery is suitable for virtually all patients whereas no more than 20-25% of patients at best will be eligible for lithotripsy and oral dissolution therapy [2]. Thus the effectiveness, permanence and safety of surgery is accompanied by short-term, but nonetheless significant, disability and loss of time from work. On the other hand, the relatively painless, non-morbid approaches trade short-term benefits for long-term cost and the chance of recurrence [6].

Short of preventing gallstones from developing at all, the ideal form of therapy would combine the short-term advantages of non-operative treatment with the effectiveness and reliability of surgery. Recent surgical advances in the management of gallstone disease suggest that this ideal may be much closer than at any time in the history of surgery and heralds a new era of minimally invasive surgery.

BIRTH OF LAPAROSCOPIC CHOLECYSTECTOMY

The introduction of laparoscopic cholecystectomy has achieved relatively minor short-term morbidity with efficacy at a reasonable cost that will probably prove to be less than either traditional surgical or non-operative therapies. Laparoscopic cholecystectomy is a natural extension of the expanding use of operative laparoscopes over the last decade. They are now routinely used in gynaecology for elective sterilization, management of ectopic pregnancies, lysis of pelvic adhesions and a variety of ovarian and uterine procedures. Earlier fibreoptic laparoscopes had the disadvantage of requiring the operator to manipulate the instrument with one hand while maintaining an eye on the eyepiece in an awkward position suspended over the operative field. The availability of videoendoscopes has allowed the laparoscope to be fitted with a videocamera or ultimately to become fully integrated with the videocamera itself as has already evolved in flexible gastrointestinal videoendoscopy [7]. The optical image is displayed on a TV monitor, thus making the operative field available to all members of the operative team rather than just the operator. Additional advantages are that the procedure can be recorded on videotape, providing a permanent record, documented on hard copy electronic photographs or transmitted remotely for teaching purposes either within or outside the hospital. The development of this technique occurred simultaneously in the USA and Europe in 1988. It evolved from a gradually expanding use of the laparoscope and other percutaneous procedures and devices in the management of cholelithiasis without removal of the gallbladder [8]. Additional surgical laparoscopic experience had already been gained in the management of appendicitis, and cholecystectomy was a natural extension of this technology [9-11]. A variety of individual surgeons including Perissat and DuBois in France, and Schultz, Reddick and McKernan in the USA began animal and human trials to test the hypothesis that videoendoscopic laparoscopic cholecystectomy could be safely performed [12-14].

Early reports in the surgical literature indicate that the technique is feasible and that the results are comparable to open cholecystectomy. The first peer-reviewed report of the technique by an American group was made by Zucker and colleagues from the University of Maryland and presented at the Society for Surgery of the Alimentary Tract during the American Gastroenterological Association meeting in San Antonio, Texas in May 1990. The results reported by this group confirmed the safety and efficacy of the procedure (Table I) and established it as an acceptable alternative to traditional open cholecystectomy [15]. Other reports have substantiated these results [13, 15–21].

TABLE I. Laparoscopic cholecystectomy: collected experience to 1/92

Number of patients	4396 (100–1518)
Operation time (min)	95 (88–118)
Laparotomy conversion (%)	4.1 (1.5–5.0)
Bile duct injury (%)	0.4 (0–2.0)
Hospital stay (days)	1 (1–7)
Recovery time (days)	8 (3–13)

References 13, 15–21.

INDICATIONS

Indications for laparoscopic cholecystectomy were initially more restricted than for open cholecystectomy but this has changed as the procedure has evolved and experience has been acquired. Patients with acute cholecystitis, significant upper abdominal adhesions, patients on anticoagulant therapy or those with significant obesity were excluded in the first reports. Many of these have subsequently become only relative contraindications. Acute cholecystitis is no longer considered prohibitive and in many cases, upper abdominal adhesions can be circumvented with judicious instrument placement. Obesity can be managed so long as the trocars are of sufficient length to transit the abdominal wall. Most surgeons remain reluctant to operate laparoscopically on patients who are taking anticoagulant therapy.

Since laparoscopic bile duct exploration is not yet a reality on a routine basis, patients with known bile duct stones may have their stones retrieved by endoscopic retrograde cholangiopancreatography (ERCP) and sphincterotomy prior to undergoing laparoscopic cholecystectomy. Precise criteria for selection of patients for preoperative ERCP, however, are still being defined.

TECHNIQUE

The procedure is evolving as different surgeons gain experience and no standardized approach has been uniformly adopted. The minimum equipment necessary for performance of the procedure include: (1) a laparoscope with video camera attachment, (2) two self-retaining or ratcheted grasping forceps, (3) blunt, atraumatic dissecting forceps, (4) a laparoscopic clip applicator, and (5) laparoscopic electrocautery scissors or laser fibre. Additionally, the operating suite must be equipped with a CO_2 insufflator, an aspiration/ irrigation apparatus and other standard components of laparoscopy/ pelviscopy sets. A host of manufacturers have devised instrument packages which contain all the required equipment and there has been an impressive proliferation of companies interested in this area.

Under most situations general anaesthesia is used, although some investigators have anecdotally reported the use of thoracic epidural and local bupivacaine instillation with excellent results. At present, several groups are prospectively evaluating different anaesthetic techniques. After adequate anaesthesia has been induced, the abdomen is widely prepared and draped. A Foley catheter is not routinely employed but may be warranted in elderly males or if a prolonged anaesthetic is anticipated. Patients with acute cholecystitis or significant intra-abdominal sepsis may benefit from an indwelling catheter to assist the anaesthesiologist in monitoring fluid status. Compression boots are used to minimize the chances of development of perioperative deep venous thrombosis. Prophylactic antibiotics are given in the form of a second generation cephalosporin. A 1cm, curvelinear incision is made in the supraumbilical area and carried down to but not through the anterior abdominal fascia. A Verres needle is inserted after palpation of the abdominal aorta. It is directed slightly to the right of the midline to minimize the chances of injury to the retroperitoneal structures. The needle is connected to a CO_2 insufflator and gas is instilled at the lowest flow setting, maintaining a cut-off pressure at approximately 10–12mmHg. Insufflation is continued until there is obvious distension of the abdomen and hepatic dullness is lost and the typical hollow sound is easily percussed in the upper abdomen. The volume of gas insufflated generally ranges from 4 to 10 litres. After the abdomen has been satisfactorily distended, the Verres needle is removed and replaced by a 10mm trocar through which the laparoscope will be inserted. Occasionally, an incision in the anterior fascia will be necessary to facilitate entry of the larger trocar. The inner sleeve is removed and the video laparoscope is inserted and the abdomen inspected. When it has been ascertained that the laparoscope is adequately positioned and there has been no intra-abdominal injury from its insertion, the flow rate of the CO_2 is increased to maintain the pneumoperitoneum. A brief visual inspection of the upper abdomen is performed and the gallbladder is located. The lateral right upper quadrant abdominal wall is then inspected from within and the optimal positions for insertion of the two 5mm trocars for access of the grasping instruments are selected. The most lateral stab wound is normally placed 4–5cm below the costal margin just medial to the anterior axillary line. A slightly more medial stab wound is placed, also 4–5cm below the costal margin, but in a location corresponding to the mid-clavicular line. The described positions should be considered merely guidelines and each patient will require trocars placed in slightly different locations depending on the position of the gallbladder. It is of paramount importance to maintain a moderate separation of these two instruments so that the operator manipulating them can move them independently without interfering with each other. The lateral grasping instrument will be used to grasp the fundus of the gallbladder and reflect it superiorly and posteriorly. If the stab wound for this trocar is too low on the abdominal wall, the angle necessary for adequate posterior tension will be awkward to maintain. The more medial instrument is used to grasp the neck of the gallbladder just above the entry of the cystic duct. Tension is maintained in an inferior and lateral direction, splaying out the duct and artery and making dissection easier. When these two trocars have been placed and the gallbladder is under appropriate tension, a 10mm stab wound is placed slightly to the right of the upper midline. This instrument should be parallel to the gallbladder in the horizontal plane to facilitate the dissection and it should be lateral to the midline so that it avoids the falciform ligament. A reducing sleeve is passed through this trocar and a 5mm blunt, atraumatic dissecting instrument is inserted to dissect the fat from the cystic duct and cystic artery and to isolate these structures (Figure 1). Ideally this instrument should be attached to the electrocautery machine so that small bleeding points can be controlled during the dissection. After the cystic duct has been isolated, the dissecting instrument and the reducing sleeve are removed and a 10mm clip applicator is introduced. A single clip is placed on the proximal (gallbladder side) cystic duct. The applicator is removed, the reducing sleeve replaced and a pair of fine curved scissors is introduced. These are used to make an incision in the anterior wall of the cystic duct through which a cholangiogram catheter is introduced. During this manoeuvre, the dissecting instrument is used to hold the neck of the gallbladder while the ratcheted grasping instrument placed through the mid-clavicular site is replaced with the cholangiogram catheter and the instrument used to pass it. A one or two

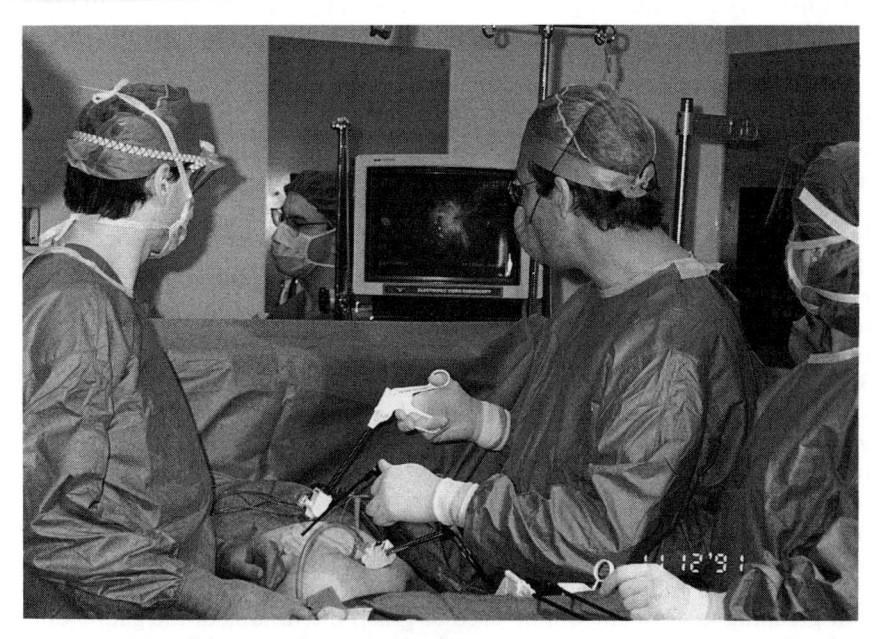

Figure 1. Surgeon manipulating dissecting forceps through upper midline trocar (right hand) and grasping forceps through lower lateral trocar (left hand) with laparoscope at umbilicus and TV monitors positioned on both sides of the operating table.

film cholangiogram is performed [22–25]. If no filling defects are found, the clip applicator is reintroduced through the midline trocar and double clips are placed on the distal (common duct portion) segment of the cystic duct. The cystic duct is then completely divided with cauterizing scissors or laser fibre.

If a stone is found on the intraoperative cholangiogram, the surgeon has two options. The first is to continue with the cholecystectomy and arrange for postoperative ERCP and sphincterotomy. The second, if the cystic duct is of adequate dimension, is to introduce an eight or nine French steerable ureteroscope through the cystic duct and advance it into the common bile duct. The stone can occasionally be retrieved by basketing. One of the potential shortcomings of this procedure is the relative difficulty in retrieving duct stones found during routine operative cholangiography. This consideration prompts the surgeon to develop a close working relationship with gastroenterological colleagues who may assist in postoperative extraction of the stones (Table II). Steerable endoscopes capable of being passed through the cystic duct are still in the developmental stage. Additionally, the development of tuneable dye lasers for laser lithotripsy of common bile duct stones continues. The laser fibre measures between 200 and 300μm and can be delivered to the stone through the working channel of an endoscope. After the cystic duct has been divided and the distal end controlled, the cystic artery is doubly clipped and divided. Care should be taken to isolate the cystic duct close to the gallbladder to prevent injury to the right hepatic artery.

TABLE II. Laparoscopic cholecystectomy: Brigham and Women's Hospital (3 March 1990 to 1 December 1991)

Preoperative ERCP	26 *(4.8%)*
Positive	77%
Negative	23%
Intraoperative cholangiography	
Performed	29 (5.1%)
positive	1 (3.4%)
Attempted	6 (1.3%)
Not indicated	525 (93.7%)
retained stones	8 (1.4%)
Postoperative ERCP/ES	*15 (2.7%)*
Retained stones	8 (53%)
Bile leak	6 (40%)
Duct injury	1 (7%)
Total ERCP involvement	*41 (7.5%)*

Having controlled the duct and the artery, the surgeon is now ready to proceed with dissection of the gallbladder from the liver bed. This can be done with a variety of instruments including electrified scissors, cutting/coagulating cautery needle or laser fibre. Proponents of laser dissection point to the minimal damage incurred in adjacent liver parenchyma, while cautery proponents point to the speed of their instrument, the greater coagulation ability and the fact that the apparent burns and charring of the liver have no significant sequelae. Dissection is continued upward while the lateral instruments are continually adjusted to maintain adequate tension on the cutting surface. When all but a few fibres of the attachments between the gallbladder and liver have been divided, the dissection is momentarily discontinued and the liver bed and the porta hepatis are reinspected to ensure that there is no bleeding from the liver bed or the artery and that there is no leak from the cystic duct remnant. This is the last time that the surgeon will be able to manoeuvre the liver superiorly using the gallbladder as a handle. When the final attachments between the gallbladder and the liver have been severed, the liver will fall back into its anatomical position and efforts to lift the liver with probes and instruments are likely to damage the hepatic capsule and incur bleeding. This is also an appropriate time to aspirate any bile or blood which has collected in the subhepatic space. When this inspection is completed, the few attachments connecting the gallbladder and the liver are divided with cautery or laser. The gallbladder is left in the suprahepatic space attached to one of the lateral grasping forceps.

At this time, the laparoscope is removed from the supraumbilical puncture site and a reducing sleeve is inserted. The video laparoscope is moved to the upper midline trocar and reinserted. This allows easy visualization of the subphrenic space and the free gallbladder. A larger grasping instrument is inserted via the supraumbilical trocar and the neck of the gallbladder is grasped. The tubing from the CO_2 insufflator is also connected to the upper midline trocar to maintain the pneumoperitoneum. Under direct vision, the gallbladder is brought back to the supraumbilical trocar. Once gently seated there, the reducing sleeve and trocar are slid out of the abdomen over the larger grasping forcep. This allows greater mobility while trying to ease the gallbladder through the abdominal wall. The large grasping forceps are used to pull the gallbladder up to the level of the skin at which point it is opened with scissors and a pool sucker is used to aspirate bile and small stones. Generally the gallbladder will have collapsed enough to allow it to be easily removed through the incision. If not, the remaining gallstones can be crushed with a Kelly clamp or the fascial incision may be slightly enlarged to allow the stones to be removed. Once the gallbladder is completely removed, the fascial incision should be closed with one or two absorbable sutures.

The pneumoperitoneum will have been lost by this point and will require a few minutes to be re-established. The subphrenic space can then be reinspected and any fluid aspirated. A final brief check for bleeding is undertaken. If none is found, the pneumoperitoneum is evacuated and all trocars are removed. Subcuticular skin sutures alone are used to close the remaining incisions. The upper midline incision, though it is 1cm in length, passes into the abdomen in an oblique fashion through the rectus and this fascial rent quickly seals itself without requiring additional sutures. 'Band-Aids' are placed over all incisions and the patient is awoken and extubated.

Approximately 15–20% of patients may be discharged from hospital on the day of operation after a 2-3 hour recovery room stay when it is clear that they are voiding without difficult and can maintain oral hydration. The remainder of patients will benefit from an overnight hospitalization (Table III). Most patients are well enough to completely resume their normal daily activities within 5 to 7 days of the procedure. There is no restriction on activity, the patients may bathe regularly, exercise and resume heavy lifting at their convenience.

TABLE III. Laparoscopic cholecystectomy: Brigham and Women's Hospital (3 March 1990 to 1 December 1991)

Patients: 560	450 Female
	110 Male
Mean age:	45.5 (17–86)
Indications: cholelithiasis	89%
acute cholecystitis	9%
other	2%
Mean operation time:	1.6 hours (0.5–6.4)
Mean hospital stay:	1.6 days (0–9)
Return to normal activities:	6 days

RESULTS AND COMPLICATIONS

The single greatest concern has been the complication rate and fears were expressed predicting an unacceptably high bile duct injury rate with this new procedure, leaving in its wake a host of benign common bile duct strictures. To date, the reported complication rate is little different from open cholecystectomy. Dubois reported two complications in his initial report of 36 cases [13], one related to bleeding from a fragile cystic artery which required laparotomy for control and one a bile leak from the gallbladder bed occurring on the second postoperative day and requiring drainage. Zucker has reported a 7% complication rate in his series including bile leak from the cystic duct and a common bile duct injury which was recognized at the time and required operative repair [15]. In our own series of 560 patients, we have seen eight bile leaks (1.4%), six of which were treated endoscopically and two of which required laparotomy and drainage for control, and three bile duct injuries (0.5%), all requiring further surgery (Table IV). These reported rates seem to be significantly higher than those reported for open cholecystectomy, but all authors acknowledge that the technique involves a learning curve and the degree of observation and reporting of complications may be far more stringent than was ever the case for open surgery. The rate of complications rapidly diminishes as surgeons acquire more experience with the technique. There is no reason to believe that late complications will be greater than following routine cholecystectomy and there is a theoretical reason to believe that abdominal wall complications such as chronic pain, symptomatic adhesions and incisional hernias will occur at a considerably lower rate than after open procedures.

TABLE IV. Laparoscopic cholecystectomy: Brigham and Women's Hospital (March 1990 to December 1991)

Patients		560
Complications		27 (4.8%)
Common bile duct		3 (0.5%)
Bile leak		8 (1.4%)
Bleeding (laparotomy)		5 (0.8%)
Biliary	1	
Abdominal wall	2	
Diaphragm	1	
Aortic injury	1	
Bowel injury		3 (0.6%)
Retained stones		8 (1.4%)
Laparotomy conversion		12 (2.1%)
Mortality		1 (0.2%)
Readmissions (30 days)		11 (2.2%)
Emergency ward visits (30 days)		7 (1.5%)

CONCLUSION

Laparoscopic cholecystectomy has emerged as a unique procedure that offers the long-term advantages of open cholecystectomy without much of the short-term morbidity. When compared to non-surgical approaches to symptomatic gallstones, it is suitable for virtually all patients rather than highly-selected groups as is the case for oral bile acid therapy or extracorporeal lithotripsy. Furthermore, it obviates the high recurrence rate seen with these techniques. Complications of bleeding and ductal injury appear to occur at a slightly higher rate than with traditional open cholecystectomy but most surgeons who have had experience with the procedure predict that these complications will become rarer as more experience is gained. We are witnessing the first major successful challenge to traditional surgical management of symptomatic cholelithiasis in 100 years and the birth of gastrointestinal laparoscopic surgery.

REFERENCES

1 Semm K. *Operative Manual for Endoscopic Abdominal Surgery*. Chicago: Year Book Medical Publishers. 1986
2 Brooks DC. Newer concepts in the management of biliary tract disease. *Surg Rounds 1989; 12(7)*: 37–48
3 Pappas TN, Slimane TB, Brooks DC. 100 consecutive common duct explorations without mortality. *Ann Surg 1990; 211*: 260–262
4 Schoenfield LJ, Lachin JM. Chenodiol (chenodeoxycholic acid) for dissolution of gallstones: The National Cooperative Gallstone Study: a controlled trial of efficacy and safety. *Ann Intern Med 1981; 95*: 257–282
5 Sackmann M, Delius M, Sauerbruch T et al. Shock-wave lithotripsy of gallbladder stones – the first 175 patients. *N Engl J Med 1988; 318*: 393–397
6 Sackmann M, Ippisch E, Sauerbruch T et al. Early gallstone recurrence after successful shock-wave therapy. *Gastroenterology 1990; 98*: 392–396
7 Sivak MV. Video endoscopy, the electronic endoscopy unit and integrated imaging. In DL Carr-Locke, *Endoscopy Update* (Baillière's Clinical Gastroenterology, International Practice

and Research) London: Baillière Tindall. 1991: 1-18
8 Kellett MJ, Russell RCG, Wickham JEA. Percutaneous cholecystolithotomy. *Endoscopy 1989; 21*: 365-366
9 Fleming JS. Laparoscopically directed appendectomy. *Aust NZ Obstet Gynecol 1985; 25*: 238
10 Gangal HT, Gangal MH. Laparoscopic appendectomy. *Endoscopy 1987; 19*: 127
11 Leahy PF. Technique of laparoscopic appendectomy. *Br J Surg 1989; 76*: 616
12 Perissat J, Collet DR, Belliard R. Gallstones: laparoscopic treatment, intracorporeal lithotripsy followed by cholecystostomy or cholecystectomy - a personal technique. *Endoscopy 1990; 21*: 373-374
13 Dubois F, Icard P, Berthelot G, Levard H. Coelioscopic cholecystectomy. Preliminary report of 36 cases. *Ann Surg 1990; 211*: 60-62
14 Reddick EJ, Olsen DO. Laparoscopic laser cholecystectomy. *Surg Endosc 1989; 3*: 50-53
15 Zucker K, Bailey RW, Gadacz TR, Imbembo AL. Laparoscopic cholecystectomy: a plea for cautious enthusiasm. *J Surg 1991; 161*: 36-44
16 Peters JH, Ellison EC, Innes J et al. Safety and efficacy of laparoscopic cholecystectomy: a prospective analysis of 100 initial patients. *Ann Surg 1991; 213*: 3-12
17 Spaw AT, Reddick EJ, Olsen DO. Laparoscopic cholecystectomy: Analysis of 500 procedures. *Surg Lap Endosc 1991; 1*: 2-7
18 Cuschieri A, Dubois F, Mouiel J et al. The European experience with laparoscopic cholecystectomy. *Am J Surg 1991; 161*: 385-387
19 Berci G, Sackier JM. The Los Angeles experience with laparoscopic cholecystectomy. *Am J Surg 1991; 161*: 382-384
20 The Southern Surgeons Club: A prospective analysis of 1518 laparoscopic cholecystectomies. *N Engl J Med 1991; 324*: 1073-1078
21 Graves HA, Ballinger JF, Anderson WJ. Appraisal of laparoscopic cholecystectomy. *Ann Surg 1991; 213*: 655-664
22 Berci G, Sackier JM, Paz-Partlow M. Routine or selective intra-operative cholangiography during laparoscopic cholecystectomy? *Am J Surg 1991; 161*: 355-360
23 Voyles CR, Petro AB, Meena AL et al. A practical approach to laparoscopic cholecystectomy. *Am J Surg 1991; 161*: 365-370
24 Reddick EJ, Olsen DO, Spaw A et al. Safe performance of difficult laparoscopic cholecystectomies. *Am J Surg 1991; 161*: 377-381
25 McEntee G, Grace PA, Bouchier-Hayes D. Laparoscopic cholecystectomy and the common bile duct. *Br J Surg 1991; 78*: 385-386

LIVER TRANSPLANTATION

P McMaster, AR Attard
Queen Elizabeth Medical Centre, Birmingham

INTRODUCTION
The 1980s have seen liver transplantation evolve from a virtual experimental procedure limited to one or two centres, to a major undertaking across the world. More than 60 centres are currently active in Europe and in 1990, the number of liver transplants performed in these centres (and in North America) was in excess of 2000. During the same period there was a marked variation in transplant rates between countries so that 5.8 transplants per million population were carried out in the UK, compared to 8.2 in Germany, 10.8 in the USA and 11.8 in France.

Increased activity has been matched by an overall improvement in results. More than three-quarters of all patients will now make a full and complete recovery after transplantation. These improved results have inevitably lowered the threshold for referral of patients with advancing liver disease, so that liver transplantation is no longer considered to be solely a 'last resort' for patients in the agonal phase of their disease. Furthermore, the indications for transplantation have broadened and previous contraindications, such as alcoholic liver disease, are no longer absolute.

Inevitably in such a complex undertaking, progress has been on many fronts. Of great importance were improvements in organ preservation and the introduction of newer immunosuppressive agents such as cyclosporin A, OKT3 and more recently FK506. Equally, there have been major improvements in the technical management of the more complex vascular problems which may be present in patients with liver disease, such as portal vein thrombosis, and the use of venous bypass during the anhepatic phase of the procedure.

Liver transplantation has, therefore, become an indispensable treatment modality in modern hepatology. However, specific problems still exist and will be the focus of much attention during the next few years. First, primary non-function and arterial thrombosis remain life-threatening complications requiring urgent re-transplantation. Secondly, despite the improvements in immunosuppression, the ideal immunosuppressive agent does not yet exist. Finally, liver transplantation has yet to make a significant impact on the survival of patients with malignant disease and post-hepatitis B cirrhosis. Transplantation in children and in patients with fulminant hepatic failure also requires special consideration. This brief paper explores some of the current areas of development and controversy.

PATIENT SELECTION AND TIMING

In the early years of transplantation, several factors, including age over 55, weight under 10kg and associated systemic disorders, such as diabetes mellitus, excluded patients from being considered for hepatic replacement. Few of these would now be considered contraindications. Table I outlines the current indications and contraindications for liver transplantation. By far the commonest indication worldwide for liver replacement is post-necrotic cirrhosis associated with chronic hepatitis B infection. In northern Europe, primary biliary cirrhosis is the commonest indication and it is in these patients that the timing of operation is particularly important.

TABLE I. Liver transplantation - more common indications and contraindications

Indications
Primary biliary cirrhosis
Postnecrotic cirrhosis
Primary sclerosing cholangitis
Alcoholic cirrhosis
Malignancy
Metabolic disorders
Acute liver failure

Contraindications
Malignancy beyond the liver
Active alcoholism
Uncorrectable major cardiac/pulmonary disease

Transplantation undertaken at the optimal time in a patient who has not entered the agonal phase of hepatic decompensation, with the attendant malnutrition and renal failure, will result in full rehabilitation in more than 90% of cases. Patients who are delayed until they develop overwhelming complications and sepsis, with multiple system failure requiring intensive care support pre-transplantation, will achieve rehabilitation in less than 50% of cases. Hence, the patient with primary biliary cirrhosis who develops progressive biochemical deterioration, with a serum bilirubin in excess of 200µmol/l, faces an uncertain future of progressive ill health with increased risk of variceal haemorrhage and sepsis. When the prognosis is estimated to be no more than 1 year to 18 months, the question of transplantation should be seriously considered. Clearly, if operation is to be undertaken it is appropriate that it is performed at the time which gives the safest option for the best chance of recovery and rehabilitation. Factors associated with a poor outcome after transplantation are listed in Table II. Although Child's grading of liver disease was originally derived from and applied to cirrhotic patients with portal hypertension undergoing portosystemic shunt surgery, it can be usefully applied to assess the risk of death in these patients. In assessing such patients, discussion between physicians and surgeons in a transplant unit is essential.

Special considerations are required in the case of children, patients with malignancy, fulminant hepatic failure, hepatitis B and alcoholic liver disease.

TABLE II. Liver transplantation – factors associated with a poor prognosis

Major risk factors
Raised bilirubin
Raised creatinine
Sepsis
Ascites
Malnutrition

Relatively less serious factors
Thrombosed portal vein
Multiple vessels
Previous surgery

LIVER TRANSPLANTATION IN CHILDREN

The diseases in paediatric patients treated with liver transplantation in Birmingham are listed in Table III. Nearly half of all paediatric transplants were performed for biliary atresia. Inborn errors of metabolism and cirrhosis from various causes were the next commonest. This is consistent with reports from other institutions with large paediatric transplant programmes.

TABLE III. Primary diagnoses in 84 children undergoing 108 transplants in Birmingham

Diagnosis	Number	%
Biliary atresia	39	46.5
Alpha-1-antitrypsin deficiency	9	10.7
Tyrosinaemia	5	5.9
Acute non-A non-B hepatitis	5	5.9
Hepatitis A	4	4.7
Others	22	26.3

Although biliary atresia is relatively uncommon, 50 cases a year are reported in the UK. Prior to 1959, the natural history of this condition was progressive liver failure and death before age 2 months. In 1959, Kasai devised the operation of hepatico-portoenterostomy, which improved the outlook of this condition. However, the procedure needs to be carried out before the age of 6 weeks and even then recurrent episodes of cholangitis will lead to progressive cholestasis and cirrhosis. Several centres have reported that prior hepatico-portoenterostomy will not adversely influence the outcome of liver replacement provided patients are referred early at the first sign of liver failure [1, 2].

Suitable donors in such small children are rarely available in the UK. The technique of segmental reduction, allowing a portion of an adult cadaveric donor liver to be harvested for implantation, gave a major spur to the development of paediatric and infant transplantation. With the adoption of the segmental technique in our own unit in 1988, results in children and infants under 10kg have improved significantly with 73% alive and well at the time of writing (Table IV). This survival rate is similar to that reported by other centres. Thus, we will consider even the smallest of infants for transplantation.

TABLE IV. Patient survival for paediatric transplants performed between 1989 and 1991

Weight (kg)	% Actuarial survival		
	1 week	1 month	1 year
<10 (n = 23)	78.3	78.3	73.6
10-30 (n = 20)	95.5	86.4	75.3
>30 (n = 15)	85.7	71.4	71.4

Hepatic artery thrombosis remains the most common (7.4-33% in some series [3, 4]) and most lethal complication (mortality 50% [5]) in paediatric transplant patients. Sepsis is an important cause of mortality in our own series. Furthermore, a potential long-term sequela of liver transplantation in children is the reported decrease in glomerular filtration rate in 85% of paediatric patients who have been on cyclosporin A for more than 1 year [6]. Close monitoring of cyclosporin levels is, therefore, an important measure in these patients.

Overall, liver transplantation in children has acceptable morbidity and mortality and will improve the quality of life. As with liver transplantation in adults, results can expect to improve with earlier referral of potential candidates, greater availability of donor organs, further technical refinements and the development of more specific and less toxic immunosuppressive agents.

LIVER TRANSPLANTATION FOR MALIGNANT DISEASE

There is considerable controversy about the role of liver transplantation for malignancy. The outcome for primary liver cancer continues to be disappointing with all too many tumours developing in cirrhotic patients and with late presentation, often stage 3 plus and with extensive nodal involvement. Results in patients with both central and peripheral cholangiocarcinoma have been dismal.

The main indications for transplantation are listed in Table V. Although liver replacement continues to be attempted in patients with extensive disease within the liver or in those with advanced cirrhosis and tumour confined to one lobe, the presence of micrometastatic lesions at the time of surgery often leads to recurrent disease. Only a third of patients will be well and disease-free at 3 years, although those transplanted for primary cirrhosis in which the tumour is an incidental finding do not usually develop recurrence.

TABLE V. Liver transplantation for malignancy – indications

'Unresectable cancer – confined to the liver'
Haemangioendothelioma
Hepatoblastoma
Hepatocellular carcinoma (fibrolamellar)
    Stage 2/3 with negative nodes
    + cirrhosis

More recently, Iwatsuki et al analysed prognostic factors for survival and recurrence following transplantation [7]. They studied 105 liver recipients with hepatoma and found that vascular invasion, tumour number, tumour shape (circumscribed or non-circumscribed) and the presence of lymph node invasion significantly affected survival. Tumour size > 5cm, multiple nodules, vascular invasion and non-circumscribed lesions were associated with recurrence.

Faced with these difficulties, surgeons in Pittsburgh adopted a very aggressive therapeutic approach to the problem, carrying out a radical en-bloc foregut excision of the liver and all adjacent vasculature and lymph nodes surrounding the coeliac axis followed by replacement with an organ cluster graft consisting of the liver, pancreas, duodenum and variable segments of proximal jejunum [8]. The preliminary results analysed at 18 months, however, continued to show a high rate of recurrent malignancy. In a further modification of the 'cluster' procedure, the liver alone was transplanted in seven patients with hepatocellular carcinoma, accepting the penalty of diabetes mellitus [9]. Of four patients with positive nodes, only one is alive at 1 year. It is therefore uncertain whether this super-radical approach will reap real benefits.

An alternative approach being adopted by several groups is one of aggressive chemotherapy after transplantation for extensive intrahepatic malignancy. Workers in Dallas have reported excellent 2 year survival and disease-free rates following aggressive chemotherapy with adriamycin and mitomycin C.

Efforts to eradicate micrometastases will remain a priority for the 1990s and the possible role of combination chemotherapy and interferon has yet to be explored. Furthermore, as with other tumours, techniques which offer better preoperative staging of disease are required.

FULMINANT HEPATIC FAILURE

Fulminant hepatic failure is a syndrome characterized by the rapid onset of jaundice, hepatic dysfunction and encephalopathy in a patient without pre-existing liver disease. Until relatively recently, this condition was considered unsuitable for hepatic transplantation because of the rapidity of onset, which leaves a very small window to find suitable donors, the somewhat unpredictable outcome and the rapid development of cerebral oedema. The aetiology of fulminant hepatic failure varies widely with hepatitis B being dominant in southern Europe and North America, and non-A non-B hepatits and paracetamol toxicity being much more common in the UK.

Liver transplantation has dramatically improved the outcome of fulminant hepatic failure, which is associated with high mortality even with intensive medical support. The combined patient survival after transplantation among all series is 68% and this approaches the survival rate of liver transplantation [10]. This represents a two- to threefold improvement in survival compared with medical treatment alone. It is therefore a major challenge for physicians treating such patients, to identify which patients are likely to die unless liver transplantation is undertaken and which are likely to survive with supportive management. Towards this end, the detailed analysis of prognostic criteria by O'Grady et al in 1989 [11] did much to clarify the position so that a series of prognostic factors will accurately predict patient outcome (Table VI). Faced with such prognostic factors giving mortality rates of over 90%, many now consider transplantation and referral to specialist centres. Delay in placing a patient on the transplant list may increase the likelihood of developing complications that might preclude liver replacement such as sepsis or multi-organ failure.

TABLE VI. Fulminant hepatic failure
– adverse prognosis (O'Grady et al [11])

Prothrombin > 6.5 (INR)

or

three of the following:

Age < 10 or > 40 years
Non-A non-B hepatitis
Drug/toxin other than paracetamol
Jaundice > 7 days
Bilirubin > 20mg/dl
Prothrombin > 3.5 (INR)

Major causes of postoperative deaths following transplantation in these patients include sepsis, neurological complications and primary graft non-function. Potential strategies for the future include hepatocyte transplantation and/or the use of hepatocyte growth factors to improve hepatic function and the more widespread use of intracerebral pressure monitoring before, during and after transplantation. In the meantime, prompt assessment of prognosis, early referral for transplantation and early recognition and aggressive management of complications remain the cornerstone of treatment.

LIVER TRANSPLANTATION FOR PATIENTS WITH HEPATITIS B

Post-necrotic cirrhosis associated with chronic hepatitis B infection remains one of the commonest causes of cirrhosis and liver transplantation is the only form of treatment that has the potential of long-term cure and rehabilitation. However, the risk of recurrence in the hepatic allograft is very high and the rate of onset and progression of the disease are greater than with the primary infection in the native liver. This may be due to the promotion of viral growth by the chronic immunosuppression, but the exact mechanism is unknown. It is interesting that the incidence of rejection in patients transplanted for chronic hepatitis B cirrhosis in our unit was lower compared to that experienced by patients transplanted for other causes of liver failure [12]. This suggests that the reduced immunity in these latter patients is not solely related to their immunosuppression therapy. This factor may also account for the higher incidence of fatal sepsis after transplantation in this group of patients.

Faced with these difficulties, several centres have used a variety of strategies for preventing recurrent hepatitis B infection after liver replacement in HBsAg (hepatitis B surface antigen) positive patients. Briefly, these have focused on the use of passive or active immunization and α-interferon, alone or in combination. Results have been disappointing. Passive immunization with small doses of specific hepatitis B human IgG has failed to influence results, while the use of larger doses to maintain the serum level of antibody in excess of 100 IU/l, has only had limited success. Furthermore, the paucity of IgG supply, cost and, in the USA, lack of FDA (Food and Drug Administration) approval for intravenous use are added problems. The development of monoclonal antibodies raised against the hepatitis B virus may solve some of these problems. Results with α-interferon have been equally disappointing and the theoretical risk of alteration of HLA Class I and II antigen expression on the liver cells by interferon may affect the incidence of rejection.

Todo et al recently reported on the results of transplantation in 59 patients who were HBsAg positive and compared the results with a control group of 38 HBsAg negative patients who all had prior hepatitis B infection and were transplanted for postnecrotic cirrhosis [13]. In summary they found that patients who were HBsAg positive pre-transplant remained so thereafter, that after 2 months mortality increased and graft function decreased in these patients and that of several therapies used to suppress the virus, none had a convincing effect on recurrence of infection. In agreement with others, the authors reported a better prognosis in patients transplanted for acute fulminant hepatitis B and those who were also infected with the hepatitis delta virus.

Another approach has been to examine the role of raised serum levels of

HBeAg and HBV.DNA on outcome after transplantation. The general consensus is that patients with smaller viral loads, indicated by the absence of HBeAg and HBV.DNA in serum preoperatively, have an improved chance of clearing HBsAg after transplantation. However, further studies are required.

Clearly one of the great challenges for the 1990s will be the more effective management of patients with chronic hepatitis B induced disease. The development of more effective antiviral agents may be the key to improved results after transplantation.

LIVER TRANSPLANTATION FOR ALCOHOLIC LIVER DISEASE
Until quite recently, alcoholic patients were considered inappropriate for transplantation. With the improved results and a greater understanding of the benefits of transplantation, alcohol induced liver damage has understandably received much attention. Studies in the USA show one year's survival of 66% in patients undergoing transplantation with very few returning to drink. It has indeed been suggested that transplantation is the 'ultimate' sobering experience!

While many patients will be unsuitable for transplantation because of cardiomyopathy, chronic cerebral alcoholic damage, myopathy and neuropathy, there may remain a significant number of alcoholic patients who merit consideration for liver replacement. From the socio-economic point of view, this represents one of the major challenges in clinical transplantation today. Current estimates are that approximately 10% of the adult population are drinking excessively with perhaps 10% of them developing significant difficulties. Even if one were to rule out more than 90% of those with alcohol induced damage, it is estimated that our current need of some 10 transplants per million population per year would rise to well over 30, which would not just swamp available facilities, but almost certainly would not be supported by the current numbers of organ donations. Increasingly, however, units are selectively accepting reformed alcoholics for transplantation.

TECHNICAL DEVELOPMENTS
A series of small but important developments over recent years has led to a significant reduction in the morbidity and mortality associated with technical problems. The introduction of venous bypass during the anhepatic phase of transplantation, combined with increased sophistication in monitoring coagulopathy and reperfusion fibrinolysis using thromboelastography, has done much to reduce bleeding problems so frequently encountered in the past. The use of aprotinin as a constant infusion to reduce the cascade sequence resulting in fibrinolysis has also been an important contribution. These considerations, together with increasing sophistication in dealing with the vascular problems associated with portal vein thrombosis and previous surgery, mean that few patients will be denied transplantation for primarily technical reasons. The ability to reconstruct the arterial and venous systems, using conduits to the aorta and inferior vena cava or portal vein, has resulted in improved results in these patients.

Nevertheless, the complexity and magnitude of liver replacement should not be underestimated and the reduced 30 day mortality, less than 5% in elective cases, must be set against the high morbidity and mortality which persists in decompensated patients with multisystem failure and sepsis where mortalities of 25% in the first 30 days continue to be recorded. Sepsis is often the terminal pathway in multisystem failure, particularly in those coming to transplantation in the agonal phase of their disease with malnutrition, hypoproteinaemia and hepatic and renal decompensation. All this emphasizes the need for optimal timing for patients undergoing transplantation.

REJECTION AND IMMUNOSUPPRESSION

It has long been held that hepatic rejection is less of a problem than with other organs such as renal and cardiac grafts. However, the introduction of protocol biopsies performed routinely at fixed intervals has clearly shown a high incidence of immunological activity within grafted patients. As many as three-quarters of patients will have a significant rejection episode following liver replacement, in spite of relatively effective induction immunosuppression protocols. Often, these histological rejection episodes are matched with modest biochemical disturbance of the organ and although often widely treated with increased immunosuppression, they may indeed resolve rapidly. Thus, although a high incidence of acute rejection is encountered, graft failure from progressive immunological destruction is uncommon. However, changes in immunosuppression may be needed. In our own unit, less than 5% of all grafts fail because of rejection.

During the course of the past decade, the standard immunosuppressive protocol for liver grafting became a combination of low dose cycolosporin A (10mg per kilogram body weight), combined with azathioprine (1.5mg per kilogram body weight) and low dose steroids. Acute rejection episodes were treated with 200mg prednisolone for 3 days, recycled if necessary, and if graft response was not adequate, conversion to the monoclonal antibody OKT3.

We have been able to demonstrate that more than 85% of patients undergoing liver grafting can have all steroids withdrawn within 3 months of transplantation, leaving patients on low dose cyclosporin A and azathioprine. Thus, the sequelae of long-standing steroid disability, such as hypertension, diabetes and osteoporosis, can be avoided. This is an important factor especially since many patients may have significant bone demineralization because of their chronic liver disease before transplantation.

The role of HLA matching in liver transplantation is still not clear. Unlike cardiac, renal and pancreatic grafting, a definite benefit for a high degree of compatibility has not been demonstrated and, on occasions, incompatible ABO grafts will succeed. Nevertheless, its role remains open to question and its influence, particularly on chronic rejection, is a matter of some study at this time.

A recent addition to the armamentarium available to control the immune response is the agent FK506. Developed in Japan in 1987, FK506 is obtained from *Streptomyces tsukubaensis*. This agent has been shown to be effective in delaying graft damage in small and large animal models and is 100 times more potent than cyclosporin A in vitro. Different toxic properties have also been demonstrated. This drug has now entered multicentre clinical trials and preliminary results show that it is indeed a potent immunosuppressive agent. Workers in Pittsburg, who used this drug initially after failed immunosuppression on standard therapy, were able to show reversal of rejection after conversion to FK506 as a rescue treatment. Both American and major multicentre European trials are now approaching completion. Inevitably, with this new patent product, there has been concern about toxic effects and the results of these trials are eagerly awaited. There can, however, be little doubt that FK506 is a potent new agent, although much work is needed before effective monitoring of blood levels will prove possible.

RESULTS

The overall quality of rehabilitation for patients undergoing liver replacement is excellent, with accelerated or catch-up growth in the majority of children. Kuchler et al [14] have demonstrated that more than 85% of patients had an excellent 'quality of life', indeed substantially better than healthy controls!

Our overall 2 year survival for semi-elective cases currently stands at 84%, although of the late complicated patients with multisystem failure, only 55% are alive and well at 2 years.

CONCLUSIONS

In recent years, liver transplantation has rapidly developed from an uncommon experimental procedure limited to a few centres, to a major international effort to support patients with advancing and decompensating liver disease. The excellent results which can be achieved with optimal timing and expert clinical management are not in doubt and the greatest emphasis must now be on obtaining suitable high quality donors at the right time to give the patient the best opportunity to make a full and complete recovery. The future role, if any, of living related donors of hepatic segments will be the focus of much debate over the next few years. New immunosuppressive agents and the prospect, in the future, of xenografting, all suggest a continuing expansion in transplant activity.

REFERENCES

1 Pettit BJ, Zitelli BJ, Rowe MI. Analysis of patients with biliary atresia coming to liver transplantation. *J Pediatr Surg 1984; 19*: 770–785
2 Millis JM, Brems JJ, Hiatt JR et al. Orthotopic liver transplantation for biliary atresia. *Arch Surg 1988; 123*: 1237–1239
3 Kalayoglu M, Strata RJ, Sollinger HW et al. Liver transplantation in infants and children. *J Pediatr Surg 1989; 24*: 70–76
4 Hoffer FA, Teele RL, Lillehei CW et al. Infected bilomas and hepatic artery thrombosis in infant recipients of liver transplants. *Radiology 1988; 169*: 435–438
5 Tzakis AG, Gordon RD, Shaw BW et al. Clinical presentation of hepatic artery thrombosis after liver transplantation in the cyclosporine era. *Transplantation 1985; 40*: 667–671
6 McDiarmid SV, Ettenger RB, Hawkins RA et al. The impairment of true glomerular filtration rate in long-term cyclosporine-treated pediatric allograft recipients. *Transplantation 1990; 49*: 81–85
7 Iwatsuki S, Starzl TE, Sheahan DG et al. Hepatic resection versus transplantation for hepatocellular carcinoma. *Ann Surg 1991; 214*: 221–229

8 Starzl TE, Todo S, Tzakis AG et al. Abdominal organ cluster transplantation for the treatment of upper abdominal malignancies. *Ann Surg 1989; 210*: 374-386
9 Tzakis AG, Todo S, Madariaga J et al. Upper-abdominal exenteration in transplantation for extensive malignancies of the upper abdomen - an update. *Transplantation 1991; 51*: 727-728
10 Starzl TE, Demetris AJ, Van Thiel D. Liver transplantation. *N Engl J Med 1989; 321*: 1014-1022
11 O'Grady JG, Gimson AE, O'Brien CJ et al. Early indicators of prognosis in fulminant hepatic failure. *Gastroenterology 1989; 97*: 439-445
12 Adams DH, Hubscher SG, Neuberger JM et al. Reduced incidence of rejection in patients undergoing liver transplantation for chronic hepatitis B. *Transplant Proc 1991; 23*: 1436-1437
13 Todo S, Demetris AJ, Van Thiel D et al. Orthotopic liver transplantation for patients with hepatitis B virus-related liver disease. *Hepatology 1991; 13*: 619-626
14 Kuchler T, Kober B, Broelsch C et al. Quality of life after liver transplantation. *Clin Transplant 1991; 5*: 94-101

UPDATE ON THE MANAGEMENT OF ULCERATIVE COLITIS

DP Jewell
Radcliffe Infirmary, Oxford

The outlook for a patient with ulcerative colitis has changed dramatically over the last 40 years – a poorly recognized success story for modern medicine amongst the more glamorous advances in, for example, cardiovascular medicine and cancer. Thus, the mortality rate of a severe attack in Oxford prior to 1952 was 37% which has fallen to a current rate of less than 1%, including patients coming to urgent surgery. This has been achieved, of course, by the introduction of corticosteroids in 1952, by improved management of fluid and electrolyte balance and nutrition, and by advances in surgical technique. Less severe attacks can mostly be readily controlled with a combination of oral and topical corticosteroids and the overall relapse rate can be reduced fourfold by long-term maintenance therapy with sulphasalazine. In addition, most patients now have access to gastroenterologists, who are well-trained in managing this disease. The advent of self-help groups (e.g. The National Association for Colitis and Crohn's Disease) has been of tremendous value in increasing patient education as well as providing support and care. The result of this 'revolution' in management has been not only a reduction in mortality and morbidity of the disease, but also an improvement in the social prognosis to a point where it differs little from the population as a whole. It is highly regrettable that the life assurance companies have not kept themselves up to date with these changes.

Nevertheless, the disease is still associated with considerable morbidity in some patients; its symptoms are embarrassing and antisocial; at least 20% of patients with a severe attack will require colectomy, and prolonged colonoscopic surveillance is required for those at high risk of developing colonic cancer. Much of the morbidity of the disease is related to the side-effects of treatment with corticosteroids and sulphasalazine as well as to chronic continuous inflammation. This chapter will review some of the new developments in medical treatment which should give even better therapeutic benefits but with fewer side-effects than the standard drugs in common use. It will not review surgical advances, such as restorative proctocolectomy, nor the present status of cancer surveillance.

CORTICOSTEROIDS

Truelove was the first to use topical corticosteroids for the treatment of active ulcerative colitis and showed that hydrocortisone (100mg in 100ml water) was more effective than a dummy enema. Since then, topical steroids have been used as retention enemas (100ml), 5ml foams, or as suppositories. Although it is uncommon to observe systemic side-effects from topical administration, the demonstration of systemic absorption after either rectal prednisolone or hydrocortisone stimulated the use of enemas containing poorly absorbed steroid compounds. These include betamethasone valerate, beclomethasone and prednisolone metasulphobenzoate, which have therapeutic activity but with minimal effect on the plasma cortisol [1]. In the UK, retention enemas of prednisolone metasulphobenzoate are available (Predenema) and are widely used.

The next logical development was the introduction of oral corticosteroids with a low systemic bioavailability. This has been achieved by developing molecules which are either poorly absorbed or cleared by first pass metabolism through the liver, or a combination of both mechanisms.

Tixocortol pivalate was the first of these new steroids. It is derived from cortisol, the 21-hydroxyl group being replaced by a thiol group esterified to pivalic acid. This compound is absorbed but is cleared by hepatic first pass metabolism such that plasma cortisol concentrations are unaffected. When given as a retention, it is as effective as rectal hydrocortisone for treating active distal ulcerative colitis [2]. However, it appears to have been much less promising when given by mouth although no formal clinical trials have been reported.

Budesonide is a non-halogenated steroid which is structurally related to 16-hydroxyprednisolone (Figure 1). It is only partly absorbed and is then cleared by first pass metabolism through the liver. This drug is being successfully developed for topical treatment of allergic rhinitis as well as asthma and has also been used as a retention enema for ulcerative colitis. A Swedish trial has compared budesonide with prednisolone-21-phosphate enemas in patients with active distal disease [3]. Both compounds seemed to give equal overall efficacy but the sigmoidoscopic and histological scores improved significantly more in the budesonide group. An oral formulation of budesonide is now available and, in open studies, appears to be effective with minimal effects on the pituitary–adrenal axis. Double-blind trials are now in progress to assess its effectiveness in both ulcerative colitis and Crohn's disease. If it is as effective as prednisolone, it should allow large doses to be given by mouth with little risk of systemic side-effects.

The third steroid compound to be developed is fluticasone, which is a fluorinated steroid. Like budesonide, it was developed for the upper respiratory tract but it is poorly absorbed from the gastrointestinal tract. In a group of patients with an ileostomy, a mean of 73% of a single oral dose was recovered in the ileostomy effluent [4]. The small amount of drug that is absorbed is cleared by first pass metabolism through the liver. Unfortunately, it has little efficacy. In one double-blind trial, it proved no better than a dummy tablet when given, over a 4 week period, to patients with mildly active distal colitis

Hydrocortisone

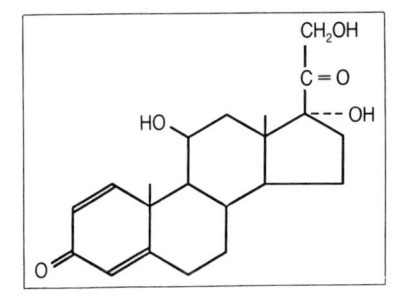

Prednisolone

Budesonide

Figure 1. The chemical structure of budesonide compared with hydrocortisone and prednisolone.

[4]. Further trials comparing it with prednisolone have also been disappointing for both ulcerative colitis and Crohn's disease.

SALICYLATES

Sulphasalazine was originally developed by the scientists of Pharmacia as a result of an idea by Dr Nana Svartz, a Swedish rheumatologist. She had conceived the idea of linking a salicylate molecule with the newly discovered sulphonamide compounds in order to treat rheumatoid arthritis. It took another 40 years to prove the drug's effectiveness in that disease but, in 1942, she reported its value in patients with ulcerative colitis [5]. Subsequent trials in the UK showed that its major role is in the maintenance of remission, an effect that continues over many years [6, 7]. It also has some benefit in treating active disease but is not so effective as corticosteroids [8]. Despite its considerable value in managing the disease, sulphasalazine has a high incidence of adverse reactions such that 10–15% of patients are unable to take it. Table I lists the major side-effects. The commonest are hypersensitivity skin rashes and the dose-related problems of headache, nausea and diarrhoea. These latter effects are, of course, worse in patients with a slow-acetylator phenotype. Most of these side-effects (including male infertility) are known to be caused by the sulphapyridine moiety and so, when it was recognized that the active ingredient was 5-aminosalicylic acid (5-ASA) [9], attempts were made to deliver 5-ASA into the colon without the sulphonamide. The hope was that greater concentrations of active drug could be given to achieve greater clinical benefit with few adverse reactions. The 5-ASA appears to act topically and therefore it cannot simply be given by mouth since it is then rapidly absorbed and excreted. Thus, two approaches have been developed (Table II).

TABLE I. Side-effects of sulphasalazine

Dose related
Nausea
Vomiting
Anorexia
Folate malabsorption
Headache
Alopecia

Non-dose related
Hypersensitivity skin rashes (occasionally with photosensitivity)
Haemolytic anaemia (Heinz bodies)
Agranulocytosis
Hepatitis
Fibrosing alveolitis, pulmonary eosinophilia
Male infertility
Colitis

The first delivers mesalazine (the official generic name for 5-ASA) to the colon either by using resin coating (delayed release) or by coating granules of 5-ASA with a semi-permeable membrane (controlled release). Both systems are pH-dependent, releasing the mesalazine when the intestinal pH reaches the values indicated in Table II. The second delivery system employs a prodrug concept, similar to sulphasalazine. Olsalazine (Dipentum) consists of two molecules of 5-ASA linked with an azo bond, whereas balsalazide is a 5-ASA molecule linked to a peptide. Both drugs behave very similarly to sulphasalazine in that they are poorly absorbed in the small intestine but release the 5-ASA in the colon as a result of bacterial azoreductases splitting the azo bond.

Many trials have now been performed to compare these new compounds

TABLE II. New salicylate drugs in ulcerative colitis

	Coating	pH
Mesalazine		
Delayed release:		
Asacol	Eudragit S	7.0
Claversal	Eudragit L	6.0
Salofalk	Methacrylic acid copolymer	6.0
Controlled release:		
Pentasa	Ethylcellulose	6.0

Prodrugs	
Olsalazine	5-ASA – 5-ASA
Balsalazide	5-ASA – 4-aminobenzoyl-β-alanine

with sulphasalazine both for the treatment of active ulcerative colitis and for maintenance therapy. The results of these studies have been recently reviewed and the overwhelming conclusion is that they are indeed as effective as sulphasalazine [10, 11]. In the maintenance studies, there has been a tendency for sulphasalazine to give greater benefit but this is not a significant difference and reflects the fact that most patients entered into these trials were already taking sulphasalazine. Therefore, they had already had a good response to the drug.

Given that these new salicylates are therapeutically active, four questions can be asked:

1 Do they have less adverse reactions than sulphasalazine?
2 Does increasing the dose give greater clinical benefit?
3 Which of the new drugs should be used?
4 What are the indications for these new compounds?

Adverse reactions

The adverse reactions associated with these new compounds have been few. The majority of patients intolerant of sulphasalazine are able to take either mesalazine or olsalazine [12, 13], confirming that omitting sulphapyridine abolishes most of the drug toxicity. The commonest side-effect of olsalazine is a loose stool seen in 10–15% of patients or, less commonly, a frank watery diarrhoea. These effects usually occur within a few days of starting the drug and gradually settle if the drug is continued. The risk of disturbing bowel function is greatly diminished if the dose is gradually increased (starting at 0.25g and building up to 1 or 2g over 7–10 days) and patients are instructed to take the drug with food. The mechanism of the diarrhoea is by inhibition of sodium absorption in the small intestine, a property which is also shared by 5-ASA alone, albeit at a higher concentration.

In published trials, few side-effects have been reported with mesalazine

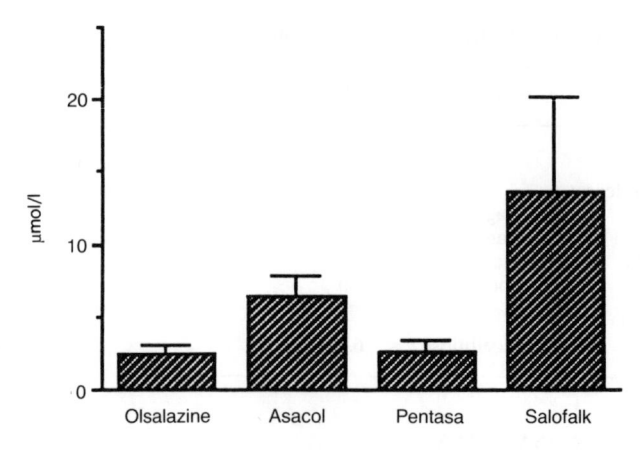

Figure 2. Serum concentrations of 5-aminosalicylic acid in patients with ulcerative colitis following oral ingestion of the new salicylate compounds. Drawn from the data of Staerk Laursen et al. *Gut 1990; 31*: 1271

although in clinical practice some patients will complain of rather non-specific malaise, headaches, nausea, and occasional diarrhoea. A few patients show obvious salicylate sensitivity with urticarial type skin rashes and diarrhoea which can be bloody leading to considerable diagnostic confusion [14].

Recently there has been concern over the potential renal toxicity of mesalazine following reports of nephrotoxicity in patients taking Asacol or Claversal [15]. Figure 2 shows that serum concentrations of 5-ASA are much higher in patients taking Asacol or Salofalk than in patients on olsalazine, reflecting the fact that the mesalazine compounds release more 5-ASA in the small intestine than the prodrug. The low concentrations associated with Pentasa are consistent with a more gradual release of 5-ASA allowing for a more complete metabolism by intestinal *N*-acetyltransferase, an enzyme which is capacity limited [16]. It seems unlikely that renal failure will be anything other than a rare complication of mesalazine therapy but patients receiving the drug should have their renal function monitored.

Dose response

Few studies have yet been done to determine the optimum dose of these new salicylate compounds. For treating active ulcerative colitis, the best study has been a trial of Pentasa conducted in North America [17]. Patients with distal disease were randomized to receive placebo 1.0, 2.0 or 4.0g. Each group contained at least 90 patients. The results showed that 1.0g was significantly better than placebo but there was little difference between 1.0 and 2.0g. A small study of olsalazine in sulphasalazine-intolerant patients who had active disease also claimed to show a dose response but the results are not very convincing given the small numbers in each group [18]. There are even fewer data available for maintaining remission. The early trials from Cardiff comparing Asacol with sulphasalazine did not show an obvious benefit in terms of reducing the relapse rate over a 4 month period when higher doses were used but this is an inferred conclusion from two distinct trials [19, 20] and may not be valid. A dose–response study using olsalazine has just been completed in Oxford and Orebro in which 200 patients have been randomized to three doses and maintained for a maximum period of one year. The data are currently being analysed.

Therefore, until further dose–response data are available, the dose schedules recommended by the pharmaceutical companies should be followed.

Which drug?

All the drugs listed in Table II have been shown to be effective therapeutic agents as indicated above. In the UK, Asacol, Pentasa, and olsalazine are all available. Only one study has been performed to compare directly these drugs and that was an open trial of olsalazine and Asacol [21]. Ninety-six patients whose ulcerative colitis was in remission were randomized to receive one or other drug for a period of one year. During this time the relapse rate was significantly lower for olsalazine ($p<0.02$) than for mesalazine. There were minimal side-effects associated with either drug. However, it is premature to conclude that olsalazine is the more effective drug on the basis of this result. A large double-blind, double-dummy trial will be needed before such statements can be made definitively. Nevertheless, the potential renal toxicity of the delayed-release mesalazine preparations needs to be remembered and these drugs are contraindicated in patients with renal impairment.

Indications for the new drugs

Sulphasalazine is a well tried drug which is cheap, effective and well-tolerated in the majority of patients. Table III shows the cost of treating a single patient for 1 month with sulphasalazine, Asacol, Pentasa, or Dipentum (olsalazine) at the recommended doses. Although hospital contracting may lower costs, it is still obvious that sulphasalazine is much cheaper. Therefore, at the present time, sulphasalazine should remain as first line therapy for maintenance of remission and the new drugs should be reserved for those who are known to be sulphonamide sensitive, young men who have not completed their family, and those who prove to be sulphasalazine intolerant.

TABLE III. Costs of treating patients for 30 days with drugs based on 5-aminosalicylic acid at the recommended doses

Sulphasalazine (Salazopyrin) 1g twice a day	£8.68
Mesalazine	
Asacol 400mg three times a day	£25.73
Pentasa 0.5g three times a day	£29.05
Olsalazine (Dipentum) 0.5g twice a day	£28.68

IMMUNOSUPPRESSIVE DRUGS

The use of azathioprine in ulcerative colitis is well established and it is used in two situations. It may be useful to maintain a remission in those patients who repeatedly relapse when corticosteroids are withdrawn [22] and two trials have demonstrated a steroid sparing-effect in patients who appeared dependent on low doses of prednisolone to control symptoms [23, 24]. However, the evidence that azathioprine is beneficial is not strong but has been recently supported by a withdrawal trial. In this study, so far only reported in abstract, patients who had responded to azathioprine and who had continued in remission were randomized to stay on the drug or to receive a dummy tablet. The relapse rate in the latter group was significantly greater than in the patients continuing on azathioprine [25].

Cyclosporin

Recent interest in immunosuppressive therapy has focused on cyclosporin. This drug was originally isolated from the fungi, *Cylindrocapa lucidum* and *Tolypocladium*, in 1972. Subsequently, the active moiety has been synthesized and has revolutionized the management of graft rejection following organ transplantation. It has also been used extensively in a variety of diseases in which immunological processes are thought to play a role. These include psoriasis, uveitis, myasthenia gravis, primary biliary cirrhosis, and rheumatoid arthritis. Cyclosporin is also being evaluated in Crohn's disease and ulcerative colitis.

Cyclosporin has a range of actions but, immunologically, it appears to act mainly on T-lymphocytes although it also affects macrophages. It binds to cyclophilin [26], a cytoplasmic protein, but the precise mechanisms whereby it exerts its effects on cell function are unknown. It reduces the activation of cytotoxic T-cells, allows activation and amplification of suppressor cells and reduces lymphocyte responsiveness to interleukin-2. However, its main effect may be the inhibition of interleukin-2 and γ-inteferon from T-cells. These cytokines are crucial for the amplification of the immune response by clonally expanding T-cells and by activating macrophages. γ-Interferon may have a particular role in ulcerative colitis since it is able to induce the expression of HLA Class II molecules by the colonic epithelial cells which do not normally express them [27]. Since cells expressing Class II molecules are potentially able to present antigen to the immune system, this could be an important mechanism for inducing chronic inflammation. There is increasing evidence that colonic epithelial cells expressing HLA-DR are able to function in this way [28] and it is of particular interest that 5-ASA is able to inhibit the induction of DR molecules on epithelial cells, at least in vitro [29]. In vivo, cyclosporin rapidly inhibits Class II expression by the colonic epithelium in patients with severe ulcerative colitis, presumably by inhibiting interferon release [30].

However, when given by mouth to patients with a severe attack, no obvious benefit has been noted although this is purely on an anecdotal basis [30]. A more promising effect has been seen when the drug has been given intravenously. Lichtiger and Present have recently reported on 15 patients with severe ulcerative colitis who had had a poor response to 10 days of intravenous corticosteroids [31]. A slow intravenous infusion of cyclosporin was then added in a dose of 4mg/kg while the steroids were continued. Eleven of these patients went into a satisfactory remission and avoided surgery, a result that was sufficiently encouraging to simulate the authors to set up a double-blind trial of intravenous cyclosporin which is now in progress. Our own experience in Oxford has been similar but relapse often occurs when the cyclosporin is stopped. Nevertheless, it has been useful to 'buy time' before surgery.

The other use for cyclosporin that is emerging is in the treatment of a resistant proctitis. Brynskov et al have reported on eight patients with a refractory distal colitis who were given cyclosporin as a daily retention enema – 5mg/kg in either olive oil or in 60ml water containing 5g sorbitol and 500mg carboxymethyl cellulose [32]. Of the eight patients, six responded very well. We have reported on a further 12 patients who had inflammation limited to the rectum and remained symptomatic despite oral and rectal steroids, oral and rectal 5-ASA, and oral immunosuppressive therapy [33]. Many of them showed the characteristic proximal constipation which had been cleared without effect on the disease. They were continued on their existing therapy but were given a daily cyclosporin enema in addition for periods which ranged from 2 weeks to 3 months. Eight of the 12 had an excellent response. Of the four whose symptoms persisted, three came to colectomy and in two the disease was found to be considerably more extensive than had been expected. In both studies, blood concentrations have been minimal suggesting poor absorption, and no side-effects related to cyclosporin have occurred. However, most patients relapse soon after stopping the enema [33].

Therefore, cyclosporin may have a role in the management of ulcerative colitis when the disease is failing to respond to standard therapy. When used systemically, it will inevitably cause side-effects of which the commonest are listed in Table IV. These are all reversible on stopping the drug with the possible exception of nephrotoxicity. Most patients show some fall in glomerular filtration rate, although this is seldom sufficient to raise the plasma creatinine. However, some studies have shown that the glomerular filtration rate does not always return to its previous value on stopping the drug. The other point to remember, if cyclosporin is to be used, is the problem of drug inter-

TABLE IV. Adverse effects of cyclosporin (decreasing order of frequency)

Paraesthesiae
Hypertrichosis
Nausea and vomiting
Gingival hyperplasia
Nephrotoxicity
Hypertension
↑ AST

action. Its elimination is increased by drugs which induce the activity of cytochrome P450, such as rifampicin, isoniazid, and phenytoin, but its elimination is reduced by erythromycin and ketoconazole. In addition, co-administration of aminoglycosides non-steroidal anti-inflammatory drugs (NSAIDs) or cotrimoxazole may cause additive effects on renal function.

If cyclosporin is to be used, blood concentrations must be monitored regularly although there is no close relation between them and the clinical response. Using a whole blood assay, the plasma concentration should be maintained at 150–400 µg/ml.

POTENTIAL DRUGS

The inflamed colonic mucosa contains increased concentrations of cytokines and inflammatory mediators which not only perpetuate the inflammatory response but may be responsible for many of the symptoms as a result of influencing epithelial function. Hence, a number of drugs which specifically inhibit some of these effector mechanisms are being developed.

Leukotriene B4 (LTB4) is one of the most potent pro-inflammatory eicosanoids synthesized by the lipoxygenase pathway of arachidonic acid metabolism. It is a powerful chemoattractant for neutrophils and has effects on both eipthelial and endothelial function. A specific lipoxygenase inhibitor, Zileuton, has been developed which has been shown to reduce the concentration of LTB4 in rectal dialysates in patients with active ulcerative colitis but has no effect on prostaglandin E2 [34]. A double-blind trial of the drug has now been performed in patients with active disease and the preliminary findings show it to be beneficial but only in patients who were not also taking sulphasalazine [35]. Undoubtedly more potent lipoxygenase inhibitors will be developed which may have greater clinical effect. Drugs which act as LTB4 receptor antagonists are also being developed as are thromboxane synthetase inhibitors.

An alternative approach to lowering the concentration of mucosal LTB4, has been to give omega-3 fatty acids such as eicosapentaenoic acid, which is a component of fish oil. These compounds compete with arachidonic acid for the lipoxygenase enzyme but produce leukotriene B5 rather than LTB4. Since LTB5 is much less inflammatory than LTB4, ingestion of fish oil may amoliorate the mucosal inflammation. However, the clinical results of fish oil given to patients with ulcerative colitis are conflicting so far and no firm conclusion can be reached as to its potential value [36, 37].

Platelet-activating factor (PAF) is another lipid mediator which is released from membrane lipids by phospholipase A2 and which is present in increased concentrations in the inflamed colonic mucosa of patients with active ulcerative colitis [38]. Its effects on colonic function can be inhibited in vitro by specific PAF receptor antagonists. A clinical trial of one such compound is now in progress in patients with active colitis.

Several other types of drug are being developed for this disease. Mast cell inhibitors are being re-explored. Disodium-cromoglycate, a known mast cell stabilizer, was without consistent effect in ulcerative colitis which was readily understandable when it was shown that intestinal mast cells differ from other mast cells. Cromoglycate has little effect on isolated intestinal mast cells [39]. However, ketotifen is much more specific and is able to influence the course of an experimental colitis in animals [40]. Finally, hydroxychloroquine is undergoing clinical trial in active ulcerative colitis. This drug has many actions which include inhibiting the movement of neutrophils and macrophages and the lysosomal processing of antigens. It is effective in an animal model of colitis [41] but in a small double-blind study of 30 patients, it was less effective than 20mg prednisolone for active distal ulcerative colitis (JM Rhodes and DP Jewell, unpublished observations). Nevertheless the initial results of another trial which is still in progress are more encouraging [42].

CONCLUSIONS
The introduction of new therapies for ulcerative colitis is continuing to improve the quality of life for those with the disease and is reducing the incidence of drug-induced side-effects. The new salicylate compounds are good examples and it is still possible that an even greater reduction in relapse rate can be achieved by using higher dosages. The promise of an oral steroid preparation with low-systemic bioavailability is exciting and will greatly improve the management of acute attacks and chronic active disease. In the meantime, the role of cyclosporin to control chronically active disease and to allow the corticosteroid dose to be reduced is being defined.

REFERENCES
1. Jewell DP. Corticosteroids for the management of ulcerative colitis and Crohn's disease. *Gastroenterol Clin North Am 1989; 18*: 21-33
2. Hanauer SB. Clinical experience with tixocortol pivalate. *Can J Gastroenterol 1988; 2*: 156-158
3. Danielsson A, Hellers G, Lyrenas E et al. A controlled randomised trial of budesonide versus prednisolone retention enemas in active distal colitis. *Scand J Gastroenterol 1987; 22*: 987-992
4. Angus P, Snook J, Reid M, Jewell DP. Oral fluticasone propionate for active distal ulcerative colitis. *Gut 1992*; in press
5. Svartz N. Salazopyrin, a new sulfanilamide preparation. A. Therapeutic results in rheumatoid arthritis. B. Therapeutic results in ulcerative colitis. C. Toxic manifestations in treatment with sulfanilamide preparations. *Acta Med Scand 1942; 110*: 557-598
6. Misiewicz JJ, Lennard-Jones JE, Connell AM et al. Controlled trial of sulphasalazine in maintenance therapy for ulcerative colitis. *Lancet 1965; i*: 185-188
7. Dissanayake AS, Truelove SC. A controlled therapeutic trial of long-term maintenance treatment of ulcerative colitis with sulphasalazine. *Gut 1973; 14*: 923-926
8. Truelove SC, Watkinson G, Draper G. Comparison of corticosteroids and sulphasalazine therapy in UC. *Br Med J 1962; ii*: 1708-1711
9. Azad Khan AK, Piris J, Truelove SC. An experiment to determine the active therapeutic moiety of sulphasalazine. *Lancet 1977; ii*: 892-895
10. Thomson ABR. New developments in the use of 5-aminosalicylic acid in patients with inflammatory bowel disease. *Aliment Pharmacol Ther 1991; 5*: 449-470
11. Ireland A, Jewell DP. Sulphasalazine and the new salicylates. *Eur J Gastroenterol Hepatol 1989; 1*: 43-50
12. Dew MJ, Harries AD, Evans BK, Rhodes J. Treatment of ulcerative colitis with oral 5-aminosalicylic acid in patients unable to take sulphasalazine. *Lancet 1983; ii*: 801
13. Ireland A, Jewell DP. Olsalazine in patients intolerant of sulphasalazine. *Scand J Gastroenterol 1987; 22*: 1038-1040
14. Austin CA, Cann PA, Jones TH, Holdsworth CD. Exacerbation of diarrhoea and pain

in patients treated with 5-aminosalicylic acid for ulcerative colitis. *Lancet 1984; i*: 917–918
15 Committee on Safety of Medicines. *Current Problems 1990; 30*
16 Pieniaszek HJ, Bates TR. Capacity-limited gut wall metabolism of 5-aminosalicylic acid, a therapeutically active metabolite of sulfasalazine in rats. *J Pharm Sci 1979; 68*: 1323–1325
17 Hanauer S, Schwartz J, Roufail W et al. Dose-ranging study of mesalazine capsules (Pentasa®) for active ulcerative colitis. *Gastroenterology 1989; 96*: A195
18 Meyers S, Sachar DB, Present DH, Janowitz HD. Olsalazine sodium in the treatment of ulcerative colitis among patients intolerant of sulphasalazine. *Gastroenterology 1987; 93*: 1255–1262
19 Dew MJ, Hughes P, Harries AD et al. Maintenance of remission in ulcerative colitis with oral preparation of 5-aminosalicylic acid. *Br Med J 1982; 285*: 1012
20 Dew MJ, Harries AD, Evans N et al. Maintenance of remission in ulcerative colitis with 5-aminosalicylic acid in high doses by mouth. *Br Med J 1983; 287*: 23–24
21 Courtney MG, Nunes DP, Bergin CF et al. A prospective trial of mesalazine vs olsalazine in the maintenance treatment of ulcerative colitis. Submitted
22 Jewell DP, Truelove SC. Azathioprine in ulcerative colitis: Final report on a controlled therapeutic trial. *Br Med J 1974; ii*: 627–630
23 Kirk AP, Lennard-Jones JE. Controlled trial of azathioprine in chronic ulcerative colitis. *Br Med J 1982; 284*: 1291–1292
24 Rosenberg JL, Wall AJ, Settles RH et al. A controlled trial of azathioprine in the treatment of chronic ulcerative colitis. *Gastroenterology 1973; 64*: 793
25 Hawthorne AB, Logan CFA, Hawkey CJ et al. Efficacy of azathioprine in maintaining remission in ulcerative colitis: a placebo-controlled withdrawal trial. *Gastroenterology 1991; 100*: A216
26 Schreiber SL. Chemistry and biology of the immunophilins and their immunosuppressive ligands. *Science 1991; 251*: 283–287
27 McDonald GB, Jewell DP. Class II antigen (HLA-DR) expression by intestinal epithelial cells in inflammatory bowel diseases of colon. *J Clin Pathol 1987; 40*: 312–317
28 Mayer L, Schlien R. Evidence for function of Ia molecules on gut epithelial cells in man. *J Exp Med 1987; 166*: 1471–1483
29 Crotty B, Hoang P, Dalton HR, Jewell DP. Salicylates used in inflammatory bowel disease and colchicine impair interferon-γ induced HLA-DR expression. *Gut 1992;* in press
30 Baker K, Jewell DP. Cyclosporin A for the treatment of severe inflammatory bowel disease. *Aliment Pharmacol Ther 1989; 3*: 143–149
31 Lichtiger S, Present DH. Preliminary report: Cyclosporin in the treatment of severe active ulcerative colitis. *Lancet 1990; 336*: 16–19
32 Brynskov J, Freund L, Thomsen OO et al. Treatment of refractory ulcerative colitis with cyclosporin enemas. *Lancet 1989; i*: 721–722
33 Winter TA, Dalton HR, Merrett MN et al. Cyclosporin A retention enemas in refractory distal ulcerative colitis and 'pouchitis'. Submitted
34 Laursen LS, Naesder J, Burkhave K et al. Selective 5-lipoxygenase inhibition in ulcerative colitis. *Lancet 1990; 335*: 683–685
35 Stenson WF, Lauritsen K, Laursen LS et al. A clinical trial of Zileuton, a specific inhibitor of 5-lipoxygenase in ulcerative colitis. *Gastroenterology 1991; 100*: A253
36 Stenson WF, Cort D, DeSchryver-Kecskemeti et al. A trial of fish oil supplemented diet in inflammatory bowel disease. *Gastroenterology 1991; 100*: A253
37 Hawthorne AB, Daneshmend TK, Hawkey CF et al. Fish oil in ulcerative colitis: final results of a controlled clinical trial. *Gastroenterology 1990; 98*: A174
38 Eliakim R, Karmelli F, Razin E, Rachmilewitz D. Role of platelet-activating factor in ulcerative colitis. *Gastroenterology 1988; 95*: 1167–1172
39 Pearce FL, Befus AD, Gauldie J, Bienenstock J. Mucosal mast cells II. Effects of antiallergic compounds on histamine secretion by isolated intestinal mast cells. *J Immunol 1982; 128*: 2481–2486
40 Eliakim R, Karmelli F, Rachmilewitz D. Ketotifen effectively prevents mucosal damage in two models of experimental colitis. *Gastroenterology 1991; 100*: A578

41 Rhodes JM, McLaughlin JE, Brown DJC et al. Inhibition of leucocyte motility and prevention of immune complex experimental colitis by hydroxychloroquine. *Gut 1982; 23*: 181-187
42 Mayer L, Turtel P, Present DH et al. Effect of hydroxychloroquine in the treatment of active ulcerative colitis: results of the open label phase of the controlled trial. *Gastroenterology 1991; 100*: A230

PRIMARY BILIARY CIRRHOSIS AND SCLEROSING CHOLANGITIS

Alastair J MacGilchrist, James M Neuberger
Queen Elizabeth Hospital, Birmingham

Primary biliary cirrhosis (PBC) and primary sclerosing cholangitis (PSC) together account for most cases of chronic cholestatic liver disease. These have always appealed to hepatologists and in the past decade have been under close scrutiny despite their rarity. This attention, fully justified by the remarkable success of liver transplantation for these conditions, has led to advances in our understanding of both their natural history and some of the immunological factors in their pathogenesis. However, the aetiology of both diseases remains unknown. Consequently, hopes for a successful medical therapy, of which many have been tried, are as yet unfulfilled.

In this review we will attempt to describe some of the more recent advances in PBC and PSC, concentrating on natural history, immunological factors, experimental treatments, and liver transplantation.

PRIMARY BILIARY CIRRHOSIS

Natural history

PBC is a rare but fascinating disease. It has an approximate incidence of 10 per million per year and prevalence of 100 per million in Europe [1], but it is almost unknown in the Third World (possibly in part due to under-reporting). Ninety per cent of cases are female. Neither of these striking epidemiological differences has unravelled the aetiology.

PBC usually presents with the typical clinical features of cholestasis, such as jaundice and pruritus, or with the complications of portal hypertension, such as ascites or bleeding oesophageal varices. Fatigue can be severe. PBC may be diagnosed when asymptomatic, following the detection of an antimitochondrial antibody (AMA) or a raised serum alkaline phosphatase. Contrary to initial reports, it is now evident that asymptomatic patients do progress, and have reduced survival compared to an age-matched population [2].

The diagnosis is made by demonstration of serum AMA and typical, or compatible, histology on liver biopsy. Occasionally, histological features will be typical of PBC in the absence of detectable AMA. The major histological features are those of non-suppurative destructive cholangitis of middle-sized intrahepatic bile ducts. Severity is graded from stages I to IV, ranging from mononuclear cell damage to the biliary epithelium, classically with granuloma formation, through portal fibrosis and eventually cirrhosis (Figure 1).

The most significant extrahepatic complication is the development of bone disease (hepatic osteodystrophy) leading to pain and fractures. The problem is osteoporosis rather than osteomalacia, and the mechanism, although poorly understood, appears to include high bone turnover. Supplements of vitamin D, calcium and fluoride are of no proven benefit. Although hepatocellular carcinoma is less frequent than in other forms of cirrhosis, there is an increased risk of other malignancies, especially carcinoma of the breast [3].

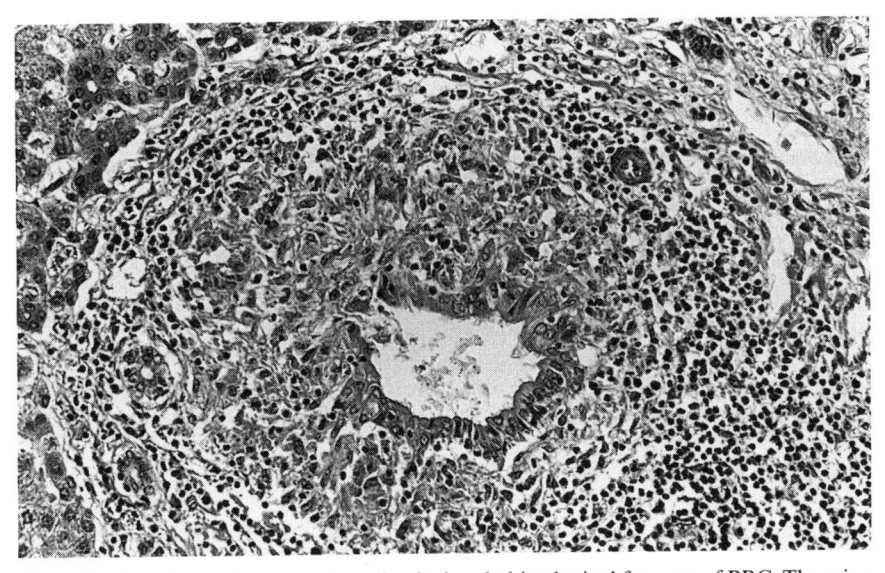

Figure 1. Liver biopsy demonstrating classical early histological features of PBC. There is a dense mononuclear cell infiltrate of the portal tract centred on the bile ductule, whose epithelium is damaged and invaded by lymphocytes.

Immunology

PBC represents something of an enigma to immunologists. Although it has several features of autoimmunity, it does not respond to immunosuppression as do other autoimmune diseases. Some of the immunological clues are well-described, for example the strong association with other autoimmune conditions such as Sjögren's syndrome, Raynaud's disease, thyroid disease and coeliac disease; the increased serum levels of immunoglobulins, especially IgM and

IgG3; the increased catabolism of complement and the increase in circulating immune complexes.

However, these features are non-specific. In contrast, PBC has a unique association with AMA, which is present in serum in over 90% of cases and is virtually diagnostic of PBC. Much recent progress has been made in discovering the antigens against which AMA are directed. Firstly, it was recognized that there were not one but many mitochondrial autoantigens, M1 to M9, of which M2, located on the inner mitochondrial membrane, is the most specific for PBC. A major breakthrough was the discovery that the M2 antigens are identical to components of the pyruvate dehydrogenase complex, including dihydrolipoamide acetyltransferase (E2) [4, 5]. These are summarized in Table I. This vital enzyme system of intermediate metabolism is ubiquitous and highly conserved in Nature.

TABLE I. Identity of the M2 antigens of PBC

	M2a	M2b	M2c	M2d	M2e
Mol. wt (kD)	68–80	60–64	50–56	43–48	36
Identity	PDC-E2	?	PDC-X	PDC-E1	PDC-E1

PDC = pyruvate dehydrogenase complex.
Data adapted from James et al *Hepatology 1989; 10*: 247.

How this antibody directed against an intracellular enzyme system common to all cells relates to the specific attack by T-lymphocytes on the biliary epithelium is still a mystery. In this regard, an intriguing clue is provided by preliminary evidence from our own group that the E2 antibody is present on the plasma membrane of isolated biliary cells from PBC but not from normal liver [6].

Another tantalizing story is the association with *Escherichia coli*. The mitochondrial antibodies recognize antigens present in many bacteria, including the rough forms of *E. coli*. In one study, this form of bacteria was detected in 100% of cases of PBC (where it comprised up to half the total *E. coli* flora) as compared to only 5% of controls [7]. However, neither the Newcastle group [8] nor ourselves (unpublished data) were able to confirm this observation, which provides an attractive, if simplistic, explanation for the autoimmune attack.

The evidence for T-lymphocyte involvement in the biliary attack of PBC is strong. In addition to the histological picture, there is a similarity to both graft-versus-host disease [9] and acute liver allograft rejection, with altered HLA Class II antigen expression on the biliary epithelium [10]. Finally, there is impairment of suppressor T-cell function.

Hopefully it will not be long before these immunological findings can be woven into a coherent story of the pathogenesis of PBC. The rate of progress in the last decade makes this a genuine possibility. In the meantime, the search for a medical therapy continues.

Medical treatment

Specific medical therapy has proved disappointing, although newer agents are under evaluation. Ignorance of the pathogenesis precludes a logical approach to therapy. The long natural history (50% survival at 10 years) makes clinical trials difficult. The end-points of such studies vary between centres. Use of surrogate markers such as bilirubin may not be valid. Death can no longer be used as the sole end-point because of the widespread use of liver transplantation.

The agents employed often have more than one mode of action, making classification difficult. One possibility is to divide them into immune-modulators (corticosteroids, azathioprine, cyclosporin A), anti-fibrotic agents (colchicine, methotrexate), and drugs which eliminate retention products of cholestasis, such as copper (penicillamine) or bile acids (ursodeoxycholic acid (UDCA).

Corticosteroids had some effect on liver chemistry in a short-term trial [11] but no long-term studies have been performed. Steroids are widely regarded as contraindicated because they exacerbate the osteoporosis. Azathioprine has at best a marginal effect, prolonging mean survival by 20 months [12]. Cyclosporin A improves symptoms, circulating chemistry and histology, but the effect on survival is unknown [13]. Nephrotoxicity and hypertension may preclude its long-term use. Colchicine improves liver function tests but not symptoms or histology, and any effect on survival is marginal and conflicting [14–16]. Methotrexate may exert a short-term benefit [17] but is hepatotoxic in the long-term. Penicillamine remains the only drug which has been proven to be of no benefit [18]! UDCA, which has few side-effects, is reported to yield good short-term results [19]. With the possible exception of UDCA, which can be tried for symptomatic relief, none of these agents should be prescribed for PBC without controlled trials.

Without a specific therapy, the physician's role in PBC is to offer symptomatic treatment and to advise on timing of referral to a transplant centre. Non-specific medical treatment is directed against the complications of portal hypertension and against the pruritus, which can be severe. It usually responds to cholestyramine. If gastrointestinal side-effects to this agent prevent its use, cholestyramine A, which substitutes aspartate for glucose in the preparation, may be better tolerated. Resistant cases may respond to UDCA, rifampicin, stanozolol or UV light.

Transplantation

However, the only therapy offering long-term improvement, or possibly cure, is orthotopic liver transplantation (OLT). Rapid advances in surgical technique and immunosuppression over the past decade have made OLT a realistic option for many patients with end-stage cirrhosis. In the UK, PBC is the most frequent indication for OLT, with a 1 year survival over 90%. Although such success precludes a controlled trial of OLT for PBC, prognostic models predicting survival in PBC have been validated [18, 20] and confirm the benefit of OLT. These models are summarized in Table II.

TABLE II. Independent prognostic factors in PBC and PSC

PBC		PSC	
European model	Mayo Clinic model	Mayo Clinic model	King's College model
Bilirubin	Bilirubin	Bilirubin	Bilirubin
Age	Age	Age	–
Haemoglobin	Haemoglobin	Haemoglobin	–
Albumin	Albumin	–	–
Ascites	Ascites	–	–
–	Prothrombin time	–	–
–	–	Inflammatory bowel disease	–
–	–	–	Alkaline phosphatase
–	–	–	Hepatomegaly
–	–	–	Splenomegaly

The critical question is when to offer a patient with PBC the option of OLT. PBC is more predictable than most other forms of cirrhosis. The prognostic models referred to above are too cumbersome for clinical use and can only be applied at presentation. Prognostic information may be gained by measuring type III procollagen peptide, a marker of hepatic inflammation/fibrosis [21] and hyaluronic acid, a marker of hepatic endothelial cell function [22]. The former is no better than more routine tests [23]. The single most useful measurement is the serum bilirubin, which remains low in the early stages and then rises exponentially. Patients should be referred for assessment to a transplant centre when the bilirubin reaches 150µmol/l [24]. However, this consideration takes no account of the patients' quality of life, nor unpredictable life-threatening complications such as variceal bleeding; clearly each case requires individual assessment. The critical point is not to delay referral until the disease is so advanced as to prejudice the chances of successful surgery.

Recurrence of PBC in the transplanted liver has been reported [25, 26], but this is controversial and to date has not been of clinical importance.

In summary, the major advances in elucidating the immunological factors in PBC have not yet been matched by proven medical therapy, and therefore OLT remains the treatment of choice, with good results from a timely operation.

PRIMARY SCLEROSING CHOLANGITIS

Natural history

PSC results from a chronic inflammatory fibrosis of the bile ducts. It is less common than PBC, and more common in men than women. Sclerosing cholangitis secondary to chronic obstruction, infection, drug toxicity or ischaemia of the biliary tree is histologically identical. The aetiology of the primary form is unknown, but any hypothesis must take account of the close association with inflammatory bowel disease (IBD).

IBD is present in at least 70% of patients with PSC [27, 28], with the proportion approaching 100% in some recent Scandinavian series [29]. Although initially recognized with ulcerative colitis, we now know that PSC can also occur with Crohn's disease of the colon [29, 30]. The clinical courses of PSC and IBD are independent of each other, and PSC can precede IBD or develop after proctocolectomy. The prevalence of PSC in patients with IBD is 5%.

PSC usually presents with features of obstructive jaundice or complications of portal hypertension. Cholangitis develops in 20%. As with PBC, fatigue is a major cause of ill health. PSC may be diagnosed at an asymptomatic stage, usually because of a raised alkaline phosphatase in patients with IBD. Although such patients may remain symptom-free for many years, the prognosis in such patients may not be as benign as once thought. In a 5 year follow-up, asymptomatic patients did have milder disease than symptomatic ones, but symptoms alone did not determine prognosis [31]. In a study of 45 asymptomatic patients over 6 years, 76% showed evidence of disease progression and 31% developed liver failure [32].

The gold standard for the diagnosis of PSC is good quality cholangiography, either percutaneous or endoscopic. This shows multiple strictures of the intrahepatic and/or extrahepatic biliary tree (Figure 2). The classical histological appearance is obliterative fibrosis of bile ductules (Figure 3), but the distribution is patchy, and liver biopsy will be diagnostic in only 50% of cases.

As with PBC, several groups have tried to develop prognostic models for PSC. The King's College group found hepatomegaly, splenomegaly, alkaline phosphatase, histological stage and age to be independent prognostic factors [33]. The Mayo Clinic group report age, bilirubin, haemoglobin and presence of IBD to be of predictive value [31]. These models are summarized in Table II. Prognostic models based on these findings have still to be tested and validated in other centres.

Patients with PSC are at considerable risk of developing a cholangiocarcinoma. The incidence of this tumour in PSC is 5 to 10% in life, rising to 40% in autopsy series [34]. The development of cholangiocarcinoma is difficult to detect. Often these tumours are not visualized on ultrasound, computed tomography (CT) scanning or angiography. Serum markers such as carcino-embryonic antigen (CEA) are unreliable. Endoscopic retrograde cholangiopancreatography (ERCP) may demonstrate increasing strictures but it is difficult to distinguish malignant narrowing from the natural progression of PSC itself. Bile cytology, although highly specific, is very insensitive.

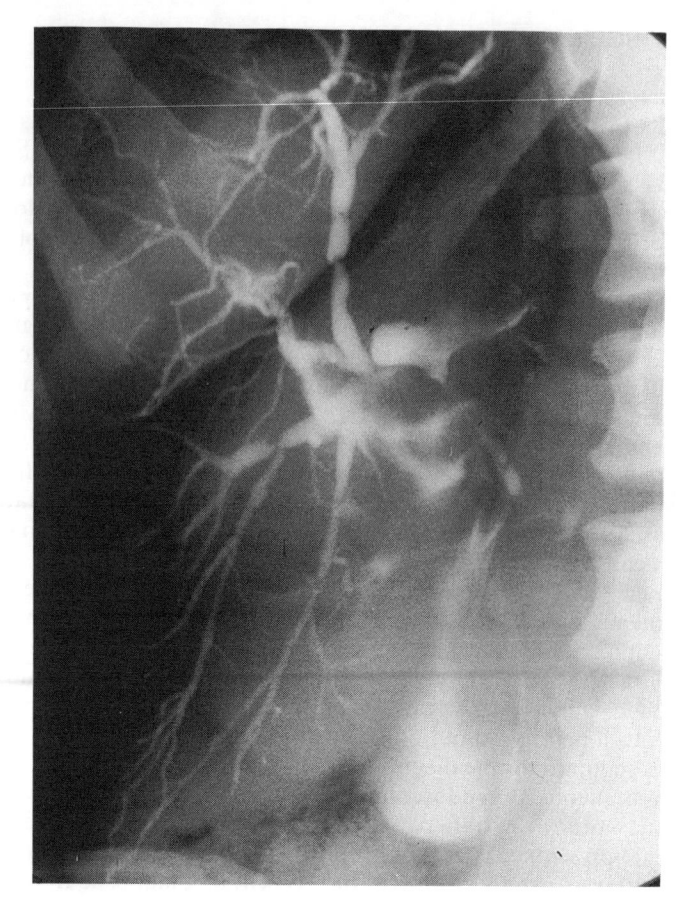

Figure 2. Cholangiogram showing multiple strictures throughout the intrahepatic biliary tree characteristic of PSC.

The prognosis once cholangiocarcinoma develops is very poor, and is not improved by medical and only rarely by surgical intervention. The mean survival is only 6 months from the time of diagnosis.

Immunology
As with PBC, there is increasing evidence that immunological factors play an important role in the pathogenesis of PSC. Most cases of PSC display HLA-B8 and HLA-DR3 phenotypes (80% and 70% respectively), a pattern present in certain organ-specific autoimmune diseases but absent in cases of IBD without PSC [35, 36]. A recent report found the HLA-DRW 52a antigen on the DR3B chain in all cases of PSC tested [37], but this has not been confirmed by others [38, 39].

Although antinuclear antibodies are present in up to 70% of patients with

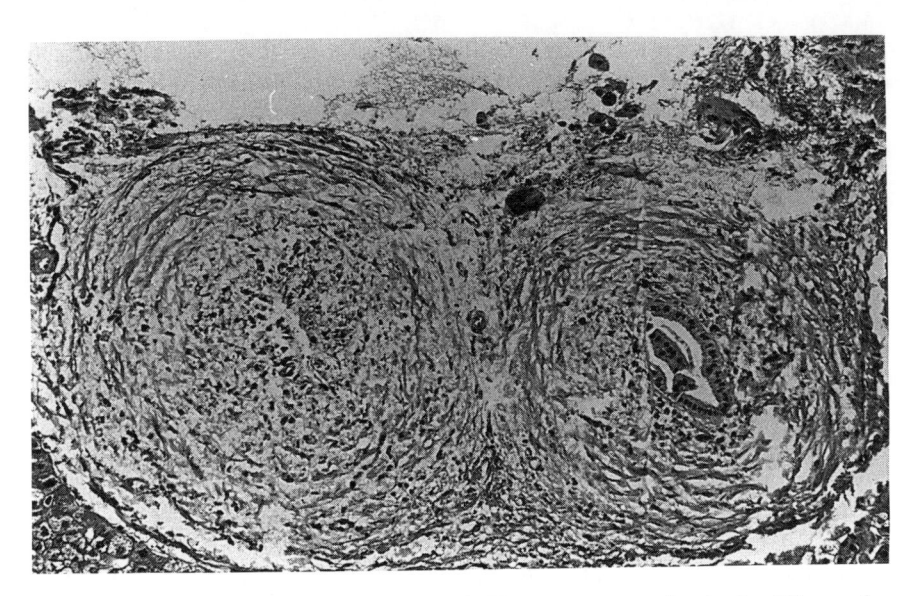

Figure 3. Liver biopsy from a patient with PSC. There are concentric whorls of fibrous tissue. The lesion on the right surrounds a damaged bile duct, whilst on the left the bile duct has already been lost (so-called 'tombstone' lesion).

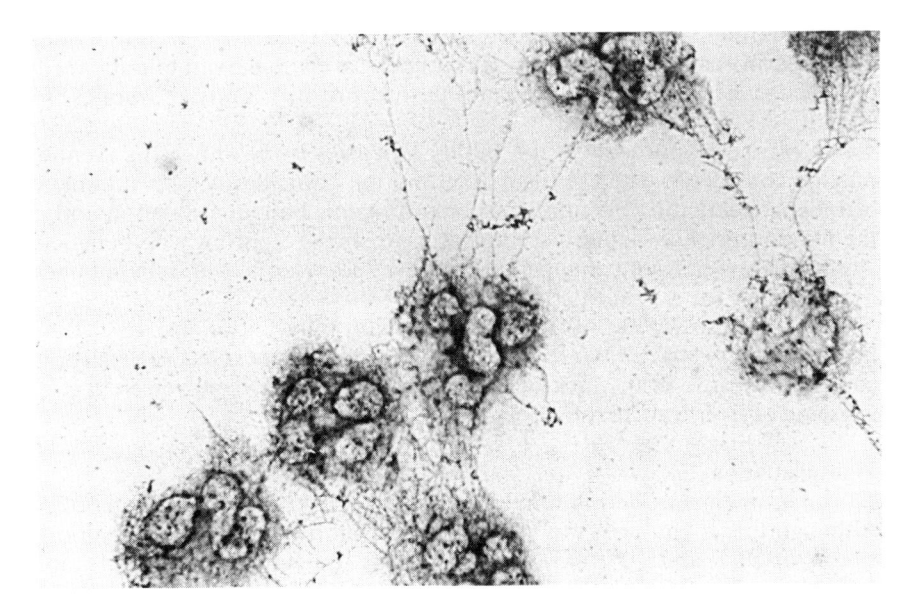

Figure 4. Peripheral blood neutrophils from a patient with PSC stained for antineutrophil cytoplasmic antibody (ANCA). The pattern of cytoplasmic granules with perinuclear accentuation and surrounding filaments is seen in the majority of patients with PSC (with or without ulcerative colitis) and is different from that seen in Wegener's granulomatosis.

PSC, there has been no specific antibody marker for PSC corresponding to AMA in PBC. However, recent work from Oxford has identified an antineutrophil nuclear antibody (ANNA) in 84% of PSC patients [40]. An antineutrophil cytoplasmic antibody (ANCA), distinct from that found in Wegener's granulomatosis, is seen in patients with PSC with or without IBD, but only rarely in other forms of liver diseases [41] (Figure 4).

Immune abnormalities occur in the cellular as well as the humoral immune system. There is a reduction in circulating T8 (suppressor) cells [42]. HLA-DR antigens, not expressed on normal bile ducts, are expressed on the bile ducts in PSC, and at an early stage [43]. Thus evidence is accumulating that the bile duct damage in PSC is immunologically mediated.

Non-surgical treatment

No specific medical therapy is of proven benefit in PSC. Judgements of treatment efficacy are hampered by the spontaneous fluctuations which characterize the clinical course, and by a dearth of controlled trials. Penicillamine was of no benefit in a controlled trial of 80 patients [44]. Uncontrolled reports of improvement with corticosteroids have not been realized. There is little enthusiasm for further trials of corticosteroids, partly because many patients have already received steroids for their colitis and partly because of the risk of worsening the osteoporosis which complicates chronic cholestasis. Clinical and biochemical improvement with UDCA has recently been reported, but only in an uncontrolled trial of 15 patients over 6 months [45]. Clearly further trials are needed before UDCA can be recommended. Cyclosporin A and colchicine are also under evaluation. Symptomatic medical measures include cholestyramine for pruritus and antibiotics for cholangitis.

Is a physical approach to the biliary strictures worthwhile? Intervention may be considered when clinical deterioration coincides with a 'dominant' extrahepatic stricture. Percutaneous or endoscopic balloon dilatation and/or the temporary endoscopic insertion of a prosthetic stent may be beneficial [46, 47]. However, such patients may improve spontaneously and the numbers are too small for a controlled trial.

The surgical resection of such strictures with biliary drainage via a Roux hepatico-enterostomy has been favoured in some centres, but is generally discouraged because of the lack of long-term benefit and the adverse effect on subsequent liver transplantation.

Transplantation

The only treatment offering long-term benefit is liver transplantation (OLT). Although this is analogous to PBC, with PSC an increasingly frequent indication for OLT, and a 1 year survival of 70–80%, the timing of surgery is more difficult than for PBC because of the erratic course in PSC. The indication is usually related to the biliary obstruction itself (jaundice, pruritus, fatigue, cholangitis) rather than to hepatocellular failure, which is a late feature. The risk of cholangiocarcinoma may prompt earlier OLT. Conversely, it can be difficult to determine whether a clinical deterioration is due to progression of

PSC or development of a cholangiocarcinoma, the latter being a contraindication to OLT because of the high risk of recurrence. As with PBC, it is clearly better to refer a deteriorating patient early than late.

There is one suggestion of cholangiographic changes suggestive of recurrent PSC in transplanted livers [48], but no reports to date of clinically significant disease recurrence. It is not known whether the risk of colorectal cancer is increased by the immunosuppression following OLT.

In summary, PSC, like PBC, is an immunologically mediated disease without any proven specific medical therapy. Liver transplantation offers a good prospect of long-term benefit or even cure, but the unpredictable clinical course and the risk of cholangiocarcinoma remain challenging problems.

ACKNOWLEDGEMENTS

The photomicrographs were kindly supplied by Dr S Hubscher, Senior Lecturer in Pathology at the University of Birmingham Medical School, the cholangiogram by Dr K Palmer, Consultant Gastroenterologist at the Western General Hospital, Edinburgh, and the illustration of the antineutrophil cytoplasmic antibody by Dr Su-Kong Lo, research fellow to Dr R Chapman, Consultant Gastroenterologist, John Radcliffe Hospital, Oxford.

REFERENCES

1. James OFW, Myszor M. Epidemiology and genetics of primary biliary cirrhosis. In Popper H, Schaffner F eds. *Progress in Liver Diseases IX*. Philadelphia: WB Saunders. 1990
2. Mitchison HC, Lucey M, Kelly P et al. Symptom development and prognosis in primary biliary cirrosis. *Gastroenterology 1990; 99*: 77–84
3. Goudie BM, Burt AD, Boyle PB et al. Breast cancer in women with primary biliary cirrhosis. *Br Med J 1985; 291*: 1597–1598
4. Coppel RL, McNeilage LJ, Surh CD et al. Primary structure of the human M2 mitochondrial autoantigen of primary biliary cirrhosis: dihydrolipoamide acetyltransferase. *Proc Natl Acad Sci, USA 1988; 85*: 7317–7321
5. Yeaman SJ, Danner DJ, Mutimer DJ et al. Primary biliary cirrhosis: identification of two major M2 mitochondrial autoantigens. *Lancet 1988; i*: 1067–1070
6. Joplin R, Lindsay JG, Johnson GD et al. Membrane dihydrolipoamide acetyltransferase (E2) on human biliary epithelial cells in primary biliary cirrhosis. *Lancet 1992; 339*: 93–94
7. Hopf U, Moller B, Stemerowicz R et al. Relation between *Escherichia coli* R (rough) forms in gut, lipid A in liver and primary biliary cirrhosis. *Lancet 1989; ii*: 1419–1422
8. Burke D, Jackson K, Freeman R et al. Primary biliary cirrhosis (PBC): No evidence to support a role for enterobacteriaceal rough (R) mutants in its aetiology. *Hepatology 1991; 14*: 62A
9. Miglio F, Pignatelli M, Mazzeo V et al. Expression of major histocompatibility complex class II antigens on bile duct epithelium in patients with hepatic graft-versus-host disease after bone marrow transplantation. *J Hepatol 1985; 5*: 182–185
10. Ballardini G, Bianelli FB, Doniach D et al. Aberrant expression of HLA-DR antigens on bile duct epithelium in primary biliary cirrhosis, relevance to pathogenesis. *Lancet 1984; ii*: 1009–1013
11. Mitchison HC, Bassendine MF, Malcolm AF et al. A pilot, double-blind controlled one year trial of prednisolone treatment in primary biliary cirrhosis. *Hepatology 1989; 10*: 420–429
12. Christensen E, Neuberger J, Crowe J et al. Beneficial effect of azathioprine and prediction of prognosis in primary biliary cirrhosis. Final results of an international trial. *Gastroenterology 1985; 89*: 1084–1091

13 Wiesner R, Ludwig J, Lindor K et al. A controlled trial of cyclosporine in the treatment of primary biliary cirrhosis. *N Engl J Med 1990; 322*: 1419-1424
14 Kaplan M, Alling D, Zimmerman H et al. A prospective trial of colchicine in primary biliary cirrhosis. *N Engl J Med 1986; 315*: 1448-1454
15 Warnes T, Smith A, Lee F et al. A controlled trial of colchicine in primary biliary cirrhosis. Trial design and preliminary report. *J Hepatol 1987; 5*: 1-7
16 Bodenheimer H, Schaffner F, Pezzullo J. Evaluation of colchicine therapy in primary biliary cirrhosis. *Gastroenterology 1988; 95*: 124-129
17 Kaplan M, Knox T. Treatment of primary biliary cirrhosis with low dose weekly methotrexate. *Gastroenterology 1991; 101*: 1332-1338
18 Neuberger J, Portmann B, Cablaria J et al. Double-blind controlled trial of D-penicillamine in patients with primary biliary cirrhosis. *Gut 1985; 26*: 114-119
19 Poupon RE, Balkau B, Eschwege E, Poupon R, UDCA-PBC study group. A multi-center, controlled trial of ursodiol for the treatment of primary biliary cirrhosis. *N Engl J Med 1991; 324*: 1548-1554
20 Dickson E, Grambsch P, Fleming T. Prognosis in primary biliary cirrhosis: model for decision making. *Hepatology 1989; 84*: 713-716
21 Babbs C, Smith A, Hunt LP et al. Type III procollagen peptide: a marker of disease activity and prognosis in primary biliary cirrhosis. *Lancet 1988; i*: 1021-1024
22 Nyberg A, Engstrom-Laurent A, Loof L. Serum hyaluronate in primary biliary cirrhosis – a biochemical marker for progressive liver disease. *Hepatology 1988; 8*: 142-146
23 Mutimer D, Bassendine M, Kelly P, James O. Is measurement of type III procollagen aminopeptide useful in primary biliary cirrhosis? *J Hepatol 1989; 9*: 184-189
24 Neuberger J. Predicting the prognosis of primary biliary cirrhosis. *Gut 1989; 30*: 1519-1522
25 Neuberger J, Portmann B, MacDougall B et al. Recurrence of primary biliary cirrhosis after liver transplantation. *N Engl J Med 1982; 306*: 1-4
26 Polson RJ, Portmann B, Neuberger J et al. Evidence for disease recurrence after liver transplantation for primary biliary cirrhosis. *Gastroenterology 1989; 97*: 715-725
27 Wiesner RH, LaRusso NF. Clinicopathological features of the syndrome of primary sclerosing cholangitis. *Gastroenterology 1980; 79*: 200-206
28 Chapman RW, Arbough BA, Rhodes JM et al. Primary sclerosing cholangitis – a review of its clinical features, cholangiography and hepatic histology. *Gut 1980; 21*: 870-877
29 Aadland E, Schrumpf E, Fauso O et al. Primary sclerosing cholangitis: a long-term follow-up study. *Scand J Gastroenterol 1987; 22*: 655-664
30 Rabinovitz M, Gavaler JS, Schade RR et al. Does primary sclerosing cholangitis occurring in association with inflammatory bowel disease differ from that occurring in the absence of inflammatory bowel disease? A study of sixty six subjects. *Hepatology 1990; 11*: 7-11
31 Schrumpf E, Fauso O, Forre O et al. HLA antigens and immunoregulatory T cells in ulcerative colitis associated with hepatobiliary disease. *Scand J Gastroenterol 1982; 17*: 187-191
32 Poryako NK, Wiesner RH, LaRusso NF et al. Patients with asymptomatic primary sclerosing cholangitis frequently have progressive disease. *Gastroenterology 1990; 98*: 1594-1602
33 Farrant JM, Hayllar KM, Wilkinson ML et al. Natural history and prognostic variables in primary sclerosing cholangitis. *Gastroenterology 1991; 100*: 1710-1717
34 Rosen CB, Nagorney DM, Wiesner RH et al. Cholangiocarcinoma complicating primary sclerosing cholangitis. *Ann Surg 1991; 213*: 21-25
35 LaRusso NF, Wiesner RH, Ludwig J et al. Prospective trial of penicillamine in primary sclerosing cholangitis. *Gastroenterology 1988; 95*: 1036-1042
36 Shepherd HA, Selby WS, Chapman RW et al. Ulcerative colitis and liver dysfunction. *Q J Med 1983; 52*: 503-513
37 Prochazka EJ, Terasaki PI, Min Sik Park DVM et al. Association of primary sclerosing cholangitis with HLA-DRW52a. *N Engl J Med 1990; 322*: 1842-1844
38 Mehal WZ, Wordsworth PB, Bell JL et al. Oligonucleotide DNA typing analysis of the HLA DRB3 locus in patients with primary sclerosing cholangitis. *Gut 1991; 32*: A839
39 Farrant JM, Doherty DG, Donaldson PT et al. HLA-DR-DQ haplotypes in primary

sclerosing cholangitis. *Gut 1991; 32*: A839
40. Snook JA, Chapman RW, Fleming K, Jewell DP. Anti-neutrophil nuclear antibody in ulcerative colitis, Crohn's disease and primary sclerosing cholangitis. *Clin Exp Immunol 1989; 76*: 30-33
41. Duerr RH, Targan SR, Landers CL et al. Neutrophil cytoplasmic antibodies: a link between primary sclerosing cholangitis and ulcerative colitis. *Gastroenterology 1991; 100*: 1385-1391
42. Whiteside TL, Lasky S, Si L, Van Thiel DH. Immunologic analysis of mononuclear cells in liver tissues and blood of patients with primary sclerosing cholangitis. *Hepatology 1985; 5*: 468-474
43. Chapman RW, Kelly P, Heryet A et al. Expression of HLA-DR antigens on bile duct epithelium in primary sclerosing cholangitis. *Gut 1988; 29*: 422-427
44. Wiesner RH, Grambsch PM, Dickson ER et al. Primary sclerosing cholangitis: natural history, prognostic factors and survival analysis. *Hepatology 1989; 10*: 430-436
45. Chazouilleres O, Poupon R, Capron J-P et al. Ursodeoxycholic acid for primary sclerosing cholangitis. *J Hepatol 1990; 11*: 120-123
46. May GR, Bender CE, LaRusso NJ, Weisner RH. Non-operative dilatation of dominant strictures in primary sclerosing cholangitis. *Am J Radiol 1985; 145*: 1061-1064
47. Johnson GK, Geenan JE, Venu RP et al. Endoscopic treatment of biliary tract strictures in sclerosing cholangitis: a larger series and recommendations for treatment. *Gastroint Endosc 1991; 37*: 38-43
48. Krom RAF. Liver transplantation at the Mayo Clinic. *Mayo Clin Proc 1986; 61*: 278-282

MALIGNANT MELANOMA

Rona M MacKie
University of Glasgow, Glasgow

INTRODUCTION
Thirty years ago cutaneous malignant melanoma was a relatively rare malignancy in the UK which commonly presented to surgical specialties at an advanced stage in its growth. At that time, the accepted management of all primary melanomas was wide surgical excision with a margin of 5cm of normal skin in all directions around the primary tumour and grafting of the deficit. In the 1960s, 5 year disease-free survival was around 50%. In 1992 the picture of cutaneous malignant melanoma has changed dramatically. The incidence of melanoma in the UK has quadrupled in the last 30 years and continues to rise at a rate of around 7% per annum. The great majority of melanomas, however, are now treated when they are small lesions less than 1cm in largest diameter. These lesions have commonly invaded less than 1mm into the underlying dermis and 5 year disease-free survival prospects for patients with such lesions is over 90%. This is not due to improved surgical or oncological techniques but to earlier diagnosis. The current agreed best practice with regard to surgical removal is to excise only one 1cm of normal skin around these smaller primary tumours and to close them directly. This rapidly changing pattern of presentation and management of melanoma makes it essential that those in medical specialties and also those in primary care are aware of both changes in clinical presentation and current management of this malignancy.

EPIDEMIOLOGY
The incidence of malignant melanoma in Scotland as recorded by the Scottish Melanoma Group is 7.1 per 100,000 for males and 10.4 per 100,000 for females for the calendar year 1989 (incidence adjusted to the 1981 Scottish population) [1]. This has risen by 80% since 1979. Figures for England and Wales for 1985 are 3.9 per 100,000 for men and 6.4 per 100,000 for women. This compares with an incidence in Scotland of 5.9 per 100,000 for men and 9.8 per 100,000 for women in 1985. Also in 1985 the incidence of melanoma in the three

Scandinavian countries, Norway, Sweden and Denmark, ranged from 6.7 to 10.4 per 100,000 for men and 9.4 to 13.4 per 100,000 for women. These figures suggest that the incidence of malignant melanoma in England and Wales is probably under-recorded. If this is not the case, then there are features in the Scottish environment and/or phenotype which result in a significantly higher incidence of malignant melanoma north of the border. Outside the UK, the trend for all countries in which accurate data are available is a steady increase. Worldwide, the rate of increase of malignant melanoma is higher than any other malignancy with the exception of lung cancer in women.

The cause of this steady increase in malignant melanoma is thought to be associated with increasing exposure of successive birth cohorts to strong sunshine [2]. Malignant melanoma is a disease of Caucasians, and the highest incidences are found in Caucasians living at low latitude in parts of the world where there are long hours of intense sunshine such as Australia. However, the actual rate of increase has been the same in temperate climates, such as the UK, as in warmer climates, and indeed greater awareness of malignant melanoma over the past 10 years in countries such as Australia appears to have coincided with a slight slowing down in the rate of increasing incidence of this malignancy. The epidemiological evidence indicates that short episodes of intense sun exposure of previously unacclimatized Caucasian skin are a greater risk factor than total hours of lifetime sun exposure. This is in contrast with the situation for non-melanoma skin cancer (basal and squamous cell carcinomas) in which total lifetime sun exposure is the major risk factor.

Malignant melanoma is excessively rare in children, but after puberty the incidence steadily rises and the age-associated incidence is highest in the over 65s. In the UK, at all age ranges prior to 75 years of age, females are more commonly affected than males with a 2:1 female to male distribution of melanoma sufferers. The reasons for this are not understood. The average age at presentation with malignant melanoma is in the early 50s and it is one of the commoner malignancies and commoner causes of death from malignancy in the third and fourth decades of life.

MOLECULAR BIOLOGY

At present the molecular mechanisms involved in malignant transformation of the melanocyte and the relationship to ultraviolet light (UV) exposure are under intense scrutiny. The two current areas of greatest activity are investigation of the roles of the ras family of oncogenes, and of the oncogene/tumour suppressor gene p53. To date three groups have reported point mutations of the N ras member of the ras family in approximately 20% of all melanoma tissue tested [3, 4]. Using the polymerase chain reaction to amplify DNA from archival paraffin processed blocks we have found that the majority of these mutations are in secondary tissue and involve codons 12/13 and 61 [5]. One group has identified mutations of Kirsten ras [6], but this has not been confirmed [7]. A recent publication using an antibody to P53 which is thought to identify the mutant protein which has oncogenic potential on fresh frozen tissue has recorded positive staining for p53 in 31 of 33 samples from secondary tissue but in very few thin early primary melanomas [8].

Thus at present molecular medicine techniques identify late events in the process of malignant transformation, and further studies are needed to identify early molecular events in tumour initiation.

PERSONAL RISK FACTORS FOR MELANOMA

The individual at risk of developing malignant melanoma is the fair-skinned, fair-haired, blue-eyed individual with skin that tans poorly and burns readily – so-called type 1 skin. Work in Scotland [9] and Denmark [10] over the past 10 years has clearly established that the most powerful phenotypic risk factor for malignant melanoma is the total number of normal non-dysplastic naevi. High counts of all melanocytic naevi (benign moles) of 2mm or greater on the skin surface correlate significantly with increasing risk of malignant melanoma of the superficial spreading and nodular varieties. Some workers, including Osterlind in Scandinavia and Green in Queensland, have observed that naevus counts on the upper arm correlate well with total body naevus counts. If upper arm naevus counts can indeed be used as an alternative to total body naevus counts, identifying at-risk individuals will be much more practical and less time-consuming.

A large case-control study carried out in Scotland in 1989 [11] established that the four most important risk factors for developing melanoma in Scotland were in descending order of importance: total number of naevi, the presence or absence of a freckling tendency, the presence of any atypical naevi (defined as greater than 5mm in diameter, with irregular pigmentation and an irregular margin or associated inflammation), and a history of severe blistering sunburn. These four risk factors have been used in a model to derive groups of individuals at lesser or greater than average risk of developing malignant melanoma and could be used to identify an at-risk section of the population at whom preventive education should be aimed (Figure 1).

The striking increase in the incidence of malignant melanoma over the past decade has been seen in both males and females. Looking at site-specific changing incidence, the greatest rate of increase in the male has been seen on the trunk, which in 1979 already was the commonest site for development of malignant melanoma in the male [1]. Since 1979, the site-specific incidence has increased from 0.8 to 2.4 per 100,000 for melanomas on the male trunk. Similarly, in females the most common site on which malignant melanoma develops, the lower leg, has become proportionally even more over-represented with the incidence rising from 1.8 per 100,000 to 4 per 100,000 over the decade 1979–89.

CLINICOPATHOLOGICAL SUBSETS

Malignant melanoma is divided into four main clinicopathological subsets. These are the superficial spreading melanoma, which is the commonest and comprises 50–60% of all melanomas in predominantly Caucasian populations, the nodular melanoma, comprising about 20%, the lentigo maligna melanoma, comprising 12–15% of most series, and the acral or acral lentiginous melanoma, comprising the remainder. In the past decade the superficial spreading melanoma has been responsible for the greatest rate of increase overall, rising

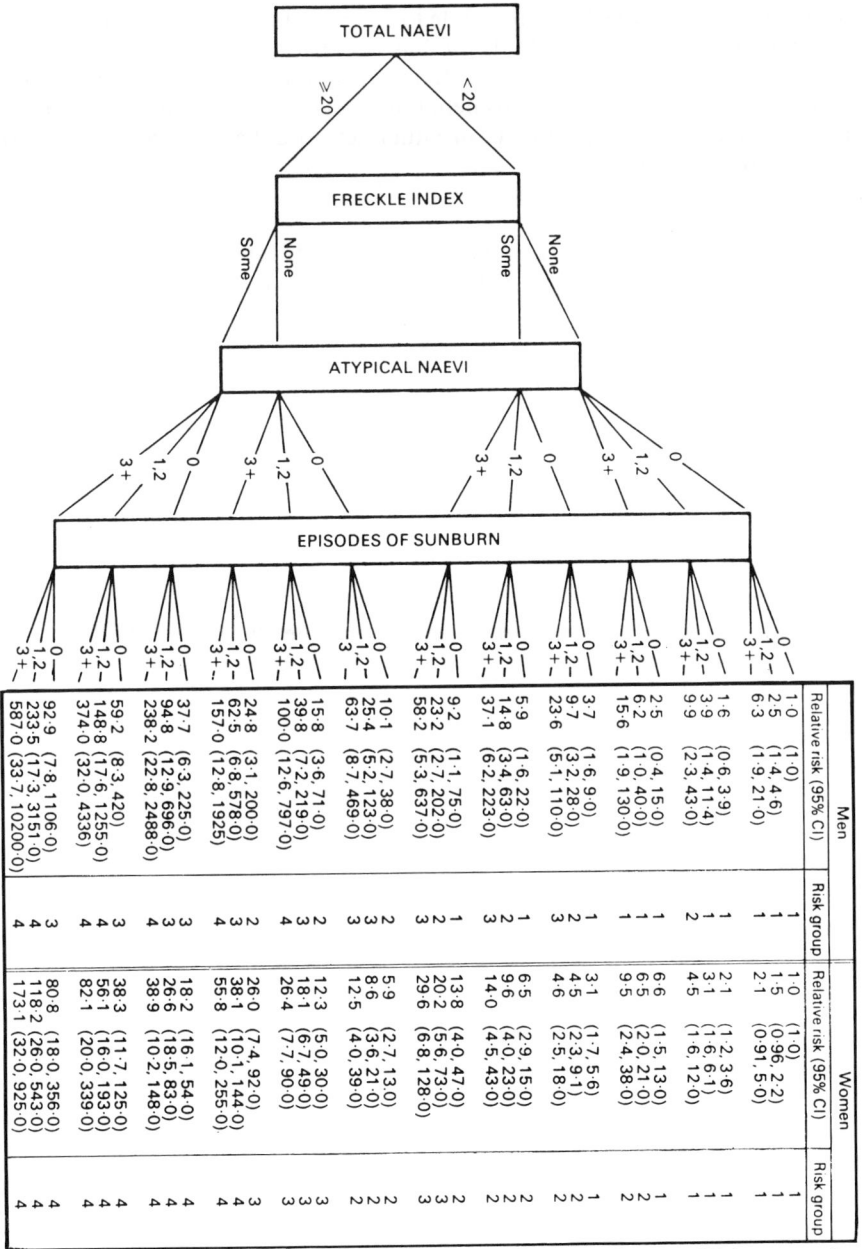

Figure 1. Flow-chart of risk factors for cutaneous malignant melanoma. Risk groups: 1 = marginally increased risk; 2 = increased risk; 3 = very increased risk; 4 = worryingly high risk. Relative risk coefficients used (for men/women, respectively): 10.1/5.9 for total naevi; 3.7/3.1 for freckles; 1.6/2.1 for atypical naevi; and 2.5/1.5 for episodes of sunburn. From MacKie et al [11] by permission of *The Lancet*.

from around 1 per 100,000 in the male to 3 per 100,000 and from 2 per 100,000 in the female to 6 per 100,000. There has also been a statistically significant but much less steep rise in the incidence of nodular and of lentigo maligna melanomas in both men and women, but no statistically significant increase in acral lentiginous melanomas in either sex in either Scotland or certain centres in the USA.

PROGNOSTIC FACTORS

In 1969–73 the work of Clark and of Breslow firmly established that the prognosis for primary cutaneous melanoma was linearly related to the level of invasion of the cells of the primary lesion into the underlying dermis. Clark defines these levels of invasion as:

level 1: intraepidermal or in situ,
level 2: only a few cells in the dermis,
level 3: a reasonable number of tumour cells filling and expanding the papillary dermis,
level 4: invasion into the reticular dermis,
level 5: invasion to fat.

Breslow used the term tumour thickness and simply measured in millimetres from the granular layer of the epidermis to the deepest invasive tumour cell. Comparison of the two techniques shows that the Breslow method is more reproducible between pathologists and is a more accurate guide to survival, but both are valuable. For example, in 1661 patients in the Scottish Melanoma Group series registered between 1979 and 1984, 5 year disease-free survival is 93% for patients with tumours less than 1.5mm thick, 72% for tumours 1.5–3.5mm thick, and only 48% for those thicker than 3.5mm [1]. These survival figures are very similar to those reported for other centres worldwide, and clearly illustrates the need to be aware of this measurement before discussing the outlook with patients and their relatives.

In the Scottish series, the second most important prognostic factor in a multifactorial analysis is presence or absence of ulceration, with a significantly poorer survival reported for patients with ulcerated lesions of the same thickness. Other features of lesser but still independent prognostic significance include the sex of the patients, with women faring better than men with lesions of the same thickness, the site of the lesion with truncal lesions carrying a poorer prognosis than limb lesions, and a number of mitoses per mm^2.

MANAGEMENT

The main form of treatment for melanoma is surgery, and the advance in the past decade has been to tailor the surgical excision margins to the thickness of the primary tumour. Thus at present margins of 1cm are recommended for lesions less than 1mm thick, of 2cm for lesions less than 2mm thick, and of 3cm for thicker lesions [12]. There is no evidence to justify the very wide excisions and even amputations of the past.

Although tumour thickness allows accurate prognostication for the individual patient, there is at present no proven adjuvant therapy, despite numerous studies of chemotherapy, immunotherapy, and biological response modifiers. At present there are a number of trials in progress using interferon, but results are not yet available. For patients with stage 2 disease (involvement of the regional lymph nodes) surgical removal of the nodes is recommended. The management of advanced (stage 3) disease is disappointing with few long-lasting responses reported with any regimen. DTIC is the single agent most commonly used with reported response rates of 20–25%, and combinations including DTIC such as BELD (bleomycin, Eldisine, lomustine and DTIC) offering slight improvement with response rates of around 40% [13]. Early dramatic responses to interleukin-2 (IL-2) have not been confirmed, and the response rate is currently around 25%, but of longer duration than that reported with chemotherapy. Because of its poor response to conventional agents, melanoma is a target for gene therapy, and at present there are pioneering studies in progress at the National Cancer Institute using tumour infiltrating lymphocyte and the gene for tumour necrosis factor (TNF).

For the majority of melanoma patients for the moment, however, the most important method of increasing survival prospects is earlier diagnosis. Both hospital physicians and general practitioners should routinely assess the skin of those at greater risk when carrying out a general medical examination, and should be reasonably confident of their ability to recognize early primary melanomas.

REFERENCES

1. MacKie RM, Hunter JAA, Aitchison TC et al. Cutaneous malignant melanoma in Scotland 1979-89. Incidence and survival. *Lancet 1992; 339*: 971–975
2. MacKie RM. Links between exposure to ultraviolet radiation and skin cancer. *J Roy Coll Phys London 1987; 21*: 91–96
3. Albino AP, Nanus DM, Mentle IR et al. Analysis of ras oncogenes in malignant and precursor lesions. *Oncogene 1989; 4*: 1363–1374
4. Bos JL. Ras oncogenes in human cancer. A review. *Cancer Res 1989; 49*: 4682–4689
5. Carr J, Burns P, MacKie RM. Point mutations of the N ras oncogene in human malignant melanoma and precursor lesions. *Br J Dermatol 1991; 125*: 478
6. Shukla VK, Hughes DC, Hughes LE et al. Ras mutations in human melanotic lesions. *Oncogene Res 1989; 5*: 121–127
7. Albino AP, Nanus DM, Davis ML et al. Lack of evidence of Ki ras codon 12 mutations in melanocytic lesions. *J Cutan Pathol 1991; 18*: 273–278
8. Stretch JR, Gatter KC, Ralfkiaer E et al. Expression of mutant P53 in melanoma. *Cancer Res 1991; 51*: 5976–5979
9. Sverdlow AJ, English J, MacKie RM et al. Benign melanocytic naevi as a risk factor for malignant melanoma. *Br Med J 1986; 292*: 1555–1559
10. Osterlind A, Tucker MA, Hou Jensen K et al. The Danish case control study of cutaneous malignant melanoma. *Int J Cancer 1988; 42*: 200–206
11. MacKie RM, Freudenberger T, Aitchison TC. Personal risk factor chart for cutaneous melanoma. *Lancet 1989; ii*: 487–489
12. Veronesi U, Cascinelli N, Adamus J et al. Thin stage 1 primary melanoma. Comparison of excision with margins of 1 or 3 cms. *N Engl J Med 1988; 318*: 1159–1162
13. Young DW, Lever RS, English JSC, MacKie RM. The use of Beld combination chemotherapy in advanced malignant melanoma. *Cancer 1985; 55*: 1879–1881

PSYCHOLOGICAL IMPACT OF SKIN DISEASE

AY Finlay
University of Wales College of Medicine, Cardiff

INTRODUCTION

Our skin provides the critical link between our 'selves' and the outside world. Skin disease therefore not only results in physical and physiological disorders of this multifunctional organ, but it can also profoundly affect our view of ourselves and the perception of us by others. Over 50% of patients referred to the dermatology outpatient clinic in Cardiff admit to their skin disease having some psychological effect on them, and many patients with chronic skin disease such as atopic eczema, psoriasis or ichthyosis, or shorter term acute disease such as severe acne, experience a major impact of their disease not only physically but also psychologically; this can have important implications in their management. The purpose of this review is to describe the relevance of the psychological impact of skin disease to clinical dermatology, and briefly summarize some of the information about this described in psoriasis, acne and eczema. The reasons why it is important to try to measure the impact of skin disease are given, and the methods being used to measure the impact of skin disease on patient's lives are outlined; recent work carried out in Cardiff using these techniques is described.

CLINICAL RELEVANCE

There are several reasons why all doctors dealing with patients with skin disease should constantly be aware of the psychological impact of the disease. First, and most fundamentally, good clinical medicine is founded on accurate and complete history taking: this history taking is neither accurate nor complete unless it includes information about the effect of the disease on patients and their lifestyles. It is unlikely that a physician will respond with appropriate management advice if the doctor does not realize that a 'minor' rash on the face is turning the patient into a recluse, or that a stable symptom-free benign eruption on the trunk is preventing a patient from continuing their favourite sport. Second, all dermatologists are forced, sometimes reluctantly, to take note of this 'secondary' aspect of disease when taking management decisions where oral therapies are considered which have some associated risks. When deciding, for example, whether to start a patient with widespread psoriasis on oral methotrexate, the risk/benefit analysis that is considered includes the clinician's subjective impression of how badly the patient's life is being affected by the disease. A third area of clinical relevance is that recording and monitoring of the psychological and practical disabling effects of a disease provides a relevant patient orientated view of the effectiveness of any management strategy. In this context it should be noted that the patients' attitude to their disease may influence the effectiveness of therapy prescribed, by affecting compliance. Finally, most patients with skin disease are very glad to have the opportunity to express and admit to their feelings about their skin disease: providing an opening for this in the consultation takes little time but may markedly improve the doctor/patient relationship.

CURRENT KNOWLEDGE
The psychological and disabling impact of many skin diseases has recently been well documented [1-3]. Until about twenty years ago there was much confusion about whether some diseases were caused by psychological problems, such as 'stress'; it is clear now that these are secondary to disease, though may play a negative feedback role in the exacerbation of some conditions such as atopic eczema.

In view of the public education compaign concerning pigmented lesions, it is not surprising that even a single lesion, affecting only 0.01% of the body surface area, can cause worry and cancerphobia, though otherwise have no immediate effect on a patient's life. Where dermatoses affect up to 20% of the body surface, as in psoriasis, eczema or acne, the psychological impact is of a different and more pervading nature, perhaps best documented in psoriasis.

PSORIASIS
In an open questionnaire, patients with psoriasis were asked 'What do you consider to be the worst feature about having psoriasis?' [4]: 87% stated embarrassment due to the appearance of the lesions. This embarrassment was sensed most when skin lesions were on exposed, or sometimes exposed, sites. The term 'embarrassment' is used to cover a variety of more subtle emotional reactions, including feeling unclean, feeling like a 'leper', and feeling that others are staring at them or avoiding them [4]. The special difficulties that psoriatics have in adjusting to highly 'visible' situations were emphasized in a study using personal construct theory, where reportary grid techniques were employed to assess the patient's interpretation of their world [5]. This study confirmed that, for example, going on a beach or going to the hairdresser may be particularly difficult for the psoriatic. In another study, when a similar open question about the worst aspect of psoriasis was posed [6], 84% of patients stated that the worst aspect of having psoriasis was the difficulty caused in establishing social contacts and relationships. This difficulty in establishing relationships was confirmed in a further study [7] which reported that 50% of patients felt that their psoriasis had inhibited their sexual relationships.

'Stigma' is a biological or social mark that separates a person off from others [8]: patients with psoriasis may experience different aspects of stigma, in particular feelings of anticipation of rejection, feelings of being flawed and oversensitivity to the opinions of others. When different physical aspects of the disease were correlated with feelings of stigmatization and despair, the strongest predictor of stigma was the presence of bleeding from scratched lesions. The clinical sign of easy bleeding from psoriatic lesions caused by the capillary loops in the elongated dermal papillae being protected by only a very thin epidermal covering, the Auspitz sign, was historically used in the diagnosis of psoriasis. It can now be recognized as a cause of great psychological distress.

There are several factors which may influence the psychological impact of psoriasis. The site of involvement is of course crucial; a small total area of involvement of only a few square centimetres on the face, hand or genital area can have profound social consequences, whereas a much large area of involvement on, say, the thighs may cause very little problems. The magnitude of the effect on a patient's life of having psoriasis is not related to the total area of involvement [9]. In a study from Cleveland in 1978 [10], women with psoriasis experienced more psychological problems than men in several areas examined, especially concerning personal relationships, stress and worry related to their condition. The time over which a patient has had psoriasis can also alter its psychological impact. The condition may initially have major effects on a patient's life, but after many years of 'learning to live' with a chronic disease, a process of adjustment may occur with reduction in concern and distress.

Practical effects on daily life

The psychological effects of having psoriasis are not simply 'self-contained' by patients, but often lead to a direct influence on many practical aspects of daily life: psychological impairment leads to social disability and hence to handicap. This disturbance of daily activities may result in a negative feedback loop with psychological problems in turn being exacerbated. The practical aspects of living affected include routine daily activities, social and leisure activities, work, study and personal relationships.

Routine daily activities most frequently made more difficult by having psoriasis include housework at home, because of scales or treatment mess, buying clothes or visiting the hairdresser. Many leisure activities may be avoided because of a 'failure of display' [1]; patients with psoriasis often hide affected skin by choice of clothes or avoidance of situations where affected areas may be exposed. Any sports activities where communal changing rooms are used are stopped and swimming is avoided (Figure 1) [11]. Living for a short time in hotels may be difficult because of scaling or because of difficulties with handling topical ointments. This 'holiday' concern may have important 'work' implications where travel is an integral part of a patient's job. Work may be affected in other ways where meeting the public is important: receptionists, shop assistants or food handlers are all at a disadvantage if psoriasis is in exposed sites, mainly because of the ignorance and reaction

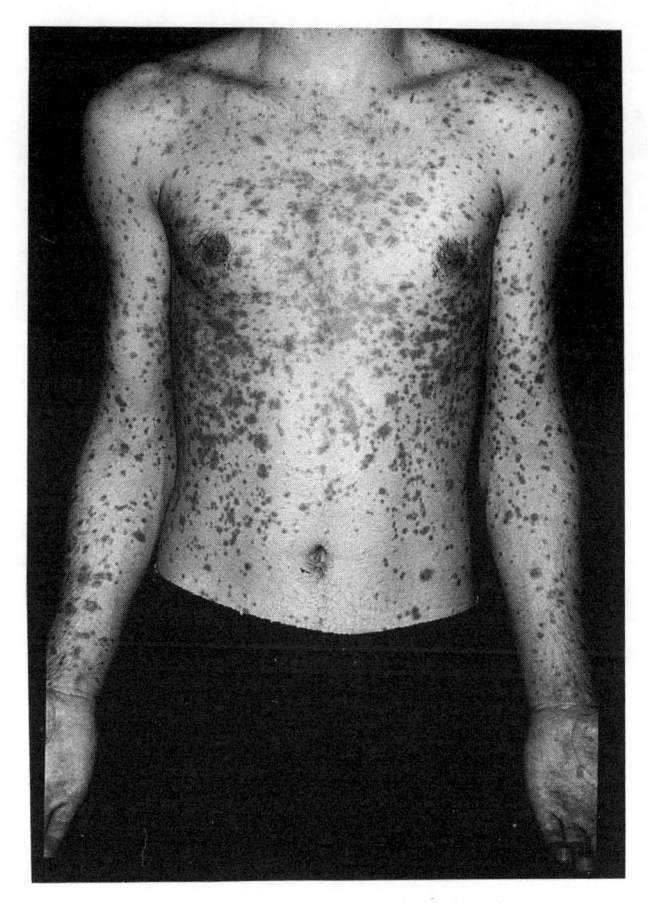

Figure 1. Widespread psoriasis preventing patient from swimming.

of others. It is the combination of this ignorance and response of strangers, along with a patient's feeling of embarrassment, that interfere with personal and social relationships. Social situations may be avoided and opportunities to make new friends reduced. These social restrictions and the inhibition of sexual relationships reported by many patients with psoriasis [7] lead to unhappiness compounding the problems of itching, discomfort and disruption caused by treatment.

ACNE AND ATOPIC ECZEMA

The experiences of having psoriasis are reflected to a certain extent in many other skin diseases, including severe acne and widespread atopic eczema (Figure 2).

The problems of having psoriasis while at work have been described above, but chronic skin disease can both alter the type of work that can be

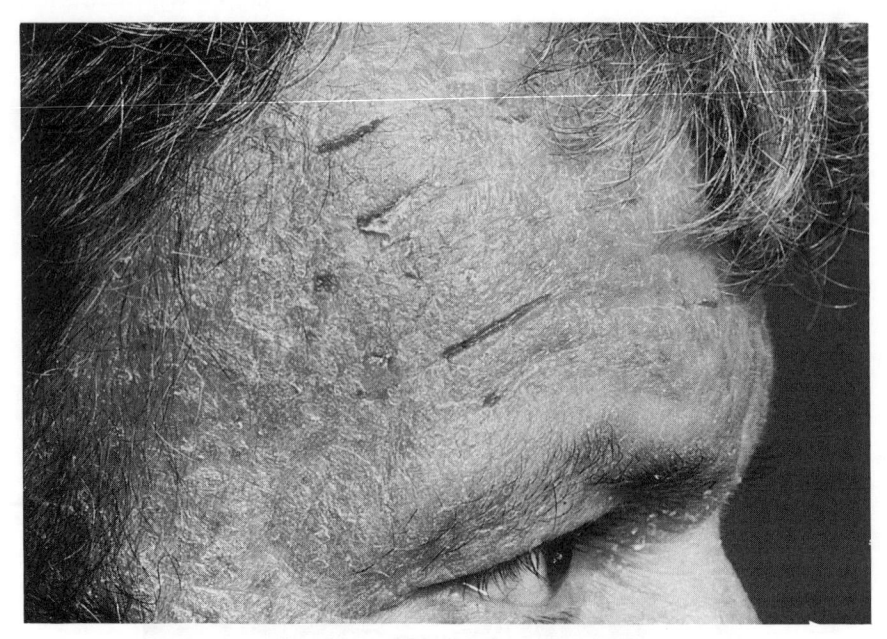

Figure 2. Severe atopic eczema of the face causing major problems at work.

carried out and, more fundamentally, reduce the ability to work at all. Entry to the armed forces, for example, may be refused if there is any history of chronic skin disease, and careers in hairdressing or surgery may be inadvisable if there is a history of persistent atopic eczema. Unemployment rates in Leeds were significantly higher in patients with acne than in matched controls (Figure 3) [12].

Atopic eczema is a good illustration of a skin disease that not only has a psychological impact on patients themselves but also on their immediate family. Having a child with severe atopic eczema can severely disturb family life, impacting on both parents whose concern is compounded by constant disturbed nights and on siblings who receive less attention than otherwise.

The various psychological effects of severe skin disease can, predictably, be at least partially alleviated by effective therapy. In acne, for example, patients with severe nodular–cystic disease become depressed and anxious; these symptoms are significantly reduced after a course of oral isotretinoin, the most effective form of therapy for severe acne [13].

MEASUREMENT OF PSYCHOLOGICAL IMPACT OF SKIN DISEASE

The importance of being able to measure the effect that skin disease has on patients' lives was recognized over two decades ago [14, 15]. The prime motivation for the methods of measurement proposed at that time was to try to broaden the basis for workers' compensation for skin disease from a measure of physical impairment to a measure of resultant social and psychological

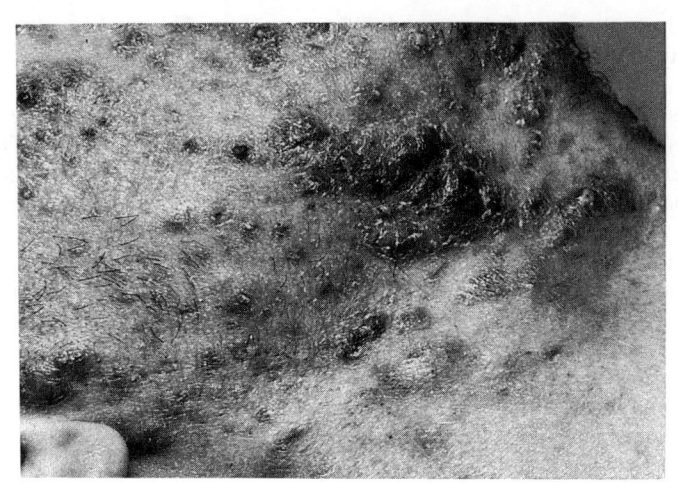

Figure 3. Patients with severe acne have a higher rate of unemployment than unaffected controls.

disability. The need for calculating financial compensation in a fair way which reflects the total impact of a condition on patient's life remains, but there are also additional important reasons for trying to objectively measure disability from skin disease. In routine clinical management a simple repeatable measure of disability would provide as useful information to the dermatologist in monitoring psoriasis as serum creatinine measurements provide the renal physician in monitoring renal failure. In clinical research a measure of dermatology disability would provide important 'consumer' orientated information to add to our physical measures of disease activity in the assessment of new forms of therapy. Similarly, measurement of dermatology disability should be at the centre of any audit of the effectiveness of the provision of dermatology care, and might more controversially provide information to aid resource allocation decisions within dermatology. There is a final political dimension to measurement of the impact that skin disease has on patients' lives; dermatology services have to compete with other areas of health care for funding, and as few patients with skin disease die, the real importance of skin disease in the community is always at risk of being underestimated. The use of broad measures of disability applicable across many branches of medicine could allow a direct comparison to be made between the 'importance' of, say, atopic eczema and rheumatoid arthritis.

There are a variety of different approaches to the measurement of the psychological and disabling affects of skin disease on the individual. Firstly 'psychological' questionnaire techniques, such as the Eysenck Personality Questionnaire, have been used in the assessment of the personality effects of acne [16]. Such validated measures provide specific information but often do not accurately reflect the wider practical consequences of the underlying psychological disturbance. Approaches which attempt to provide this broader view include the use of disease specific questionnaires such as the Psoriasis Disability Index [9] or the Acne Disability Index [17] and more general health measures such as the UK Sickness Impact Profile [18].

The Psoriasis Disability Index is a short (15 question) questionnaire covering the areas of patients' lives most frequently affected by this disease. The use of this index in an audit of the value of inpatient therapy has demonstrated both that inpatient management with topical therapy of severe psoriasis does result in a significant alleviation of disability [9], and that those few patients in whom further additional therapy is required can be identified.

The Psoriasis Disability Index has been validated against the much more detailed (136 question) UK Sickness Impact Profile (UKSIP) [18]. The advantages of the use of such wider measures include the gathering of more detailed information concerning the effect of disease on patients, and the provision of comparative data between different skin diseases and diseases of other systems. The level of disability in patients with psoriasis as measured by the UKSIP is greater than in patients with hypertension but of a similar level to that experienced by patients with angina.

Both the UKSIP and a compact disease-specific measure of eczema disability have been used as part of the assessment of the effectiveness of oral cyclosporin in the treatment of severe atopic dermatitis [19]. This double-blind placebo-controlled study demonstrated that there was a dramatic improvement in quality of life in patients taking cyclosporin; some improvement persisted at follow-up in those patients who took placebo following active therapy.

A different approach to estimating how badly a patient's life is affected by their skin disease is to pose hypothetical questions concerning the financial 'value' placed on their disease [17]. Most acne patients would prefer to have their acne cured rather than be given £500, but a few would prefer the gift: such questions can identify patients whose lives are not significantly affected by their disease. The use of Quality Adjusted Life Years (QALYs) [20] would be another possible approach applicable to dermatology, though little work in this field has yet been published. From the clinical point of view what would perhaps be helpful would be a compact simple 'Dermatology Disease Disability Index' for daily use in the clinic: we are currently developing such a tool.

CONCLUSION

It is clear that skin disease does have a major psychological impact resulting in a wide range of effects on social life, work life and personal relationships. An understanding of these effects is frequently of direct clinical relevance in taking appropriate management decisions. New methods of measuring the effects of skin disease on patients' lives are being evolved and have been used in several common skin conditions. An important clinical goal for the dermatologist should be to recognize and alleviate dermatology disability.

REFERENCES

1. Ryan TJ. Disability in dermatology. *Br J Hosp Med 1991; 46*: 33–36
2. Jowett S, Ryan T. Skin disease and handicap: an analysis of the impact of skin conditions. *Soc Sci Med 1985; 20*: 425–429
3. Meding B, Swanbeck G. Consequences of having hand eczema. *Contact Dermatitis, 1990; 23*: 6–14
4. Stankler L. The effect of psoriasis on the sufferer. *Clin Exp Dermatol 1981; 6*: 303–306
5. Dooley G, Finlay AY. Personal construct systems of psoriatic patients. *Clin Exp Dermatol 1990; 15*: 401–405
6. Jobling RG. Psoriasis – a preliminary questionnaire study of sufferers' subjective experience. *Clin Exp Dermatol 1976; 1*: 233–236
7. Ramsay B, O'Reagan M. A survey of the social and psychological effects of psoriasis. *Br J Dermatol 1988; 118*: 195–201
8. Ginsberg IH, Link BG. Feelings of stigmatization in patients with psoriasis. *J Am Acad Dermatol 1989; 20*: 53–63
9. Finlay AY, Kelly SE. Psoriasis – an index of disability. *Clin Exp Dermatol 1987; 12*: 8–11
10. Roenich RK, Roenich HH. Sex differences in the psychological effects of psoriasis. *Cutis 1978; 21*: 529–533
11. Savin JA. Patients' beliefs about psoriasis. *Trans St John's Hosp Dermatol Soc 1970; 56*: 139–142
12. Cunliffe WJ. Acne and unemployment. *Br J Dermatol 1986; 115*: 386
13. Rubinow DR, Peck GL, Squillace KM, Gantt GG. Reduced anxiety and depression in cystic acne patients after successful treatment with oral isotretinoin. *J Am Acad Dermatol 1987; 17*: 25–32
14. Robinson HM. Measurement of impairment and disability in Dermatology. *Arch Dermatol 1973; 108*: 207–209
15. Sauer GC. A guide to the evaluation of permanent impairment of the skin. *Arch Dermatol 1968; 97*: 566–569
16. Lim C-CL, Tan T-C. Personality, disability and acne in college students. *Clin Exp Dermatol 1991; 16*: 371–373
17. Motley RJ, Finlay AY. How much disability is caused by acne? *Clin Exp Dermatol 1989; 14*: 194–198
18. Finlay AY, Khan GK, Luscombe DK, Salek MS. Validation of Sickness Impact Profile and Psoriasis Disability Index in psoriasis. *Br J Dermatol 1990; 123*: 751–756
19. Finlay AY, Salek M, Khan G et al. Quality of life improvement in cyclosporin treated atopic dermatitis patients – a double blind cross over study. *Br J Dermatol 1991; 125*: Supplement 38, 16
20. Editorial, Quality of Life. *Lancet 1991; 338*: 350–351

IMMUNOLOGY AND THE SKIN

PS Friedmann
Royal Liverpool University Hospital, Liverpool

INTRODUCTION
Situated at the interface between the 'milieu intérieur' and the external world, the skin is exposed to a wide variety of physical, chemical and microbial assaults. Apart from the capacity to repair injuries, another vital function of skin is participation in immune defence. The immune function of skin presumably evolved to deal with microbes including viruses, fungi and parasites, such as the scabies mite, that succeed in breaching the outer physical barrier to penetrate the epidermis. The antimicrobial immune response in skin is closely reflected in the allergic contact hypersensitivity response. This is a delayed hypersensitivity response characterized by the infiltration of CD4+ T-lymphocytes into the dermis and also the epidermis.

The contact hypersensitivity system has been used to study mechanisms involved in the immune response. In this account, some of the known cellular mechanisms that underlie the immune response will be described. Then some observations will be presented on the integrated physiological response of the immune system.

INDUCTION OF IMMUNE RESPONSE (AFFERENT PHASE)
Activation of the immune system by antigen requires firstly the presence of antigen presenting cells in the periphery. In the skin, antigen presenting cells are Langerhans' cells (LCs), mesenchymal, bone-marrow-derived members of the macrophage family. They are recognized by the presence of a formalin-resistant membrane adenosine triphosphatase (ATPase), a specific cytoplasmic organelle – the Birbeck granule, membrane antigens including CD1 (T6) and Class II major histocompatibility (MHC) determinants. As part of their function in antigen presentation, they appear to pick up antigen that enters through the epidermis, and 'process' it by associating it with Class II MHC molecules on the cell surface. When antigen is painted onto skin it penetrates through the barrier of stratum corneum to the viable cell layer. This induces changes in LCs including loss of activity of ATPase associated with formation of

many coated pits following by formation of numerous Birbeck granules [1]. Once in this state, LCs appear temporarily unable to process another antigen. Thus, guinea pigs exposed on the same site to a second antigen failed to become sensitized and furthermore, were unresponsive to subsequent sensitization through normal skin.

Over the next 12 to 24 hours, antigen-bearing LCs are seen in the dermis [2] and their numbers in epidermis diminish [3–5]. They appear in the draining lymph node within 24 hours and their numbers are proportional to the dose of antigen applied [6, 7]. It has been suggested that the emigration of LCs from the epidermis to the lymph node is a response induced only by antigenic substances [8] but more recent evidence indicates that emigration of LCs occurs to a variable extent following contact with irritant substances too (personal observation).

It appears that the vital initial encounter between antigen-bearing LCs and T-lymphocytes occurs in the regional lymph nodes. Antigen-bearing LCs migrate via the lymphatics to reach the paracortical areas of regional lymph nodes (Figure 1). In this site, they interact with CD4+ helper/inducer T-lymphocytes. Activation of T-cells by antigen-bearing LCs involves a combination of interactions in which the initial event is probably the binding of the T-cell receptor to the complex of antigen/MHC Class II. This is followed by binding of other adhesion molecules – lymphocyte function associated antigen (LFA-1) on the T-cell to intercellular adhesion molecule-1 (ICAM-1) on the LC, and probably also CD2 on the T-cell to LFA-3 on the LC.

Binding of the T-cell receptor to its target causes a transient rise in the affinity of LFA-1 ensuring tighter and, therefore, more stable contact between the cells [9]. The signal to initiate T-cell proliferation, expression of receptors for interleukin-2 (IL-2) and other changes are mediated via the phosphoinositide/calcium second messenger pathway, activated both by the T-cell

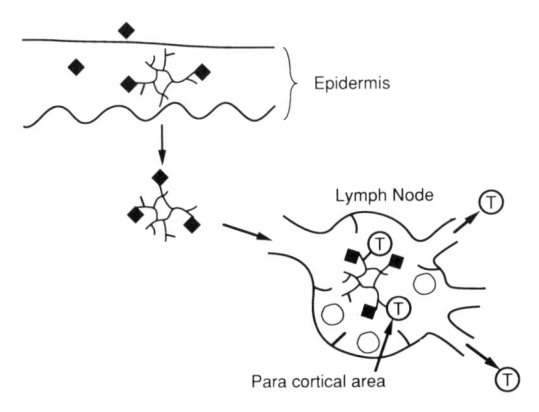

Figure 1. Induction of the immune response: antigen penetrating through the epidermis is transported by Langerhans' cells to the paracortical areas of the regional lymph node. T = T-lymphocyte. (Reproduced from reference 19 with permission of Blackwell Scientific Publications.)

receptor and LFA-1 interactions with their ligand [9, 10]. Interleukin-1 from the LC provides an essential additional or second activation signal.

Upon stimulation by appropriate antigen-bearing presenting cells, there is activation and clonal proliferation of T-lymphocytes specifically committed to that antigen, with the induction of immunological memory. At a certain stage of clonal expansion these cells leave the lymph node and enter the circulation. Once this occurs, the altered (increased) reactivity or state of sensitization can be detected by the inflammatory response that develops at sites of encounter with that antigen. This can be shown experimentally by sensitization and challenge with compounds such as dinitrochlorobenzene (DNCB).

In the skin of mice there is a second population of dendritic cells characterized by the presence of the Thy-1 surface antigen and the lack of Class II MHC antigens. These cells appear to be part of the T-cell lineage as they contain T-cell receptor genes that have undergone rearrangement prior to active expression [11, 12]. Thy-1^+ cells can present antigen in a way that preferentially activates suppressor T-cells resulting in inhibition of the immune response to that antigen [13]. Thy-1^+ cells have no human homologue.

EXPRESSION OF IMMUNE SENSITIVITY (EFFERENT PHASE)

Basically, upon secondary encounter with antigen, T-cells are activated again, presumably after recognition of specific target antigen presented by LCs in association with HLA-DR. An interesting question that arises is how T-cells in the intravascular compartment can 'see' the antigen (Figure 2). It is unknown just how many T-cells have to participate in the initiation of the reaction – but theoretically just one should be enough. The statistical likelihood of a chance encounter between the appropriate T-cell and its antigen must be very low. Therefore, there must be initial processes, independent of T-cells, which non-specifically increase cellular traffic and hence, the efficiency of immune surveillance.

Evidence is accumulating that this is indeed the case. Such recruitment mechanisms have been studied in skin following application of chemical compounds, antigenic or irritant, in people known either to be sensitive or non-sensitive to the substance. From 2 to 4 hours after application of antigens such as nickel sulphate or irritants such as anthralin, the number of LCs in the superficial dermis increases [5; Friedmann et al, personal observation]. From 2 to 4 hours onwards, dermal microvascular endothelial cells show increased expression of adhesion molecules. Thus, immunocytochemical staining for ICAM-1 shows increase both in intensity and numbers of vessels stained, compared with untreated skin [14]. Similarly, ELAM-1 (endothelial cell adhesion molecule) and VCAM-1 (vascular cell adhesion molecule) appear on endothelial cells from 4 to 8 hours onwards [14]. From 8 hours onwards, epidermal keratinocytes express ICAM-1 and also tumour necrosis factor alpha (TNF-α) with increasing intensity [5, 14, personal observation]. Also from 8 hours on, lymphocytes and macrophages begin to appear around dermal vessels. These events can occur regardless of whether people are sensitized or not, after contact with antigenic or irritant compounds. In other

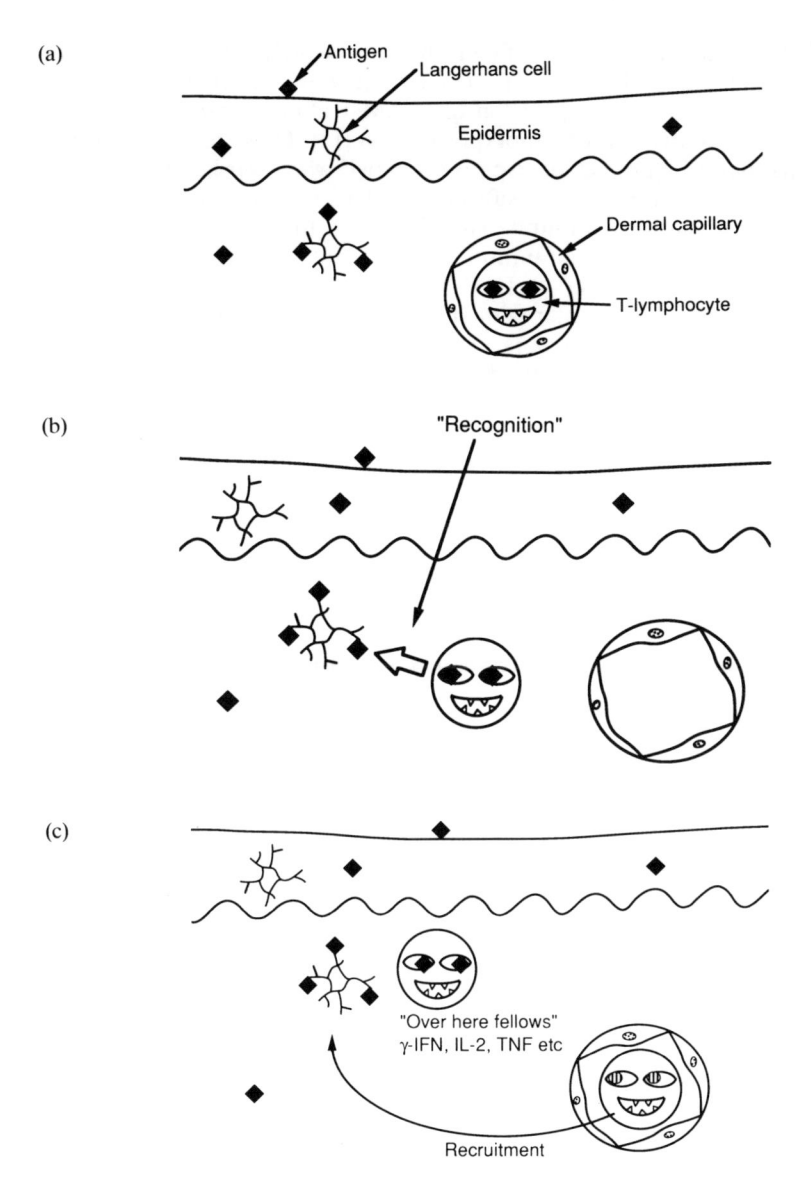

Figure 2. Elicitation of the secondary response to antigen. (a) Antigen is taken into the dermis by Langerhans' cells; T-cells specific for the antigen pass through the circulation. (b) Recognition of the antigen requires physical encounter between T-cell and Langerhans' cell bearing antigen. (c) Recruitment of other cells in a non-specific way – open invitation to the 'party'. (Reproduced from reference 19 with permission of Blackwell Scientific Publications.)

words, there are general, non-specific mechanisms which are not the result of signals from T-cells. This is supported by the observation that cultured keratinocytes will turn on expression of ICAM-1 after in vitro exposure to antigen such as pentadecyl catechol (poison ivy) [15]. These mechanisms are thus the first part of a protective response initiated whenever keratinocytes or endothelial cells 'sense' foreign substances. The response is designed to recruit T-cells to perform immune surveillance – the adhesion molecules potentiate attachment and emigration of T-cells into the tissues. Cytokines such as TNF-α and interleukin-8 (IL-8), which appears later, are chemotactic for T-cells. Following encounter with substances to which the subject is *not* sensitized, or even irritants, there is a small and transient infiltration with T-cells in the dermis. This infiltration subsides over 24–48 hours unless the specific interaction occurs between a T-cell and its specific antigen. If this recognition event occurs, the T-cell is stimulated to release various cytokines, the most important of which appears to be gamma interferon (γ-IFN). Thus, inoculation of rats with a monoclonal antibody to γ-IFN reduced by 50–90% the migration of lymphocytes into reactions [16] (Figure 2c). However, IL-2, TNF-α and probably many others may also be involved. This recruits more cells including monocytes and other lymphocytes. The end-product is an increased infiltration by T-cells and macrophages, and inflammation with increased blood flow (erythema) and vascular permeability (oedema) which develops over 48–72 hours. This is of course recognized clinically as allergic contact eczema.

Having considered some of the molecular and cellular mechanisms underlying the immune response, some aspects of how they work in an integrated and coordinated way will now be considered. Firstly the nature of the dose–response relationships in the immune system was examined using a system of experimental contact sensitization with the antigen dinitrochlorobenzene (DNCB).

Five groups of healthy subjects received an initial dose of DNCB applied to the forearm on a circular area 3cm in diameter. This was to induce sensitivity. The doses applied were 1000, 500, 250, 125 and 62.5μg. Four weeks later a series of challenge doses was applied on standard 1cm diameter patch-test discs. The responses were evaluated after 48h both clinically and by measurement of the skin thickness with calipers. From the observations it became clear that as for most physiological systems, the human immune system exhibits responses which are proportional to the log of the stimulus [17–19]. First, simply using the clinical assessment of the response to challenge to decide that sensitivity was detectable, the proportions of sensitized subjects showed a sigmoid relationship with the log of the sensitizing dose. Thus, 500μg of DNCB sensitized 100% of people (Figure 3). The next point was that as sensitizing dose increased, not only were more people made clinically sensitive, they were sensitized to a greater degree. The responses to challenge plotted against log of challenge dose are represented by curves which are the lower portions of sigmoid dose–response curves (Figure 4). The upper portions could not be explored satisfactorily because blisters developed and the measurement system breaks down.

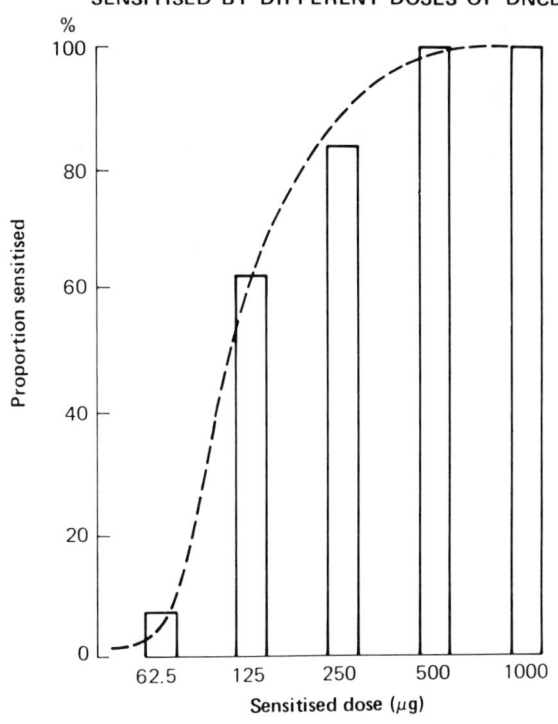

Figure 3. Effect of sensitizing dose on proportion of subjects showing clinically detectable sensitivity to dinitrochlorobenzene (DNCB). (Reproduced from reference 18 with permission of Karger, Basel.)

Since the immune response exhibits classical log dose–response relationships, it is logical that the underlying events, including the expression of adhesion molecules and cytokines that follow encounter with 'foreign' substances, also exhibit dose responses. In other words, the higher the concentration of applied compound the greater will be the expression of these recruitment mechanisms. There is no direct evidence for this yet but it is supported by the following observations [20, 21]. Individuals sensitive to two different antigens were challenged simultaneously with a series of dilutions of each antigen separately and also in combination [20]. The two individual antigen dilution series gave dose–response curves that exhibited a threshold concentration below which there was no clinically detectable response. For the dilution series in which the two antigens were combined at each site, the threshold was shifted to a much more dilute strength. In other words, summation or even synergy of two sub-threshold concentrations had occurred, greatly increasing the efficiency of recruitment of passing T-cells, and hence ensuring that one or both antigens were recognized. The identical phenomenon was seen when one of

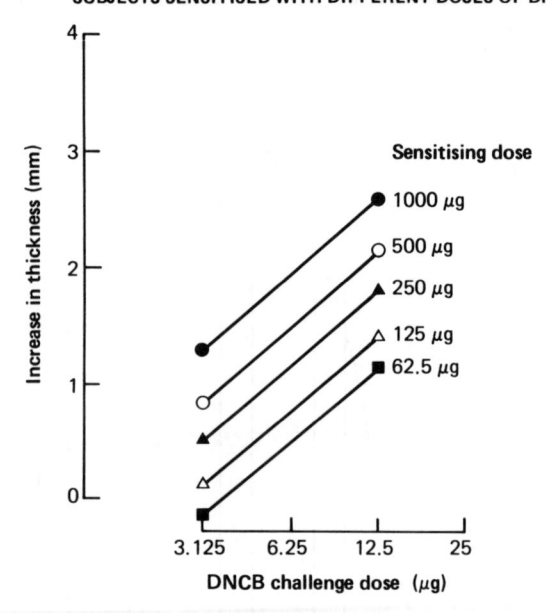

Figure 4. Degree of reactivity elicited by challenge with DNCB. Curves are the calculated slopes of dose–response curves. (Reproduced from reference 18 with permission of Karger, Basel.)

the antigens was replaced by an irritant compound [21]. Again, antigen and irritant in combination gave clear positive responses at concentrations well below the clinical threshold for either alone.

In conclusion, the skin provides a highly effective contribution to the body's defences. Not only does it form a physical barrier to invasion by microbes, but if the barrier is breached, the mechanisms for initiating immune sensitization via Langerhans' cells are present. Also, there are tissue elements able to 'sense' foreign substances and, by expressing the adhesion molecules and cytokines that attract T-cell traffic, immune surveillance mechanisms are recruited.

REFERENCES

1 Hanau D, Fabre M, Lepoittevin JP et al. ATPase and morphologic changes induced by UVB on Langerhans cells in guinea pigs. *J Invest Dermatol* 1985; *85*: 135–138
2 Carr MM, Botham PA, Gawkroger DJ et al. Early cellular reactions induced by dinitrochlorobenzene in sensitized human skin. *Br J Dermatol* 1984; *110*: 637–641
3 Silberberg-Sinakin I, Thorbecke GJ, Baer Rl et al. Antigen-bearing Langerhans cells in skin, dermal lymphatics and in lymph nodes. *Cell Immunol* 1976; *25*: 137–151
4 Bergstresser PR, Toews GB, Streilein JW. Natural and perturbed distributions of Langerhans cells: Responses to ultraviolet light, heterotopic skin grafting and dinitrofluorobenzene sensitization. *J Invest Dermatol* 1980; *75*: 73–77

5 Sterry W, Kunne N, Weber-Matthiesen K et al. Cell trafficking in positive and negative patch-test reactions: Demonstration of a stereotypic migration pathway. *J Invest Dermatol 1991; 96*: 459–462
6 Macatonia SE, Edwards AJ, Knight SC. Dendritic cells and the initiation of contact sensitivity to fluorescein isothiocyanate. *Immunology 1986; 59*: 509–514
7 Kinnaird A, Peters SW, Foster JR, Kimber I. Dendritic cell accumulation in draining lymph nodes during the induction phase of contact allergy in mice. *Int Arch Allergy Appl Immunol 1989; 89*: 202–210
8 Botham PA, Rattray NJ, Walsh ST, Riley EJ. Control of the immune response to contact sensitizing chemicals by cutaneous antigen-presenting cells. *Br J Dermatol 1987; 117*: 1–9
9 Dustin ML, Springer TA. T-cell receptor cross-linking transiently stimulates adhesiveness through LFA-1. *Nature 1989; 341*: 619–624
10 Wacholtz MC, Patel SS, Lipsky PE. Leukocyte function-associated antigen 1 is an activation molecule for human T cells. *J Exp Med 1989; 170*: 431–448
11 Kuziel WA, Takashima A, Bonyhadi M et al. Regulation of T cell receptor gamma-chain RNA expression in murine Thy-1$^+$ dentritic epidermal cells. *Nature 1987; 328*: 263–266
12 Stingl G, Gunther KC, Tschachler E et al. Thy-1$^+$ dentritic epidermal cells belong to the T-cell lineage. *Proc Natl Acad Sci (USA) 1987; 84*: 2430–2434
13 Okamoto H, Kripke ML. Effector and suppressor circuits of the immune response are activated in vivo by different mechanisms. *Proc Natl Acad Sci (USA) 1987; 84*: 3841–3845
14 Griffiths CEM, Barker JNWN, Kunkel S, Nickoloff BJ. Modulation of leucocyte adhesion molecules, a T-cell chemotaxin (IL-8) and a regulatory cytokine (TNF-α) in allergic contact dermatitis (rhus dermatitis). *Br J Dermatol 1991; 124*: 519–526
15 Griffiths CEM, Nickoloff BJ. Keratinocyte Intercellular Adhesion Molecule-1 (ICAM-1) expression precedes dermal T lymphocyte infiltration in allergic contact dermatitis (Rhus dermatitis). *Am J Pathol 1989; 135*: 1045–1053
16 Issekutz TB, Stoltz JM, Van Der Meide P. Lymphocyte recruitment in delayed type hypersensitivity. *Clin Exp Immunol 1988; 73*: 70–75
17 Friedmann PS, Moss C, Schuster S, Simpson JM. Quantitative relationships between sensitising dose of DNCB and reactivity in normal subjects. *Clin Exp Immunol 1983; 53*: 709–711
18 Friedmann PS, Moss C. Quantification of contact hypersensitivity in man. In Maibach HI, Lowe NJ eds. *Models in Dermatology Vol 2*. Basel: Karger 1985: 275–281
19 Friedmann PS. Graded continuity, or all or none – studies of the human immune response. *Clin Exp Dermatol 1991; 16*: 79–84
20 McLelland J, Shuster S, Matthews JNS. 'Irritants' increase the response to an allergen in allergic contact dermatitis. *Arch Dermatol 1991; 127*: 1016–1019
21 McLelland J, Shuster S. Contact dermatitis with negative patch tests: the additive effect of allergens in combination. *Br J Dermatol 1990; 122*: 623–630

CONNECTIVE TISSUE DISEASES AND THE SKIN

Neville R Rowell
University of Leeds, Leeds

The connective tissue diseases are considered to include discoid (DLE) and systemic lupus erythematosus (SLE), localized and generalized morphoea, systemic sclerosis, Sjögren's syndrome and rheumatoid arthritis [1]. The skin manifestations of these diseases are too large a subject for the space available so I would like to discuss a facet which has interested me for over 30 years. This is the nature of what are now called subsets. Physicians have in the past been divided into 'lumpers' and 'splitters'. With experience I have changed from being a 'lumper' to a 'splitter'. Why have I done this and why is it important? I believe that defining subsets is helpful in diagnosis, in prognosis, in understanding the pathogenesis, in conducting meaningful research and in comparing treatment regimens. I propose to support my thesis by confining the discussion to a consideration of lupus erythematosus and systemic sclerosis.

Lupus erythematosus can be divided into DLE, a cutaneous disorder which may be localized to the head and neck or widely disseminated over the body, and SLE which is a multisystem disease in which the skin is involved at some time in 80% of patients. In the 1960s Dr (now Professor) Beck and I studied patients with DLE in an attempt to show that if investigated fully they showed similar features to patients with SLE [2]. This proved to be correct (see Table I); 55% had laboratory abnormalities and this together with the knowledge that the cutaneous lesions and histological appearances could be identical, that patients with SLE may have typical lesions of DLE, and that patients with DLE may later develop SLE seemed to be strong evidence that DLE and SLE are variants of the same disease. But there is considerable evidence that this is not so simple. The risk of conversion from DLE to SLE appeared to be small and a 15 year follow-up of the same patients confirmed that the risk was only 6.5% [3]. This is important for patients with DLE and their physicians to know as many fear that there is a high risk of developing SLE. Patients with disseminated DLE had an increased risk (22%) compared with those with DLE confined to the head and neck (1.2%). However, the presence of laboratory abnormalities did not appear to predispose to the development of SLE and the majority of patients with DLE exposed to ultraviolet light, trauma or physical or mental stress did not convert to SLE. Immunohistologically, immunoglobulins and complement do not occur in the uninvolved light-exposed skin in DLE unlike SLE. Finally the age and sex distribution is markedly different in SLE [4] and DLE [5]. In DLE two females are affected for every male and in SLE the female:male sex ratio is 8:1. I believe that DLE and SLE are separate entities with different genetic backgrounds and support for this view has been provided by HLA typing [6]. Patients with DLE and haematological and immunological abnormalities are not patients with SLE in disguise. Those patients who convert from DLE to SLE and those patients with SLE and discoid lesions must have the genetic predisposition for both conditions. DLE patients without the predisposition to SLE will not convert whatever environmental factors they are exposed to. Studies of the age at onset in DLE suggest that there are at least three genotypes of DLE related to age of onset [5], and histocompatibility typing is consistent with this [6]. From the practical point of view there appears to be an increased risk of conversion of DLE to SLE in HLA B8 females developing DLE between the ages of 15 and 40.

TABLE I. Features of a personal series of patients with discoid and systemic lupus erythematosus

	Lupus erythematosus	
	Discoid	Systemic
No. of patients	120	40
ESR 20mm/h	20%	85%
Globulin > 3g%	29%	76%
Antinuclear factor	35%	86%
Precipitating antibodies	4%	38%
False + serology	5%	22%
Rheumatoid factor	15%	37%
Direct Coombs' test	2.5%	15%
Leucopenia	12.5%	37%
Thrombocytopenia	5%	21%

DLE itself is not a homogeneous disease. In addition to subsets by age at onset there are also clinical subsets with differing distribution between the sexes and with different prognoses. The classical scaling erythematous discoid rash, usually on the light-exposed areas of the face, ears and hands, may be associated with similar lesions in the scalp resulting in permanent localized scarring alopecia. Although the cutaneous lesions may last for years 50% eventually clear completely [7]. Subsets with a good prognosis include a rosaceous type and lesions on the trunk and limbs, but preauricular tumid lesions and chilblain lupus affecting mainly the ears, fingers and toes last indefinitely. The preauricular variety occurs in males and the chilblain type in females, which provides further evidence for a genetic predisposition.

These subsets run true over the years. The only constant immunological association occurs in Rowell's syndrome [8, 9] in which lesions of DLE or SLE are associated with erythema multiforme-like lesions: patients have speckled antinuclear factor, anti-La and rheumatoid factor. Other clinical subsets include a telangiectatic variety, hyperkeratotic LE, nodular LE and lupus profundus (panniculitis).

A subset of LE midway between discoid and lupus erythematosus has been termed subacute cutaneous LE [10]. Patients have non-scarring papulosquamous or annular polycyclic lesions particularly on the neck, upper trunk and upper arms. About half the patients fulfil the criteria of the American Rheumatism Association for SLE. Anti-Ro and anti-La antibodies are frequent; the course is relatively benign and most patients respond to sunscreens, topical corticosteroids and oral antimalarials. There is an increased frequency of HLA B8 and DR3, the latter associated particularly with patients with the annular type and anti-Ro antibody [11]. The features of this subset are similar to those of antinuclear negative SLE and the annular rash resembles that of neonatal LE which is associated with anti-Ro and to a lesser extent anti-La or anti-U1 RNP antibodies.

In SLE clinical cutaneous subsets are less easy to define than immunological subsets. The classical rash is less scaly than that of DLE and the erythema is usually more symmetrical over the nose and cheeks in a butterfly distribution. Photosensitivity is a feature in 33–75% according to the amount of sunshine and although lesions can occur anywhere on the skin surface they are more likely in light-exposed areas. Almost any type of rash may occur. Lesions may be bullous (bullous LE), erythema multiforme-like, urticarial, macular, purpuric, vasculitic, papular or nodular (sometimes containing mucin within the dermis). Sclerosis is uncommon and calcinosis is rare. Vascular lesions include reticulate telangiectatic erythema on the fingers, palms and soles, dilated nail fold capillaries with ragged cuticles, periungual digital necroses resembling those seen in rheumatoid arthritis, peripheral gangrene, livedo reticularis with or without ulceration, atrophie blanche, leg ulcers and pyoderma gangrenosum. There may be transitory reddening of the scalp with diffuse alopecia and breaking of the hair giving an unruly appearance. The nails may show a variety of changes including splinter haemorrhages and striate leuconychia. Cutaneous subsets include the erythema multiforme syndrome already mentioned in DLE, the association of livedo reticularis with cerebral vasculitis and urticarial vasculitis with complement deficiency.

Immunological subsets can be identified and some are shown in Table II. None are as specific as the erythema multiforme syndrome. In addition thrombotic subsets are associated with the presence of antiphospholipid antibodies especially with the LE anticoagulant and with anticardiolipin antibodies. In our experience the anticoagulant occurs in 14% of unselected patients with SLE, half of whom have thrombotic episodes [12]. In SLE defining subsets also has prognostic value. Patients with renal [13] and cerebral involvement do badly; on the whole patients with predominately cutaneous or articular involvement do much better. Males have a poorer prognosis than females [13, 14].

TABLE II. Antibody subsets in systemic lupus erythematosus

DNA	Nephritis
Sm	Nephritis. Highly specific for SLE
Red cells	Haemolytic anaemia
Platelets	Thrombocytopenia
Neurones	Central nervous system disease
U1 RNP	Mixed connective tissue disease
Histone	Drug induced lupus
Ro	Subacute cutaneous LE
	Antinuclear antibody (ANA) negative LE
	Neonatal LE
	SLE and homozygous C2 and C4 deficiency
	SLE/Sjögren's overlap

Can we define subsets in scleroderma? Firstly let me say that morphoea, either localized in the form of plaques or linear lesions, or generalized over the whole skin surface, is a different disease from systemic sclerosis although sometimes lesions of both may occur rarely in the same patient. In morphoea, Raynaud's phenomenon and systemic involvement are usually absent and over the years lesions almost invariably resolve. Systemic sclerosis (SS) is preceded by Raynaud's phenomenon in more than 95% of cases, and the skin changes are associated with involvement of internal organs such as the gastrointestinal tract, lungs and kidney [15]. As in SLE, females predominate (4 females to 1 male) and the prognosis is worse in males [16, 17]. Classification has always been controversial in this disease but undoubtedly the most important prognostic feature apart from sex is the degree of cutaneous involvement. The recent agreement by workers from around the world [18] suggests that in the present state of our knowledge there appear to be two distinct subsets (Table III) which have been called limited cutaneous systemic sclerosis (lSSc) and diffuse cutaneous systemic sclerosis (dSSc). In the former there is usually a long history of Raynaud's phenomenon with skin involvement confined to the face, fingers, hands, forearms and feet, whereas

TABLE III. Classification of systemic sclerosis

Limited cutaneous systemic sclerosis
Long history of Raynaud's phenomenon
Peripheral skin involvement
Calcification, telangiectasia, late onset of pulmonary hypertension
Anticentromere antibody positive 70–80%

Diffuse cutaneous systemic sclerosis
Short interval (1 year) between the onset of Raynaud's phenomenon and the development of skin changes
Truncal skin involvement as well as peripheral
Pulmonary fibrosis, gastrointestinal disease, myocardial involvement, renal failure
Scl 70 antibody positive 30%
Anticentromere antibody negative

the diffuse subset is a more rapidly developing disorder with a short interval between the onset of Raynaud's phenomenon and cutaneous changes. The latter occur on the trunk as well as the peripheral parts of the body. In the limited form anticentromere antibody predominates, whereas Scl 70 is almost specific to the diffuse variety, although these two antibodies are not mutually exclusive [19].

In my experience these two clinical patterns seem to be laid down from the start of the patient's illness and do not alter. Nor do the antibodies appear to alter significantly during the course of the disease. Although familial cases are rare, abnormalities of serum proteins and antinuclear antibodies occur frequently in first degree relatives of patients with systemic sclerosis [20]. HLA typing shows an increase of DR2, DR3 and DR5 with this disease, DR2 and DR5 being associated particularly with mild disease and anticentromere antibodies [21]; HLA B8 is more frequent in the severely involved patients [22]. No relationship between HLA type and Scl 70 antibodies has been described. Like SLE the age and sex specific onset rates are in favour of genetic predisposition [23]. I believe that in the course of time clinical and immunological subsets and probably organ distribution will be related to specific genetic factors.

Thus in both diseases subsets, both clinical and immunological, can be recognized. These tend to run true. Evidence has been produced to indicate that such subsets may be related to specific genetic factors and only those with such factors get the disease. Patients with overlapping features either have the genotype for more than one disease or a particular gene may predispose to more than one disease.

For clinicians it is important to recognize subsets in order to give an accurate diagnosis to patients. Their recognition also is important when evaluating various types of treatment. Patients with subsets with a good prognosis should not be grouped with patients with a poor prognosis. Patients in clinical trials should come from the same subsets. Finally further study of subsets will lead to better understanding of the pathogenesis of disease.

This limited survey of relatively uncommon conditions has implications for many other disorders which up to now may have been considered to be homogeneous. Although the aetiology of most diseases is multifactorial, genetic factors frequently play a primary role not only in aetiology but also in prognosis.

REFERENCES

1. Rowell NR, Goodfield MJD. The connective tissue diseases. In Champion RH, Burton JL, Ebling FJG, eds. *Textbook of Dermatology*, 5th edn. Oxford: Blackwell Scientific Publications. 1992: 2163-2294
2. Beck JS, Rowell NR. Discoid lupus erythematosus. *Q J Med 1966; 35*: 119-136
3. Millard LG, Rowell NR. Abnormal laboratory test results and their relationship to prognosis in discoid lupus erythematosus. *Arch Dermatol 1979; 115*: 1055-1058
4. Burch PRJ, Rowell NR. Systemic lupus erythematosus. *Am J Med 1965; 38*: 793-801
5. Burch PRJ, Rowell NR. Lupus erythematosus. Analysis of the sex – and age – distributions of the discoid and systemic forms of the disease in different countries. *Acta Derm Venereol 1970; 50*: 293-301

6 Millard LG, Rowell NR, Rajah SM. Histocompatibility antigens in discoid and systemic lupus erythematosus. *Br J Dermatol 1977; 96*: 139–144
7 Rowell NR. The natural history of lupus erythematosus. *Clin Exp Dermatol 1984; 9*: 217–231
8 Rowell NR, Swanson-Beck J, Anderson JR. Lupus erythematosus and erythema-multiforme-like lesions. *Arch Dermatol 1963; 88*: 176–180
9 Parodi A, Drago EF, Varaldo G et al. Rowell's syndrome. *J Am Acad Dermatol 1989; 21*: 374–377
10 Sontheimer RD, Thomas JR, Gilliam JN. Subacute cutaneous lupus erythematosus. *Arch Dermatol 1979; 115*: 1409–1415
11 Sontheimer RD, Stastory P, Gilliam JN. Human histocompatibility associations in subacute cutaneous lupus erythematosus. *J Clin Invest 1981; 67*: 312–316
12 Rowell NR, Tate GM. The lupus anticoagulant in systemic lupus erythematosus. *Acta Derm Venereol 1989; 69*: 111–115
13 Wallace DJ, Podell T, Weiner J et al. Systemic lupus erythematosus – survival patterns. *JAMA 1981; 245*: 934–938
14 Kellum RE, Haserick JR. Systemic lupus erythematosus. *Arch Intern Med 1964; 113*: 200–207
15 Rowell NR. Systemic sclerosis. *J Roy Coll Phys London 1985; 19*: 23–30
16 Rowell NR. The prognosis of systemic sclerosis. *Br J Dermatol 1976; 95*: 57–60
17 Medsger TA, Masi AT, Rodnan GP et al. Survival with systemic sclerosis (scleroderma). *Ann Intern Med 1971; 75*: 369–376
18 Leroy EC, Black C, Fleischmajer R et al. Scleroderma (systemic sclerosis): classification, subsets and pathogenesis. *J Rheumatol 1988; 15*: 202–205
19 Jarzabek-Chorzelska M, Blaszcyzyk M, Kolacinska-Strasz Z et al. Are ACA and Scl 70 antibodies mutually exclusive? *Br J Dermatol 1990; 1202*: 201–208
20 Pereira S, Black C, Welsh K et al. Autoantibodies and immunogenetics in 30 patients with systemic sclerosis and their families. *J Rheumatol 1987; 14*: 760–765
21 Black CM, Welsh K, Maddison PJ et al. HLA antigens, autoantibodies and clinical subsets in scleroderma. *Br J Rheumatol 1984; 23*: 267–275
22 Hughes P, Gelsthorpe K, Doughty RW et al. The association of HLA-B8 with visceral disease in systemic sclerosis. *Clin Exp Immunol 1978; 31*: 351–356
23 Burch PRJ, Rowell NR. Autoimmunity. Aetiological aspects of chronic discoid and systemic lupus erythematosus, systemic sclerosis and Hashimoto's thyroiditis. *Lancet 1963; ii*: 507–513

AGEING AND THE SKIN

Katharine L Dalziel
University Hospital, Nottingham

THE SKIN AS A MODEL OF AGEING
The accessibility of skin for clinical observation and as a source of tissue for cell culture makes this organ particularly suitable for the study of ageing. In the 1960s Hayflick and Moorhead used human skin fibroblasts to demonstrate that the replicative capacity of cultured cells is finite and is inversely proportional to the age of the donor [1, 2]. More recently, much of the exciting work on mechanisms of cellular senescence (as reviewed by Goldstein [3]), such as the roles of tumour-suppressor genes, proto-oncogenes etc., has also utilized the cultured human skin fibroblast. Despite the difficulty of correlating in vitro findings with cellular senescence in vivo, these models are gradually defining the processes of cellular ageing. It may then prove possible to alter or influence these processes both in diseases characterized by premature ageing, such as progeria and cutis laxa [4], and in 'normal' physiological ageing.

INTRINSIC AND EXTRINSIC FACTORS IN SKIN AGEING
Ultraviolet light (UV) is the most important extrinsic factor in producing the changes which we recognize as an aged appearance in skin. Skin exposed to UV for decades shows the changes of photoageing, i.e. deep wrinkling, thickening, yellowing of white skin and patchy hypo- and hyper-pigmentation. Dysplastic and neoplastic epidermal lesions such as solar keratoses, basal and squamous cell carcinomas arise on this background of UV damage. These appearances are much grosser than those seen in skin protected from UV where subtle changes such as drying, fine wrinkles, loss of elasticity and a range of benign neoplasms comprise the features of 'intrinsic' skin ageing [5]. The facial appearance of an elderly individual will depend on the degree of photodamage and other factors such as skin type (as defined by the ability to tan in response to UV [6]), facial animation patterns [7], smoking [8], etc. It is interesting that individuals who look a lot older than their biological age are also said to be physiologically older in other body systems [9].

The histological changes of photoageing are most noticeable in the dermis

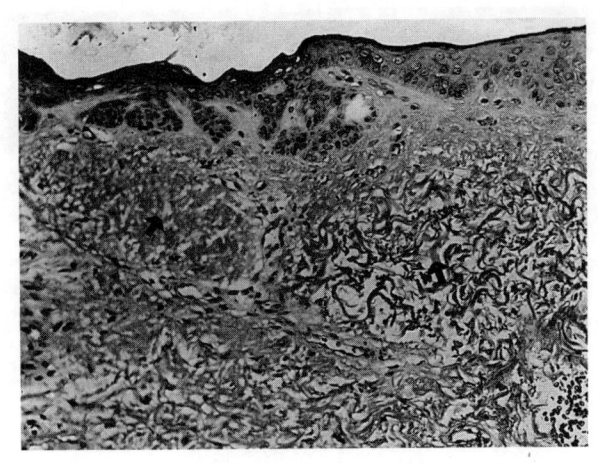

Figure 1. Histology of aged sun-exposed facial skin showing a thin epidermis with mild cellular atypia. Nodular and fragmented aggregates of solar elastotic tissue are present in the dermis (arrows)

as 'solar elastosis' in which aggregates of abnormal elastotic material accumulate (Figure 1). The mechanism by which this material is formed and its exact biochemical nature is still unclear although the structure of normal elastic tissue is being better defined [10] and estimates of elastin synthesis within a tissue can be made by measuring the amount of elastin messenger-RNA present [11]. Elastases, which are capable of degrading elastic tissue, are produced by cells such as neutrophils and macrophages and are themselves inhibited by plasma proteins such as α_2-macroglobulin and α_1-protease inhibitor [10]. It seems likely that a loss of normal homeostatic control of elastin synthesis and degradation occurs in solar elastotic tissue and recent research developments should help to clarify this.

Solar elastosis is manifest clinically by deep wrinkles, nodules of elastotic material and the so-called cutis rhomboidalis nuchae (Figure 2). Within the elastotic areas, follicular dilatation and blockage may be seen as large comedones, and sebaceous hyperplasia is common producing small pearly-white papules with a central punctum.

ULTRAVIOLET LIGHT, AGEING AND CARCINOGENESIS IN SKIN
In addition to causing the changes of photoageing, UV is incontrovertibly linked with the development of certain types of skin cancer, particularly basal cell and squamous cell carcinoma [12]. Predisposing factors for these non-melanoma skin cancers (NMSC) include a tendency to burn in the sun (skin types 1 and 2), outdoor occupation and geographic location [13]. In white populations, the incidence of NMSC rises steadily as the equator is approached [14]. The latent period between the years of maximum sun exposure and the development of skin cancer may be several decades. UV induces

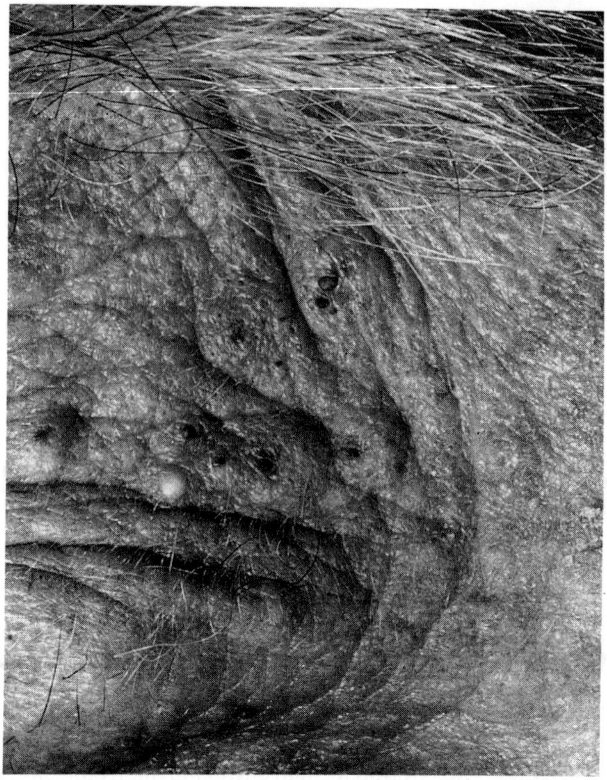

Figure 2. Solar elastotic skin near the eye showing characteristic deep wrinkles and large comedones.

structural changes in cellular deoxyribonucleic acid (DNA) [15] but specific protection and repair mechanisms exist within cells to minimize the effects of this [16]. The failure of these repair mechanisms is important in the development of NMSC. This is dramatically demonstrated by the inherited disease known as xeroderma pigmentosum (XP) in which there is a defect in excision repair of UV-induced DNA damage [17]. Individuals with the severe forms of XP develop multiple skin cancers in light-exposed areas from an early age. The repair genes involved in certain subtypes of XP are now being defined, opening the way to future therapeutic options [18]. Reduced DNA synthesis occurs in senescent cells in culture and there is evidence that this is more than just a passive process [19]. Although there is no direct evidence that human skin fibroblasts lose their ability to repair UV-induced DNA damage it is possible that reduced DNA synthesis in ageing cells contributes to the appearance of non-melanoma skin cancer in ageing, sun-exposed skin.

Even in temperate climates NMSC is extremely common and the incidence is rising steadily [20]. There is evidence from the USA that NMSC is the commonest form of human cancer [21] and official incidence figures for

NMSC in the UK are probably underestimated by up to a factor of four [22]. Since NMSC is still predominantly a disease of the elderly, the rising incidence is compounded by the demographic shift towards an older population. This has major implications for the provision of dermatological, radiotherapy and plastic surgery services in the forthcoming decades.

The rising incidence of NMSC appears to be associated with alterations in social attitudes to sunshine and tanning. Patterns of dress have altered radically since the Second World War, a sun-tan has become associated with health and attractiveness and many more people are able to take regular 'sunshine' holidays. In the USA there has been a shift of population towards the sun-belt and sun-bed usage is common [23]. In countries such as Australia which have extremely high rates of NMSC, public awareness campaigns have been implemented combining advice on reducing UV exposure with information on the use of high factor sunblocking agents [24].

There is now considerable concern that increased UV exposure will result from ozone depletion compounding the existing rises in melanoma and NMSC. Using predictions for future ozone depletion, various figures have been estimated for the anticipated rise in the incidence and deaths from skin cancer [25]. It is particularly worrying that recent evidence shows that ozone depletion is worse than previously predicted, particularly over temperate areas such as Europe and North America [26].

SKIN DISEASES IN THE ELDERLY

Skin disease is very common in the elderly population with a majority of individuals having at least one significant skin problem [27]. The elderly are susceptible to virtually any dermatosis but certain diseases are most common in, or present specific problems for, this age group. The commonest symptoms are xerosis (dry skin) and pruritus and no convincing theories exist to completely explain these problems. Several specific skin diseases of the elderly seem to relate to the alterations in immune function which occur as a function of ageing. Of the various types of eczematous dermatitis, seborrhoeic dermatitis has been described in up to 10.5% of a population aged 50-91 years [27]. Although seborrhoeic dermatitis occurs in the so-called 'seborrhoeic' areas, it is not related to increased sebum secretion, which is reduced in the elderly [28]. A causal role for the pityrosporum yeast in dandruff and seborrhoeic dermatitis has been proposed and the disease responds well to imidazole antifungal agents [29]. It is possible that ageing changes in immune-surveillance may be an aetiological factor in seborrhoeic dermatitis and this has been supported by the observation that severe seborrhoeic dermatitis is seen in some individuals infected with the HIV virus [30].

The recrudescence of varicella infection as herpes zoster occurs most commonly in the elderly with two-thirds of cases seen in individuals over 50 years [31], an incidence rising 10 per 1000 in octogenarians [32]. Reduced cell-mediated immunity appears to be a factor even in otherwise healthy old people developing herpes zoster since they show a delayed immune response to the virus [33].

Autoantibodies occur more frequently in the elderly and self-antigens become more reactive in this age group [34]. Bullous pemphigoid is an autoimmune disease which is virtually confined to the elderly [35] although other autoimmune blistering diseases occur throughout adult life. Tense blisters arise on pruritic urticated erythematous skin. Histology shows subepidermal blisters and immunofluorescence demonstrates the deposition of IgG and complement at the dermo-epidermal junction. These antibodies are pathogenic and circulating IgG autoantibodies which react with normal skin are usually detectable.

An interesting phenomenon which may be immune-mediated is the 'autosensitization' dermatitis which is seen most commonly in the elderly. This reaction occurs in individuals with an established localized eczematous dermatitis such as an allergic contact eczema around a leg ulcer. Patches of eczema occur at distant sites and this may become confluent and generalized [36]. The pathophysiology of this reaction is not defined. Some conceptualize it as an autoimmune reaction to tissue antigens released from the damaged skin whilst others feel that it represents a generalized non-specific hyperirritability of the skin [37].

Treatment of skin disease in the elderly presents particular problems. Bathing and care of hair and nails is difficult for a significant proportion of the very aged [27]. Many will find it impossible to apply topical therapies unaided and systemic therapies may be necessary to control widespread eczema or psoriasis [38]. The increased number of medications taken by the elderly predispose them to drug eruptions which may go undiagnosed and may persist for a considerable time following withdrawal of the offending drug.

SOCIAL IMPACT OF AGEING SKIN
An attractive appearance is perceived as being associated with positive personality characteristics [39] and maintaining a youthful appearance is considered attractive. Since it is mainly photodamage which causes the changes we perceive as an aged appearance, preventing or reversing photoageing has excited much interest, not least from the cosmetic and pharmaceutical industries. Emollients (moisturizers) have long been recognized to temporarily improve dry, wrinkled skin and many are now promoted as improving the appearances of ageing. In the last decade high factor sunblocking agents have proliferated. There is evidence from animal experiments that these agents reduce both solar elastosis and the risk of UV-induced squamous cell carcinoma in mice [40, 41]. It is difficult to extrapolate this to the human situation although high factor sunblockers do appear to be useful in conditions such as xeroderma pigmentosum, and it is reasonable to assume that they will protect against solar damage if used long-term. Theoretical problems with these agents include contact allergic reactions and reduced cutaneous vitamin D metabolism [42].

Topical retinoic acid (an anti-acne drug) is the first agent shown to be capable of at least partially reversing UV-induced skin changes. Animal experiments have been followed by human studies which show that topical retinoic acid can improve facial wrinkles and patchy pigmentary change and cause a 'rosy' appearance [43]. At the time of writing retinoic acid is not licensed for this indication but this has not stopped it being widely used, particularly in the USA. Retinoic acid has been shown to have multiple actions on epidermal maturation, collagen and elastic tissue [44]. These changes have mainly been demonstrated in studies using short-term high-dose retinoic acid under occlusion and it is not clear how these findings relate to its low-dose long-term usage. Retinoic acid causes an irritant erythema and may photosensitize. It is therefore combined with sunblockers and emollients [45]. The beneficial effects are only maintained by continued usage and there is no knowledge of the consequences of using it over a period of many years.

Interest in ageing skin is therefore multifaceted. Much research remains before we understand the mechanisms of specific skin diseases in the ageing population. Problems such as dry, itchy skin which cause misery in the elderly are common and should be much more actively treated with simple emollients. Therapeutic approaches towards preventing and reversing the ravages of solar damage are areas of intensive research, with the goal of maintaining a youthful appearance. The epidemic of skin cancer which is already underway could be halted and reversed by changing attitudes to sun exposure and the importance of this is underlined by recent evidence on increased UV exposure due to ozone depletion.

REFERENCES

1 Hayflick L, Moorhead PS. The serial cultivation of human diploid cell strains. *Exp Cell Res 1961; 25*: 585–592
2 Hayflick L. The limited in vitro lifetime of human diploid cell strains. *Exp Cell Res 1965; 37*: 614–636
3 Goldstein S. Replicative senescence: the human fibroblast comes of age. *Science 1990; 249*: 1129–1133
4 Fazio MJ, Olsen DR, Uitto JJ. Skin aging: lessons from cutis laxa and elastoderma. *Cutis 1989; 43*: 437–444
5 Leyden JJ. Clinical features of ageing skin. *Br J Dermatol 1990; 122 S35*: 1–3
6 Harber LC, Bickers DR. In *Photosensitivity Diseases: Principles of Diagnosis and Treatment*. Philadelphia: BC Decker. 1989: 387
7 Ellis DA, Masri H. The effect of facial animation on the aging upper half of the face. *Arch Otolaryngol Head Neck Surg 1989; 115(6)*: 710–713
8 Kadunce DP, Burr R, Gress R et al. Cigarette smoking: risk factor for premature facial wrinkling. *Ann Intern Med 1991; 114*: 840–844
9 Borkan GA, Norris AH. Assessment of biological age using a profile of physical parameters. *J Gerontol 1980; 35(2)*: 177–184
10 Uitto J, Fazio MJ, Olsen DR Cutaneous aging: molecular alterations in elastic fibers. *J Cut Ageing Cos Dermatol 1988; 1(1)*: 13–26
11 Olsen DR, Fazio MJ, Shamban AT et al. Cutis laxa: reduced elastin gene expression in skin fibroblast cultures as determined by hybridizations with a homologous cDNA and an exon 1-specific oligonucleotide. *J Biol Chem 1988; 263*: 6465–6467
12 Epstein JH. Photocarcinogenesis, skin cancer, and aging. *J Am Acad Dermatol 1983; 9*: 487–502
13 Vitaliano PO, Urbach F. The relative importance of risk factors in non-melanoma carcinoma. *Arch Dermatol 1980, 116*: 454–456
14 Bickers DR, Harber LC, Kopf A. Non-melanoma skin cancer and melanoma. In Harber LC, Bickers DR, eds. *Photosensitivity Diseases*. Toronto: BC Decker. 1989: 315–330
15 Thompson LH. Dissecting human DNA repair. *Photodermatology 1987; 4*: 63–65

16 Lambert WC, Hanawalt PC. DNA repair mechanisms and their biologic implications in mammalian cells. *J Am Acad Dermatol* 1990; 22: 299–308
17 Lehman AR, Bridges BA. Sunlight-induced cancer: some new aspects and implications of xeroderma pigmentosum. *Br J Dermatol* 1990; 122(S35): 115–119
18 Tanaka K, Miura N, Satokata I et al. Analysis of a human DNA excision repair gene involved in group A xeroderma pigmentosum and containing a zinc-finger domain. *Nature* 1990; 348: 73–76
19 Liu S-C, Meagher K, Hanawalt PC. Role of solar conditioning in DNA repair response and survival of human epidermal keratinocytes following UV irradiation. *J Invest Dermatol* 1985; 85: 93–97
20 Glass AG, Hoover RN. The emerging epidemic of melanoma and squamous cell skin cancer. *JAMA* 1989; 262(15): 2097–2100
21 Rogers GS, Gilchrest BA. Environmental influences on skin ageing. *Br J Dermatol* 1990; 122 S35: 55–60
22 Lloyd Roberts D. Incidence of non-melanoma skin cancer in West Glamorgan, South Wales. *Br J Dermatol* 1990; 122 (3): 399–403
23 NIH consensus development conference: sunlight, ultraviolet radiation and the skin: program and abstracts. May 8–10 1989, Bethesda, Md. Washington, DC, Department of Health and Human Services: 65–66
24 Marks R. Freckles, moles, melanoma and the ozone layer: a tale of the relationship between humans and their environment. *Med J Australia.* 1989; 151: 611–613
25 Moan J, Dahlback A, Larsen S et al. Ozone depletion and its consequences for the fluence of carcinogenic sunlight. *Cancer Res* 1989; 49: 4247–4250
26 United Kingdom Stratospheric Ozone Review Group. *Stratospheric Ozone 1991*. London: HMSO
27 Beauregard S, Gilchrest BA. A survey of skin problems and skin care regimens in the elderly. *Arch Dermatol* 1987; 123: 1638–1643
28 Burton JL, Pye RJ. Seborrhoea is not a feature of seborrhoeic dermatitis. *Br Med J 1983;* 286: 1169–1170
29 Ford GP, Farr PM, Ive FA, Shuster S. The response of seborrhoeic dermatitis to ketaconazole. *Br J Dermatol* 1984; 111: 603–607
30 Goodman DS, Teplitz ED, Wishmer A et al. Prevalence of cutaneous disease in patients with acquired immunodeficiency syndrome (AIDS) or AIDS related complex. *J Am Acad Dermatol* 1987; 17(2): 210–220
31 Oxman MN. Varicella and herpes zoster. In Fitzpatrick TB, Eisen AZ, Wolff K et al, eds. *Dermatology in General Medicine*. New York: McGraw Hill. 1987: 2314–2335
32 Hope-Simpson RE. The nature of herpes zoster: a long term study and a new hypothesis. *Proc R Soc Med 1965;* 58: 9–20
33 Sørensen OS, Haahr S, Møller-Larsen A et al. Cell-mediated and humoral immunity to herpes virus during and after herpes zoster infections. *Infect Immunol* 1980; 29: 369–375
34 Thoman ML, Weigle WO. The cellular and subcellular basis of immunosenescence. *Adv Immunol* 1989; 46: 221–261
35 Korman N. Bullous pemphigoid. *J Am Acad Dermatol* 1987; 16(5): 907–924
36 Epstein WL. Autosensitisation dermatitis. In Fitzpatrick TB, Eisen AZ, Wolff K et al, eds. *Dermatology in General Medicine*. New York: McGraw Hill. 1987: 1383–1384
37 Roper SS, Jones HE. A new look at conditioned hyperirritability. *J Am Acad Dermatol* 1982; 7: 643–650
38 Dalziel KL. Aspects of cutaneous ageing. *Clin Exp Dermatol 1991;* 16: 315–323
39 Kligman AM, Graham JA. The psychology of appearance in the elderly. *Dermatol Clin* 1986; 4: 501–507
40 Kligman LH, Akin FJ, Kligman AM. Prevention of ultraviolet damage to the dermis of hairless mice by sunscreens. *J Invest Dermatol* 1982; 78: 181–189
41 Kligman LH, Akin FJ, Kligman AM. Sunscreens prevent ultraviolet photocarcinogenesis. *J Am Acad Dermatol* 1980; 3: 30–35
42 Matsuoka LY, Wortsman J, Hanifan N et al. Chronic sunscreen use decreases circulating concentrations of 25-hydroxyvitamin D. *Arch Dermatol* 1988; 124: 1802–1804
43 Weiss JS, Ellis CN, Headington JT et al. Topical tretinoin in the treatment of aging skin.

J Am Acad Dermatol 1988; 19: 169-175
44 Roberts L. Questions raised about anti-wrinkle cream. *Science 1988; 239*: 564
45 Goldfarb MT, Ellis CN, Vorhees JJ. Topical tretinoin: its use in daily practice to reverse photoageing. *Br J Dermatol 1991; 122 S35*: 87-91

INFESTATIONS – RECOGNITION AND MANAGEMENT

DA Burns
Leicester Royal Infirmary, Leicester

INTRODUCTION

Humanity has been plagued by a variety of ectoparasites since time immemorial, and louse and scabies infections are still common and troublesome in our so-called 'developed' countries. Total eradication of these cutaneous passengers seems unlikely in the foreseeable future, in spite of the development of effective insecticides, because little attempt is made to mount a concerted effort to eliminate the common ectoparasites. Our present ectoparasite control activities are those of containment of the problem, rather than complete eradication.

LOUSE INFECTION

Head lice [1, 2]

The head louse (*Pediculus humanus capitis*) is transmitted by head to head contact with another infected individual. It is a cosmopolitan louse, not only in its geographical distribution, but also in its social preference. Major surveys of the distribution of head lice in the UK earlier this century demonstrated that head lice were principally a problem in the lower social classes in industrial conurbations. However, in recent years the head louse has moved to the country, and climbed the social ladder; it is now quite common in rural areas and amongst the upper echelons of society.

Head louse infection is encountered most frequently in children, and in girls more often than boys. An affected individual complains of an itchy scalp, and head louse infection should be suspected in any child complaining of persistent scalp pruritus. Examination will reveal the empty egg-cases (nits) attached to hair shafts, usually in greatest number on the hair above the ears and in the occipital region. Intact eggs are attached to the hair close to the surface of the scalp, and are usually more difficult to see. Repeated parting of the hair will usually reveal adult lice or louse nymphs. Keratin casts around the hair shafts may be mistaken for nits, but louse egg-cases can easily be rec-

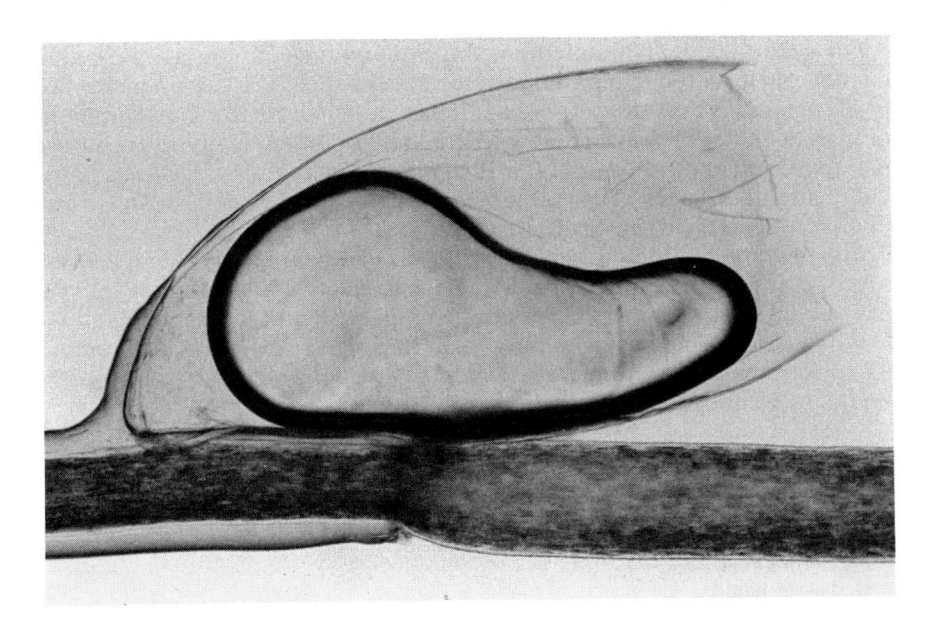

Figure 1. Empty egg-case ('nit').

ognized by microscopic examination (Figure 1). Occasionally, inflammatory papules and excoriations are present on the nape of the neck, and rarely, usually in the presence of a heavy infection of long duration, there may be a more generalized non-specific itchy eruption of tiny papules accompanied by excoriations. Head louse infection may also be accompanied by scalp impetigo, and in these circumstances the hair is often matted together in an unpleasant tangle with pus and exudate.

Head louse infection is not difficult to recognize, but problems may arise in deciding whether head lice have been completely eradicated by treatment. The presence of nits indicates that infection has been present, and the position of the nits on the hair shafts will provide some idea of the duration of the infection. For example, if nits are found on the ends of shoulder-length hair then the infection has been present for many months. However, the presence of adult lice or louse nymphs on the scalp provides the only absolute evidence of ongoing infection.

Treatment [2–6]
The ideal pediculicide should produce rapid demise of adult insects, and preferably also have significant ovicidal activity. The acetylcholinesterase-inhibiting insecticides malathion and carbaryl have provided the mainstay of treatment for head louse infection in the UK for several years. They replaced gamma-benzene hexachloride (lindane) in the 1970s, following evidence of the emergence of resistance to the organochlorine insecticides [7]. More recently, synthetic pyrethroids have been added to the pediculicide armamentarium.

For maximum benefit malathion and carbaryl preparations should be left on the scalp for several hours. Lotion preparations should be used in preference to shampoos, as the latter expose the insects to relatively low concentrations of insecticide for a brief period, and are therefore more likely to encourage the development of resistance. It is the policy of most Health Districts in the UK to alternate the use of malathion and carbaryl every 3 years, in an attempt to discourage development of resistance.

Although most currently employed pediculicides have good ovicidal activity, not all eggs are killed, and it is preferable to repeat treatment after an interval of 7–10 days. All members of an affected family should be treated.

When treating patients who have scalp impetigo or extensive excoriations it is preferable to use a preparation with an aqueous base, such as Derbac-M liquid, as alcohol-base preparations will irritate.

TABLE I. Treatment of head lice: proprietary pediculicides

Malathion
  Prioderm lotion
  Derbac-M liquid
  Suleo-M lotion

Carbaryl
  Carylderm lotion
  Clinicide lotion
  Suleo-C lotion
  Suleo-C shampoo
  Derbac shampoo

Pyrethroids
  Lyclear creme rinse
  Full Marks shampoo
  Full Marks lotion

Malathion [7–10]. Malathion is an excellent pediculicide, and also has good ovicidal activity. It is adsorbed on to keratin, a process which takes about 6 hours, and confers residual protective effect against reinfection for approximately 6 weeks. Proprietary preparations containing malathion are shown in Table I.

Carbaryl [11]. Carbaryl is also an efficient pediculicide and ovicide. It does not, however, confer any residual protective effect against reinfection. Proprietary preparations containing carbaryl are listed in Table I. There is evidence which suggests that these proprietary preparations are not of equal pediculicidal and ovicidal activity, and this variation in effectiveness appears to be determined to some extent by the components of the bases used in these preparations [12]. The variation in insecticidal activity is particularly noticeable when short application times are employed.

Synthetic pyrethroids. The development and use of this group of insecticides has recently been reviewed by Taplin and Meinking [13]. Synthetic pyrethroids have been developed from pyrethrins, which are naturally occurring insecticides produced by plants of the genus *Chrysanthemum*. They are photostable, rapidly biodegraded, and have low mammalian toxicity. Permethrin and phenothrin are the synthetic pyrethroids present in proprietary preparations available in the UK (Table I). After use of permethrin, residual insecticidal activity may persist for up to 6 weeks.

Clothing lice (body lice) [1, 2]

The clothing louse is the louse of abject poverty. Its hosts in 'developed' countries are vagabonds and down-and-outs who have one set of clothing which is never removed and never cleaned, and who rarely wash themselves. It lives in the clothing, attaching its eggs to the material, and only moves on to the body to feed.

An individual with clothing louse infection usually, but not invariably, itches, because they have developed hypersensitivity to louse salivary antigens. Their skin is covered in excoriations, and is often hyperpigmented (vagabond's disease). The hyperpigmentation is a post-inflammatory phenomenon. If the diagnosis of clothing louse infection is suspected, it is the clothing and not the patient which should be examined to detect lice (Figure 2).

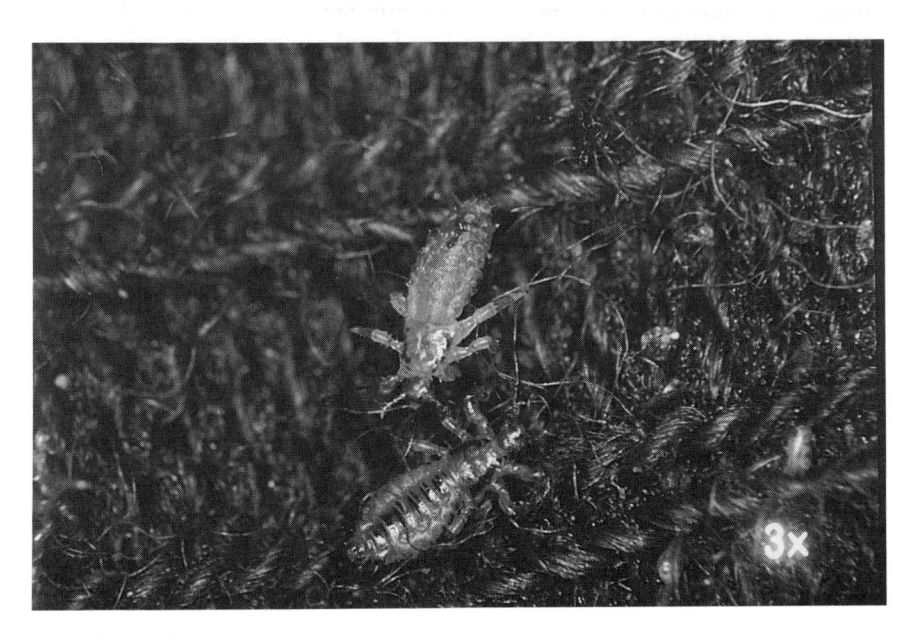

Figure 2. Clothing lice.

Treatment
It is the clothing, not the patient, which requires treatment. High temperature laundering of underclothes, and dry-cleaning of outer clothing, will kill lice and eggs. If the clothing is placed in a tumble-dryer for 15 minutes the lice and eggs will also be eradicated [14].

In countries where clothing lice are an endemic problem, insecticides are used to treat clothing. Malathion dusting powder [15, 16] and permethrin [17] are used for louse control.

Crab lice (pubic lice) [1, 2]
Phthirus pubis, the crab louse, is a parasite adapted to living in hair of a particular density. It will colonize scalp margins, eyelashes, beard hair, and hair on any part of the trunk and limbs, but it does not favour the main mass of scalp hair. It is transmitted by close physical contact, usually during sexual activity. The crab louse is a relatively sedentary insect during the day, but is quite active at night [18].

Itching is the main symptom of crab louse infection, and this is usually most troublesome at night. Examination will reveal the lice clinging to hair with their powerful claws, and their eggs cemented to hair shafts. In heavy infections there may also be quantities of red-brown louse faeces on the skin. Another sign of crab louse infection is the presence of spots of blood on the underwear. Young children are sometimes affected, usually as a result of contact with infected parents, and lice will be found around the margins of the scalp and on the eyelashes. When children are affected the question of whether this is a manifestation of sexual abuse may be raised, but perfectly normal close physical contact between parents and children is quite adequate to explain transmission.

When the eyelashes are affected the louse eggs are readily seen attached to the hair (Figure 3).

Treatment [6, 19, 20]
Preparations containing lindane, malathion, carbaryl or pyrethroids may be used in the treatment of crab louse infection. Alcohol-base preparations may be irritant when applied to the scrotum, and aqueous preparations such as Quellada lotion or Derbac-M liquid are preferable. In view of the frequent involvement of other hairy areas of the body, in addition to the pubic region, it is advisable to treat the whole of the trunk and limbs, and preferably the scalp. Treatment should be repeated after an interval of 7–10 days. All sexual contacts should also be treated.

Treatment of eyelash infection [21, 22]. A variety of methods have been suggested for the treatment of infection of the eyelashes, including white soft paraffin, physostigmine eye ointment, 10–20% fluorescein, and cryotherapy. Any of the previously mentioned insecticide preparations may be used to treat crab lice on the eyelashes, but alcohol-base preparations are irritant if inadvertently introduced into the eye, and aqueous preparations such as Derbac-M liquid or Quellada lotion are the treatment of choice. The preparation should be

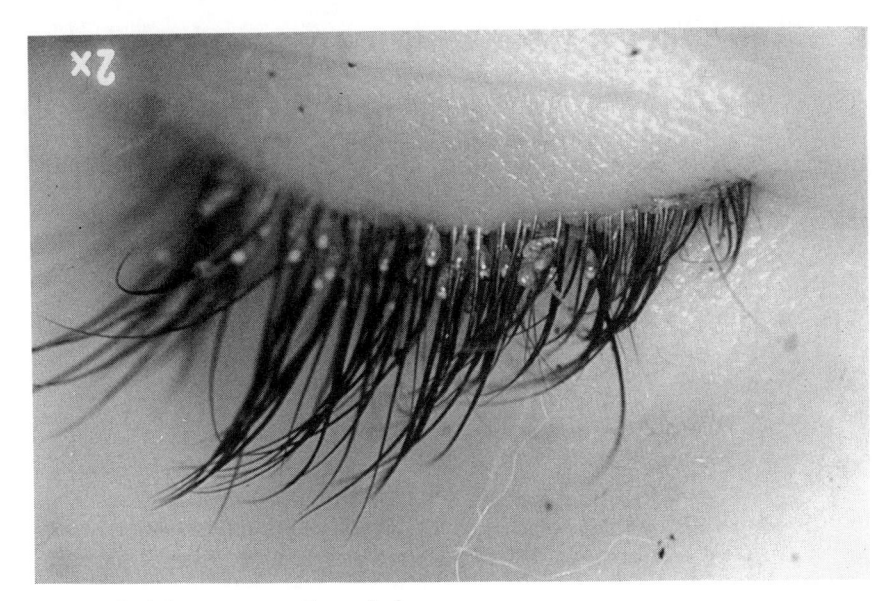

Figure 3. Crab louse eggs on the eyelashes.

smeared over the eyelids and lashes, and the treatment repeated 7–10 days later. If a young child is being treated, wait until he or she is asleep before attempting this.

SCABIES [23, 24]

Scabies is acquired by close physical contact with another infected individual. Hand-holding is probably a common means of transmission. Female scabies mites burrow in the epidermis, and lay eggs which occupy the burrow behind them. Initially the host is unaware of the presence of the mites, but after a period of 4–6 weeks develops hypersensitivity to mite allergens, principally mite faeces, and begins to itch. Itching is continuous, but tends to be worse at night. The scratching of the host destroys burrows, and serves to keep the mite population in check.

Scabies can affect any age group, although it occurs most commonly in children and young adults. Its not infrequent occurrence in the elderly should not, however, be forgotten, as it is often misdiagnosed in this age group.

There are two primary signs of scabies infection: the presence of burrows and a rash of tiny inflammatory papules. Scabies burrows are superficial, tortuous tracks, sometimes several millimetres long (Figure 4), which may be found on the sides of the fingers, in the web-spaces between the fingers, around the wrists, on the insteps of the feet, and sometimes on the palms and soles. In babies, burrows may be found on the head and neck, but do not occur in this area in older children and adults. Burrows are also seen much

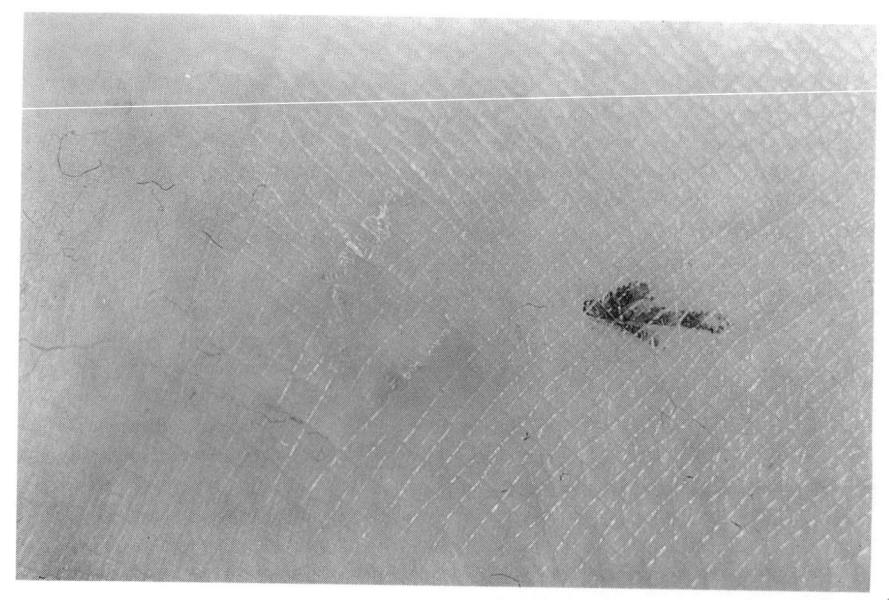

Figure 4. Typical scabies burrow.

more frequently on the palms and soles in children than in adults, and they also commonly occur on the trunk in babies and in the elderly.

The appearance of the scabies rash coincides with the onset of pruritus. The eruption is composed of small inflammatory papules which tend to be grouped around the axillary folds, scattered across the abdomen, particularly in the region of the umbilicus, and also scattered over the thighs (Figure 5). This distribution immediately suggests scabies to the experienced dermatologists, who will then embark on a hunt for burrows. Having discovered a burrow, this is gently scraped off the skin, and the scrapings examined microscopically for mites and eggs.

This unadulterated clinical picture may, however, be clouded by secondary phenomena which are the result of itching – eczematization, excoriations and secondary infection – and these features may mislead the unwary, and lead to inappropriate treatment.

Treatment [6, 23, 24]
There are several currently available scabicides, and the choice of preparation is usually determined by the particular preference of the dermatologist, the age of the patient, or the degree of secondary eczematization. If secondary eczematization is severe, a non-irritant scabicide should be used. Whatever preparation is used, it should be applied from the neck to the toes, preferably with a 5cm paint brush, and by someone other than the patient. Instruction leaflets are a great help in explaining the treatment regimen.

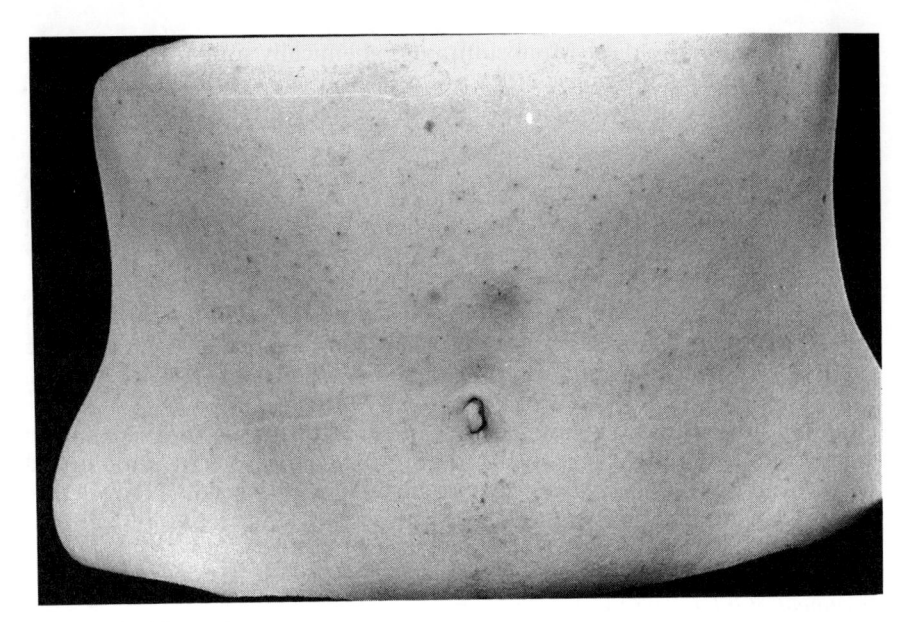

Figure 5. Scabies rash.

Benzyl benzoate. This has been in use as a scabicide since 1937, and is very effective. Its only drawback is that it is irritant, but this is not usually a problem unless it is used excessively. Most treatment regimens employ two or three applications of 25% benzyl benzoate emulsion either within a 24 hour period, on successive days, or each application separated by an interval of a week. It is important to stress to patients that this preparation should not be used more than the recommended number of times, otherwise they may develop troublesome irritant dermatitis.

Gamma-benzene hexachloride (lindane). A single application, washed off after 24 hours is usually recommended, but it has been demonstrated that shorter application times (12 or 6 hours) produce an equivalent cure rate. Although there have been several reports of adverse neurological effects, principally seizures, following the use of lindane, in the majority of these cases toxicity was associated with excessively long application times, frequent repeated use, use in children whose epidermal barrier function was compromised by pre-existing skin disease, or accidental ingestion. If used correctly it is safe, and adverse reactions are rare.

A number of anecdotal reports suggest that scabies resistant to lindane is being encountered with increasing frequency.

Monosulfiram (Tetmosol). A 25% solution in industrial methylated spirit is diluted with two or three parts of water to form an emulsion immediately prior to use, as the resulting suspension is not stable. It is applied once daily on 2 or 3 consecutive days. Monosulfiram is chemically similar to disulfiram (Antabuse), and an Antabuse-effect, with flushing, tachycardia and nausea, may occur if alcohol is ingested during, or soon after, treatment.

Malathion. Malathion 0.5% in an aqueous base is marketed in the UK as Derbac-M liquid, for the treatment of louse infection and scabies. It should be left on the skin for 24 hours, and a higher cure rate is obtained if a second treatment is applied after an interval of a few days.

Permethrin. Although not yet available in the UK, 5% permethrin cream (Elimite) has been available in the USA for some time, and is an effective scabicide. It is employed as a single application, washed off after 8–12 hours.

Itching does not resolve immediately after treatment, and it is helpful to provide patients with a topical antipruritic such as crotamiton and hydrocortisone (Eurax-Hydrocortisone) cream to use on residual itchy areas. All members of the family of a patient with scabies, and close physical contacts, should also be treated.

Treatment of infants and young children
The irritant effects of benzyl benzoate, and the potential neurotoxicity of lindane have led some authors to recommend avoidance of these preparations in infants. However, the irritancy of benzyl benzoate can be lessened by dilution with two or three parts water, and lindane appears to be safe unless prolonged application times and frequent, repeated applications are employed. Monosulfiram and aqueous malathion are also useful in the treatment of scabies in children. If burrows are present on the head and neck in babies, these may be treated with crotamiton (Eurax) cream.

Scabicides in pregnancy
The safety of currently available scabicides when used during pregnancy has not been critically assessed, but there does not appear to be any evidence that any has been responsible for adverse effects.

Crusted (Norwegian) scabies [23, 24]
Whereas in classical scabies the mite population on an infected individual is relatively small (an average of 12 adult females), in crusted scabies there may be millions of mites and eggs on the skin. The appellation 'Norwegian' for this type of scabies is derived from the first description of this condition in Norwegian lepers. This massive multiplication of the mite population occurs in situations where the host is mentally retarded, has impaired sensation, cannot respond to itching because of paralysis or arthropathy, or is immunosuppressed as a result of either disease or therapy.

The appearance is of massive crusting on the hands and feet, and often on other parts of the body. This scale is teeming with mites and eggs. The appearance may be mistaken for psoriasis or hyperkeratotic eczema, but the diagnosis is readily confirmed by examining skin scrapings by microscopy.

Because patients with crusted scabies shed scale containing large numbers of mites and eggs into their environment, they may be responsible for outbreaks of the commoner type of scabies in those around them.

Treatment
The treatments used in ordinary scabies are usually effective in crusted scabies, although several applications of a scabicide may be necessary.

Institutional outbreaks of scabies [6, 24–26]
Outbreaks of scabies in residential homes for the elderly are a frequent occurrence, and their eradication may prove extremely difficult. Similar problems occasionally occur in hospitals. The source of the outbreak is usually an individual with severe scabies, often of the crusted variety.

If this situation is encountered it is important to request the help of a dermatologist to determine the source of the problem, and to advise on appropriate treatment. If the outbreak is in a residential home, all residents should be examined, and if a case of severe scabies or crusted scabies is discovered that individual should be isolated until effectively treated. All residents in the home should be treated with a scabicide, preferably on two occasions separated by an interval of a few days. All the nursing staff and their families should also be treated. As an additional precaution all communal areas, such as sitting-rooms, should be sprayed with an acaricide; the Environmental Health Department will assist with this. Ordinary laundering of bedding is sufficient.

If, following this procedure, the problem persists, then the whole process must be repeated. If there is any doubt about the efficacy of a scabicide in these circumstances, then an alternative should be used.

REFERENCES
1. Alexander JO'D. Infestation with Anoplura – lice. In *Arthropods and Human Skin*. Berlin: Springer-Verlag. 1984: 29–55
2. Burns DA. Lice (Phthiraptera). In Champion RH, Burton JL, Ebling FJG, eds. *Textbook of Dermatology*, 5th edn, Vol. 2. Oxford: Blackwell Scientific Publications. 1991: 1281–1287
3. Altschuler DZ, Kenney LR. Pediculicide performance, profit and the public health. *Arch Dermatol 1986; 122*: 259–261
4. Meinking TL, Taplin D, Kalter DC, Eberle MW. Comparative efficacy of treatments for pediculosis capitis infestation. *Arch Dermatol 1986; 122*: 267–271
5. Rasmussen JE. Pediculosis: treatment and resistance. In: *Advances in Dermatology* Vol. 1. Chicago: Year Book Medical Publishers. 1986: 109–125
6. Burns DA. The treatment of human ectoparasite infection. *Br J Dermatol 1991; 125*: 89–93
7. Maunder JW. Resistance to organochlorine insecticides in head lice and trials using alternative compounds. *Medical Officer 1971; 125*: 27–29
8. Maunder JW. Use of malathion in the treatment of lousy children *Community Medicine 1971; 126*: 145–147
9. Taplin D, Castillero PM, Spiegel J et al. Malathion for treatment of *Pediculus humanus* var *capitis* infestation. *JAMA 1982; 247*: 3103–3105
10. Urcuyo FG, Zaias N. Malathion lotion as an insecticide and ovicide in head louse infestation. *Int J Dermatol 1986; 25*: 60–62
11. Maunder JW. Clinical and laboratory trials employing carbaryl against the human head louse, *Pediculus humanus capitis* (de Geer). *Clin Exp Dermatol 1981; 6*: 605–612

12 Burgess I. Carbaryl lotions for head lice – new laboratory tests show variations in efficacy. *Pharmaceutical J 1990; 245*: 159–161
13 Taplin D, Meinking TL Pyrethrins and pyrethroids in dermatology. *Arch Dermatol 1990; 126*: 213–221
14 Maunder JW. Pediculosis corporis; an updating of attitudes. *Environ Health 1983; May*: 130–132
15 Hayes WJ Jr, Mattson AM, Short JG, Witter RF. Safety of malathion dusting powder for louse control. *Bull WHO 1960; 22*: 503–514
16 Barnes WW, Eldridge BF, Greenberg JH, Vivona S. A field evaluation of malathion dust for the control of body lice. *J Econ Entomol 1962; 55*: 591–594
17 Scholdt LL, Rogers EJ Jr, Gerberg EJ, Schreck CE. Effectiveness of permethrin-treated military uniform fabric against human body lice. *Milit Med 1989; 154*: 90–93
18 Burgess I, Maunder JW, Myint TT. Maintenance of the crab louse, *Pthirus pubis*, in the laboratory and behavioural studies using volunteers. *Community Med 1983; 5*: 238–241
19 Orkin M, Maibach HI. Treatment of today's pediculosis. In Orkin M, Maibach HI, eds. *Cutaneous Infestations and Insect Bites*. New York: Marcel Dekker. 1985: 213–217
20 Kalter DC, Sperber J, Rosen T, Matarasso S. Treatment of pediculosis pubis. *Arch Dermatol 1987; 123*: 1315–1319
21 Couch JM, Green WR, Hirst LW, De La Cruz ZC. Diagnosing and treating *Phthirus pubis* palpebrarum. *Surv Ophthalmol 1982; 26*: 219–225
22 Burns DA. The treatment of *Pthirus pubis* infestation of the eyelashes. *Br J Dermatol 1987; 117*: 741–743
23 Alexander JO'D. Scabies. In *Arthropods and Human Skin*. Berlin: Springer-Verlag. 1984: 227–292
24 Burns DA. Scabies. In Champion RH, Burton JL, Ebling FJG, eds. *Textbook of Dermatology* 5th edn, Vol 2. Oxford: Blackwell Scientific Publications. 1991: 1300–1307
25 Carslaw RW, Dobson RM, Hood AJK, Taylor RN. Mites in the environment of cases of Norwegian scabies. *Br J Dermatol 1975; 92*: 333–337
26 Burns DA. An outbreak of scabies in a residential home. *Br J Dermatol 1987; 117*: 359–361

MOLECULAR BIOLOGY – NEW INSIGHTS INTO GENETIC DISEASE

ID Young, GS Cross
Interdisciplinary Centre for Medical Genetics, City Hospital, Nottingham

INTRODUCTION

During the last 10 years dramatic progress has been made in molecular biology with direct implications for medicine in general and clinical genetics in particular. In 1980 only a handful of the 3000 single-gene entities recognized at that time had been characterized at the molecular level. By the end of 1990 molecular defects had been identified in over 200 different single-gene disorders [1] including many of the most common and distressing chronic conditions of childhood and adult life such as cystic fibrosis [2] and Duchenne muscular dystrophy [3]. For disorders in which specific molecular defects have not been identified, molecular genetics may still have something to offer. Over 80 genetic disorders can now be studied in families indirectly by analysing restriction fragment length polymorphisms (RFLPs) generated by DNA markers known to be closely linked to the relevant locus [1].

These new developments, which were first labelled the 'new genetics' by Comings in 1980 [47], have greatly enhanced knowledge and understanding of the underlying nature and genesis of inherited disease. At the DNA level mutations have been found to consist most commonly of nucleotide substitutions and deletions, with insertions and duplications accounting for much smaller proportions of recognized gene defects [1]. CG dinucleotides appear to be particularly prone to spontaneous point mutation and account for 35% of all known single base-pair substitutions causing inherited human disease [5]. This may be a reflection of the ease with which methylated cytosine residues are deaminated. Small deletions are generally found closely adjacent to direct repeat sequences [6], which suggests that they are probably generated by slippage during DNA replication (the DNA strands slip out of alignment and a small segment is excised). Various other mechanisms may be responsible for the generation of larger deletions. These include intrachromosomal looping and unequal crossing-over during meiosis or mitosis.

Perhaps it is not surprising that heterogeneity at the molecular level has been found to be the rule rather than the exception, and the discovery of locus heterogeneity in conditions such as adult polycystic kidney disease and retinitis pigmentosa has emphasized the need for caution when applying these new innovative techniques in a clinical setting. The possibility that genes at up to four loci may be implicated in tuberous sclerosis [7] serves as a salutary reminder that the concept of one gene – one protein – one disease is likely to be a gross over-simplification.

Research in molecular biology has thrown up some rather unexpected findings regarding how genes are inherited and the ways in which they are expressed. Fundamental to genetic counselling is an understanding of the basic modes of inheritance. Traditionally these are considered under the headings of chromosomal, single-gene and multifactorial, and whilst this remains a valid sub-division, it has emerged that inheritance is not as simple or straightforward as was once imagined. These new observations are of direct relevance for genetic counselling and it is with these particular aspects of the 'new genetics' that this paper is concerned.

PARENTAL ORIGIN OF GENETIC DISEASE

A first step in establishing the underlying cause of a genetic disease is to try to identify the parent in whom the original disease-inducing mutational event occurred. Until recently, available information was limited to circumstantial evidence which pointed towards maternal meiosis as the culprit for most chromosomal abnormalities and paternal gametogenesis as the likely source of most single-gene mutations. This circumstantial evidence largely took the form of observed parental age effects in that disorders resulting from non-disjunction, such as Down's syndrome (trisomy 21), show an association with advanced maternal age, whereas a paternal age effect is observed for new mutations in several Mendelian disorders such as achondroplasia, Apert's syndrome and Marfan's syndrome.

These parental age effects are consistent with fundamental differences in meiosis in male and female. In the male, spermatogenesis commences at puberty by which time the primordial germ cells have undergone approximately 30 cell divisions during the formation of mature stem-cell spermatogonia. These then undergo further mitotic division with some daughter cells persisting as the stem-cell population whereas others undergo further mitotic and subsequent meiotic divisions resulting in mature spermatozoa. The stem-cell spermatogonia population continues to divide at an estimated rate of approximately 23 cell divisions per annum [8]. Effectively this means that a sperm produced by a 30 year old male, this being close to the mean paternal age in the UK, will have undergone up to 400 cell divisions in its lifetime. If it is acceptable to extrapolate further, this number will have risen to almost 1000 for sperm produced by a 55 year old man. The observed paternal age effect is consistent with the concept that most new mutations arise due to copy error in mitosis.

In contrast, the formation of a mature ovum in the female is thought to involve approximately only 21 cell divisions [8]. Oogenesis occurs during foetal life and ceases by the time of birth when the mature oocyte reaches the diplotene stage of prophase in meiosis I, i.e. before homologous chromosomes have separated. The oocyte then enters a potentially lengthy stage of maturation arrest (dictyotene), with meiosis being completed at ovulation and fertilization. It is assumed that during this long period of suspended animation environmental agents may disturb the cytodynamic structure and function of the resting oocyte thereby predisposing to abnormal subsequent separation of the paired homologous chromosomes.

Molecular studies have largely confirmed that when non-disjunction results in a chromosome abnormality, the error has usually occurred during maternal meiosis I. Table I shows that this holds true for the common autosomal trisomies (13, 18 and 21) and for the triple X syndrome (XXX). Curiously, however, over 50% of males with Klinefelter's syndrome (XXY) have inherited their additional X chromosome from their father, and in Turner's syndrome (XO) it is the paternal sex chromosome which has been lost in almost 80% of cases.

TABLE I. Parental origin of de novo chromosome abnormalities resulting from non-disjunction or anaphase lag

Chromosome abnormality	No. of cases	Parental origin Paternal	Maternal
Trisomy 13	20 [9]	3 (15%)	17 (85%)
Trisomy 18	20 [10]	1 (5%)	19 (95%)
Trisomy 21	68 [11]	8 (12%)	60 (88%)
	193 [12]	9 (5%)	184 (95%)
45, XO	34 [13]	27 (79%)	7 (21%)
47, XXX	28 [14]	2 (7%)	26 (93%)
47, XXY	35 [15]	20 (57%)	15 (43%)
49, XXXXX	5 [16]	0	5 (100%)
49, XXXXY			

The story becomes even more curious if de novo chromosome deletions are considered (Table II). For example, provisional results suggest that when a child has Wolf's syndrome (4p−) as a result of a de novo deletion, this deletion will usually have occurred on the paternally derived number 4 chromosome. It may well be relevant that this is the site of the locus for Huntington's chorea, a disease in which the age of onset is influenced by the sex of the transmitting parent. Similar skewing of the parental origin is observed for de novo constitutional deletions associated with Wilms' tumour and two dysmorphic conditions – the Prader–Willi and Angelman syndromes.

For single-gene disorders, knowledge of the parental origin of new mutations is limited. However, for both neurofibromatosis and retinoblastoma it has been shown that germline mutations usually occur during spermatogenesis rather than oogenesis (Table II). Strangely, neither of these disorders shows a paternal age effect. This suggests that these mutations occur in mature spermatozoa rather than stem-cell spermatogonia. Alternatively mutations for these conditions may occur equally commonly in spermatogenesis and oogenesis, but only be expressed if they originate from the male. This is considered further in the section on genomic imprinting.

TABLE II. Parental origin of de novo single-gene mutations and micro-deletions

	No. of cases	Parental origin	
		Paternal	Maternal
Single-gene disorder			
Neurofibromatosis	14 [17]	12	2
Retinoblastoma	14 [18]	13	1
Micro-deletion			
4p− (Wolf's syndrome)	7 [19]	7	0
11p13 (Wilms' tumour)	8 [20]	7	1
15q11-13 (Angelman syndrome)	26 [21]	0	26
15q11-13 (Prader-Willi syndrome)	24 [22]	21	3

PREMUTATION

One of the most intriguing denouements and striking successes of molecular genetics in recent years has been the elucidation of the basic defect in the fragile X syndrome. This, the most common cause of inherited mental retardation, has long been a puzzle for clinical and molecular geneticists alike. The disease is characterized under the light microscope by the presence of a fragile site at the end of the long arm of the X chromosome (Xq27.3) in a proportion of cells from affected males and carrier females. Males with the full-blown syndrome are severely retarded with a prominent lower jaw, large ears and post-pubertal macro-orchidism. Approximately one-third of female carriers are mildly retarded.

Usually this disorder shows straightforward X-linked inheritance, but for some time it has been apparent that in many families unaffected male ancestors must have carried the gene and transmitted it to their offspring. This bizarre and almost unprecedented phenomenon can now be explained. It has emerged that the fragile X mutation consists of an increase in the size of a region in the first exon of the fragile X mental retardation (FMR-1) gene. A long CGG trinucleotide repeat sequence is thought to be responsible for this variation [23]. In a normal X chromosome there are on average 40 copies of this CGG triplet and these are inherited in a stable fashion. Normal transmitting males have from 55 to 125 copies, although some may have up to 200. This constitutes the clinically silent 'premutation'. Affected males generally have a much greater number of trinucleotides. This 'full mutation' is highly unstable and is often seen as a smear of multiple bands on a Southern blot [24] (Figure 1). Carrier females may have a premutation or full mutation size band in addition to their normal band (Figure 1). Some carrier females have

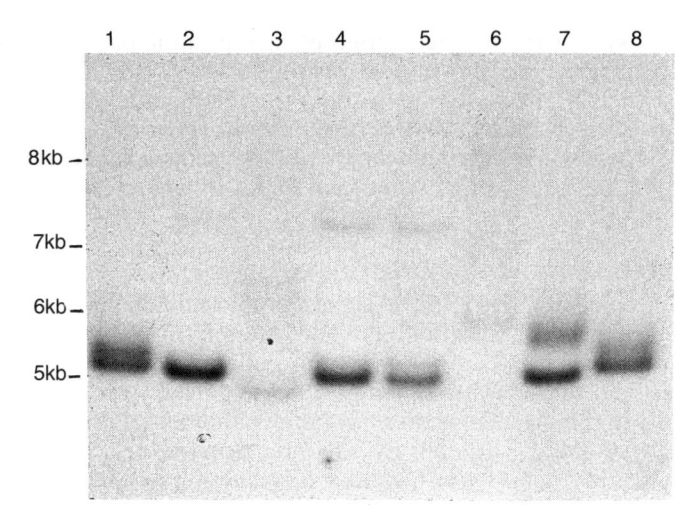

Figure 1. Fragile X affected males and carrier females. An autoradiograph of a Southern blot after hybridization with OX1.9, a probe detecting the mutable region of the FMR-1 gene.
Lanes 2 and 4: normal males - with normal size 5.1kb band.
Lanes 1, 7 and 8: female carriers - each with an additional larger band.
Lanes 3 and 6: affected males - with smears.

The faint upper bands in the normal male tracks are the result of partial enzymic digestion of the DNA, not the result of mutations. The DNA used for lane 3 was extracted from chorionic villi during prenatal diagnosis for the woman in lane 1 whose previous affected son is shown in lane 6.

We are grateful to Dr Kay Davies for providing the OX1.9 probe (Molecular Genetics Group, Institute of Molecular Medicine, John Radcliffe Hospital, Oxford).

a smear. Almost 50% of females who carry the full mutation have some degree of mental retardation, with a much lower incidence in carriers of the premutation.

In view of these observations it is now believed that the FMR-1 'premutation' is generated by an increase in the number of CGG triplets, although it is not known whether this is a consequence of amplication or of an insertion. It is believed that size increases in this region occur during meiosis in a female. The transition to a full mutation appears to need a premutation step as mothers of affected children are always carriers of either a premutation or a full mutation. The smear observed on a Southern blot is thought to be a manifestation of somatic instability of the full mutation leading to many different length mutations in the cells of the affected individual being studied.

The concept of premutation ('delayed' or 'unstable' mutation) has been proposed in humans before, notably in the context of ectrodactyly [25], but it is only with its very recent demonstration in the FMR-1 gene that a role for premutation in human disease has been established. It seems likely that unstable DNA in other genes may be the underlying explanation for several apparent idiosyncrasies of genetic diseases such as anticipation in myotonic dystrophy and variable expression in tuberous sclerosis and adult polycystic kidney disease [26]. A role for methylation in the premutation/full mutation mechanism is suggested by the observation that expression of the fragile X phenotype is associated with methylation of DNA sequences closely adjacent to the FMR-1 gene, in contrast to normal males in whom this region is not methylated [27].

MOSAICISM

The term mosaicism refers to the existence in an individual of two cell lines with differing genetic constitutions. The mosaicism may be limited to somatic or gonadal tissues or be present in both ('gonosomal' mosaicism).

Chromosomal mosaicism has long been recognized in humans but it is only recently that molecular studies have shown that mosaicism at the single-gene level may also be a relatively common occurrence. Confirmation of gonadal (germline) mosaicism has been forthcoming in several conditions, most notably Duchenne muscular dystrophy (DMD) [28]. Figure 2 shows analysis of the gene known to be defective in DMD, i.e. the dystrophin gene, in several members of a family containing a single affected case (lane 2). There is clear evidence of an altered dystrophin gene in the affected boy and it is equally clear that this is not present in the mother's blood (lane 4). However, this is present in blood from one of his sisters (lanes 1 and 3). The only possible explanation for this is that the mother must be a gonadal mosaic.

Analysis of deletions in the dystrophin gene, defects in which cause both Duchenne and Becker muscular dystrophy, has revealed that gonadal mosaicism is a relatively common occurrence. Several females have been identified [24] who do not show a deletion in DNA obtained from blood, yet have had more than one child showing the deletion, e.g. an affected son and a carrier daughter. Families have also been identified in which a healthy unaffected male has transmitted a deletion to more than one daughter [30]. For DMD observations have suggested that the risk to the brother of an affected deletion positive male whose mother is deletion negative is approximately 1 in 14, or 1 in 7 if he inherits the same X chromosome [28]. This is obviously consistent with the premise that gonadal mosaicism underlies a very significant proportion of apparently isolated 'new' mutations.

Somatic mosaicism may also be a common phenomenon and given the vast number of mitotic events occurring in the human organism it seems entirely reasonable to postulate that during pre- and postnatal life 'virtually the entire repertoire of known mutations must occur within all normal individuals' [31]. Segmental neurofibromatosis is a likely candidate, which should soon be confirmed or refuted with the recent discovery of the neurofibromatosis gene [32]. One confirmed example is provided by osteogenesis imperfecta (OI). A family has been reported in which a father with mild OI had a son with lethal disease [33]. Biochemical and molecular analysis of type I collagen from these individuals showed that the father was mosaic for the mutation which was present in non-mosaic form in the deceased son. Therefore mosaicism in a parent with the full-blown disease in

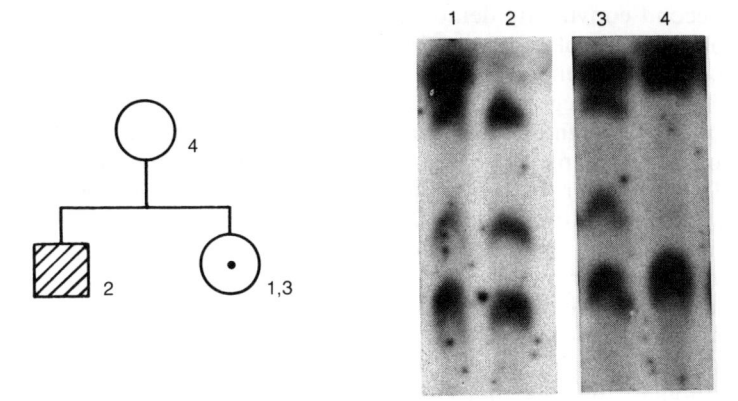

Figure 2. Germline mosaicism in a Duchenne muscular dystrophy family. An autoradiograph of a Southern-blotted pulsed field electrophoresis gel following hybridization to a dystrophin cDNA probe.

The affected boy (lane 2) has a deletion which has resulted in the absence of the top band and the appearance of 2 new bands. These extra bands are not present in the lymphocyte DNA of his mother (lane 4) who has the normal pattern. The extra bands are present, however, in the boy's sister (lanes 1 and 3), indicating that she also has inherited the deletion.

a child is another possible explanation for both anticipation and variable expression where the severity of a disease increases dramatically from parent to child.

GENOMIC IMPRINTING

The patient and confused(!) reader who has followed the story so far may well be hoping that there is a simple underlying unifying hypothesis which might help explain some of the curious observations outlined in the previous pages. Regrettably no immediate assistance is at hand, but one relatively new concept, genomic imprinting, does go a long way towards explaining some of the recently discovered vagaries of human inheritance.

It has always been assumed that genes inherited from each parent exert equal effects. Studies in mice indicate that whilst this is usually so, there are notable exceptions. Two particular pieces of evidence have shown that the expression of certain genes and chromosome segments depends on the parental origin of the genetic material. In other words the gene has a memory or 'imprint' based on whether it has passed through a paternal or maternal meiosis [34]. The first piece of evidence is based on the observed effects when all nuclear genes in an embryo are derived from only one parent [35]. If the male is the sole contributor, the embryo fails to develop normally although the placenta and membranes appear relatively normal. Conversely an embryo with two sets of maternally derived chromosomes results in an apparently healthy embryo, but with very poor extra-embryonic development. Both conditions are lethal. An analogous situation in humans is that of the complete hydatidiform mole which is derived exclusively from two paternal sets of haploid chromosomes.

The second convincing demonstration of genomic imprinting in mice is based on the study of embryos which have received both copies of a specific chromosome segment or arm from one particular parent (uniparental disomy). For some segments this has no effect: for others the result is lethality or the mouse is significantly abnormal [36]. Comparable situations have been noted in humans. Two children with cystic fibrosis have been described both of whom inherited two copies of their healthy carrier mother's cystic fibrosis allele on chromosome 7. Both children were unusual in showing quite marked short stature which is attributed to the absence of paternally imprinted genes for all or part of chromosome 7 [37, 38]. More recently a young man who inherited both number 14 chromosomes from his mother has been reported. He was of above average intelligence but had several physical abnormalities including short stature, hydrocephalus and small testes [39].

It is thought that the molecular mechanism responsible for imprinting involves differential DNA methylation during gametogenesis [40], an observation consistent with the known role of methylation in rendering one X chromosome inactive in somatic cells in the female. Methylation of cytosine nucleotides in the regulatory regions of genes renders the gene inactive by preventing the binding of transcription activators.

Imprinting and parental origin

Almost identical deletions of chromosome 15q11-13 are seen in over 50% of children with the Prader-Willi and Angelman syndromes. These deletions are derived almost exclusively from the father in the Prader-Willi syndrome and from the mother in Agelman syndrome. This suggests that loss of the same region from the paternal or maternal chromosome 15 has a totally different effect. Confirmation that this is likely to be due to genomic imprinting comes from analysis of this region of chromosome 15 in children with these syndromes who do not have cytogenetic or molecular deletions. Some of these children have been found to show uniparental disomy with both number 15 chromosomes being maternally derived in the Prader-Willi syndrome [41] and paternally derived in Angelman syndrome [42]. This suggests that it is the lack of a particular parental chromosome which results in a specific phenotypic effect.

The skewed parental origin sex ratio for chromosome loss in foetuses and children with Turner's syndrome [13] indicates that the maternal X may be more essential for embryonic survival than the paternal sex chromosome contribution. This is in keeping with the original studies in mice which showed that the maternal chromosome complement was particularly important for embryonic development.

Finally, the apparently exclusive paternal origin of de novo 4p deletions [19] correlates with existing hypotheses that the parental age effect in Huntington's chorea, the gene for which is located on chromosome 4p, is mediated via genomic imprinting [43, 44]. Another very unusual feature of Huntington's disease is that the clinical features are no more severe in homozygotes than in patients with only one copy of the abnormal gene [45]. While it is not immediately obvious how these facts interrelate, it does appear that there is something very unusual about the way in which genes at and adjacent to the Huntington's locus are expressed.

Imprinting and the fragile X syndrome
In 1987, in an attempt to explain the peculiar inheritance of the fragile X syndrome, Laird [46] proposed that the mutation locally blocks reactivation prior to oogenesis of a previously inactive X chromosome. In affected patients this imprinted region would then be more methylated and therefore less active than in a normal chromosome. Although the subsequent discovery of a premutation appears to contradict Laird's hypothesis, the discovery that expression of the fragile X mutation is associated with hypermethylation in and around the FMR-1 gene [27], coupled with the long-standing observation that expression only occurs if the gene is transmitted through a female meiosis, suggests that imprinting plays a significant role in fragile X expression. Whether the increase in the number of CGG triplets associated with disease expression is a cause or an effect of the associated changes in methylation remains to be resolved.

Imprinting and oncogenesis
Over the last few years much has been learned about underlying mechanisms in oncogenesis, particularly for childhood tumours which may sometimes have a constitutional genetic contribution such as retinoblastoma and Wilms' tumour. Two events are required for the development of these tumours. One of these may be constitutional (i.e. inherited) and the other somatic, or both may be somatic as in sporadic unilateral tumours. The first event is believed to be a mutation in the retinoblastoma gene on chromosome 13q14 or in a Wilms' tumour gene, one of which is located on chromosome 11p13. These normally act as tumour suppressors, by acting as brakes on normal cell turnover. If this mutates then the cell is primed to undergo malignant change following a second mutational event involving the normal homologue. This second event may consist of a point mutation, deletion or non-disjunction or any other mechanism which leads to loss of the normal homologue or homozygosity for the mutant allele [47, 48].

In the section on parental origin reference was made to the preferential paternal origin of new constitutional retinoblastoma mutations [19] and deletions of 11p13 in Wilms' tumour [20]. While this may simply be a reflection of the greater number of mitoses in spermatogenesis, the absence of a paternal age effect for these disorders suggests that alternative explanations should be sought. One such possible explanation is genomic imprinting with the paternally inherited allele being preferentially expressed.

For retinoblastoma supporting evidence is conflicting since parental allele loss in sporadic tumours is random [18], although in osteosarcoma, which is due to mutation at the same locus, there is a strong bias towards retention of the paternal allele [49]. This implies that the primary mutation usually occurs on the paternally derived chromosome followed by unmasking or 'liberation' of this mutation by loss of the normal homologue. In Wilms' tumour there is firm evidence that maternal alleles are preferentially lost in both sporadic and bilateral tumours [50]. This strongly suggests that expression of maternal and paternal alleles at the Wilms' tumour locus on chromosome 11p13 differs, with the most plausible explanation for this being genomic imprinting. If imprinting is found to be a significant factor in other malignancy, as has recently been shown to be the case for familial glomus tumours [51], then this will rapidly become a subject of major importance in clinical medicine.

CONCLUSION
In this relatively brief review of a complex and rapidly expanding subject, an attempt has been made to outline some of the more surprising recent observations and discoveries. In the short term these are of greatest relevance for clinical geneticists and others involved in genetic counselling, but in the long term there is good reason to believe that these new developments shall impose themselves on every branch of clinical and laboratory medicine. For example, susceptibility to insulin-dependent diabetes mellitus may well be associated with polymorphisms located at the imprinted region of chromosome 11p15 which houses the insulin and insulin-like growth factor II genes [52]. If gene therapy for conditions such as diabetes mellitus becomes a reality, as is likely given the recent demonstration of growth hormone activity following injection of genetically engineered myoblasts into mice [53], then everyone involved in clinical practice will have to become familiar with the intricacies of the 'new genetics'. It is hoped that this short introduction will go some way towards achieving that end.

REFERENCES
1 Cooper DN, Schmidtke J. Diagnosis of genetic disease using recombinant DNA. Third edition. *Hum Genet 1991; 87*: 519–560
2 Rommens JM, Iannuzzi MC, Kerem BS et al. Identification of the cystic fibrosis gene: chromosome walking and jumping. *Science 1989; 245*: 1059–1065
3 Koenig M, Hoffman EP, Bertelson CF et al. Complete cloning of the Duchenne muscular dystrophy (DMD) cDNA and preliminary genomic organisation of the DMD gene in normal and affected individuals. *Cell 1987; 50*: 509–517
4 Comings DE. Prenatal diagnosis and the 'New Genetics'. *Am J Hum Genet 1980; 32*: 453–454
5 Cooper DN, Krawczak M. The mutational spectrum of single base-pair substitutions causing human genetic disease: patterns and predictions. *Hum Genet 1990; 85*: 55–74
6 Krawazak M, Cooper DN. Gene deletions causing human genetic disease: mechanisms of mutagenesis and the role of the local DNA sequence environment. *Hum Genet 1991; 86*: 425–441
7 Haines JL, Short MP, Kwiatkowski DJ et al. Localisation of one gene from tuberous sclerosis within 9q32–9q34, and further evidence for heterogeneity. *Am J Hum Genet 1991; 49*: 764–772
8 Vogel F, Rathenerg R. Spontaneous mutation in man. In Harris H, Hirschhorn K, eds. *Advances in Human Genetics 5*. New York: Plenum Press. 1975: 223–318
9 Hassold T, Jacobs PA, Leppert M, Sheldon M. Cytogenetic and molecular studies of trisomy 13. *J Med Genet 1987; 24*: 725–732
10 Kupke KG, Muller U. Parental origin of the extra chromosome in trisomy 18. *Am J Hum Genet 1989; 45*: 599–605
11 Petersen MB, Schinzel AA, Binkert F et al. Use of short sequence repeat DNA polymorphisms after PCR amplification to detect the parental origin of the additional chromosome 21 in Down syndrome. *Am J Hum Genet 1991; 48*: 65–71
12 Antonarakis SE, Lewis JG, Adelsberger PA et al. Parental origin of the extra

chromosome in trisomy 21 as indicated by analysis of DNA polymorphisms. *N Engl J Med* 1991; *324*: 872-876
13 Hassold T, Benham F, Leppert M. Cytogenetic and molecular analysis of sex-chromosome monosomy. *Am J Hum Genet* 1988; *42*: 534-541
14 May KM, Jacobs PA, Lee M et al. The parental origin of the extra X chromosome in 47, XXX females. *Am J Hum Genet* 1990; *46*: 754-761
15 Jacobs PA, Hassold TJ, Whittington E et al. Klinefelter's syndrome: an analysis of the origin of the additional chromosome using molecular probes. *Ann Hum Genet* 1988; *52*: 93-109
16 Deng HX, Abe K, Kondo I et al. Parental origin and mechanism of formation of polysomy X: an XXXXX case and four XXXXY cases determined with RFLPs. *Hum Genet* 1991; *86*: 541-544
17 Jadayel D, Fain P, Upadhyaya M et al. Paternal origin of new mutations in Von Recklinghausen neurofibromatosis. *Nature* 1990; *343*: 558-559
18 Zhu X, Dunn JM, Phillips RA et al. Preferential germline mutation of the paternal allele in retinoblastoma. *Nature* 1989; *340*: 312-313
19 Quarrell OWJ, Snell RG, Curtis MA et al. Paternal origin of the chromosomal deletion resulting in Wolf-Hirschhorn syndrome. *J Med Genet* 1991; *28*: 256-259
20 Huff V, Meadows A, Riccardi VM et al. Parental origin of de novo constitutional deletions of chromosomal band 11p13. *Am J Hum Genet* 1990; *47*: 155-160
21 Webb T, Clayton-Smith J, Malcolm S, Pembrey M. Cytogenetic studies in Angelman syndrome - implications for the family. *Clin Genet* 1991; *40*: 379
22 Nicholls RD, Knoll JH, Glatt K et al. Restriction fragment length polymorphisms within proximal 15q and their use in molecular cytogenetics and the Prader-Willi syndrome. *Am J Med Genet* 1989; *33*: 66-77
23 Verkerk AJMH, Pieretti M, Sutcliffe JS et al. Identification of a gene (FMR-1) containing a CGG repeat coincident with a breakpoint cluster region exhibiting length variation in fragile X syndrome. *Cell* 1991; *65*: 905-914
24 Hirst MC, Nakahori Y, Knight SJL et al. Genotype prediction in the fragile X syndrome. *J Med Genet* 1991; *28*: 824-829
25 Auerbach C. A possible case of delayed mutation in man. *Ann Hum Genet* 1956; *20*: 266-269
26 Sutherland GR, Haan EA, Kremer E et al. Hereditary unstable DNA: a new explanation for some old genetic questions? *Lancet* 1991; *338*: 289-292
27 Bell MV, Hirst MC, Nakahori Y et al. Physical mapping across the fragile X: hypermethylation and clinical expression of the fragile X syndrome. *Cell* 1991; *64*: 861-866
28 Bakker E, Veenema H, Den Dunnen JT et al. Germinal mosaicism increases the recurrence risk for 'new' Duchenne muscular dystrophy mutations. *J Med Genet* 1989; *26*: 553-559
29 Wood S, McGillivray BC. Germinal mosaicism in Duchenne muscular dystrophy. *Hum Genet* 1988; *78*: 282-284
30 Darras BT, Francke U. A partial deletion of the msucular dystrophy gene transmitted twice by an unaffected male. *Nature* 1987; *329*: 556-558
31 Hall JG. Somatic mosaicism: observations related to clinical genetics. *Am J Hum Genet* 1988; *43*: 355-363
32 Wallace MR, Anderson LB, Savlino AM et al. A *de-novo Alu* insertion results in neurofibromatosis type 1. *Nature* 1991; *353*: 864-866
33 Wallis GA, Starman BJ, Zinn AB et al. Variable expression of osteogenesis imperfecta in a nuclear family is explained by somatic mosaicism for a lethal point mutation in the α1 (I) gene (COLIAI) of type I collagen. *Am J Hum Genet* 1990; *46*: 1034-1040
34 Monk M. Genomic imprinting. Memories of mother and father. *Nature* 1987; *328*: 203-204
35 Surani MAH, Barton SC, Norris ML. Influence of parental chromosomes on spatial specificity in androgenetic ↔ parthenogenetic chimaeras in the mouse. *Nature* 1987; *326*: 395-397
36 Cattanach BM, Kirk M. Differential activity of maternally and paternally derived chromosome regions in mice. *Nature* 1985; *315*: 496-498
37 Spence JE, Perciaccante RG, Greig GM et al. Uniparental disomy as a mechanism for human genetic disease. *Am J Hum Genet* 1988; *42*: 217-226
38 Voss R, Ben-Simon E, Avital A et al. Isodisomy of chromosome 7 in a patient with cystic

fibrosis; could uniparental disomy be common in humans? *Am J Hum Genet 1989; 45*: 373-380
39 Temple IK, Cockwell A, Hassold T et al. Maternal uniparental disomy for chomosome 14. *J Med Genet 1991; 28*: 511-514
40 Sapienza C, Peterson AC, Rossant J, Balling R. Degree of methylation of transgenes is dependent on gamete of origin. *Nature 1987; 328*: 251-254
41 Nicholls RD, Knoll JHM, Butler MG et al. Genetic imprinting suggested by maternal heterodisomy in non-deletion Prader-Willi syndrome. *Nature 1989; 342*: 281-285
42 Malcolm S, Clayton-Smith J, Nichols M et al. Uniparental paternal disomy in Angelman's syndrome. *Lancet 1991; 337*: 694-697
43 Reik W. Genomic imprinting: a possible mechanism for the parental origin effect in Huntington's chorea. *J Med Genet 1988; 25*: 805-808
44 Ridley RM, Frith CD, Farrer LA, Conneally PM. Patterns of inheritance of the symptoms of Huntington's disease suggestive of an effect of genomic imprinting. *J Med Genet 1991; 28*: 224-231
45 Wexler NS, Young AB, Tanzi RE et al. Homozygotes for Huntington's disease. *Nature 1987; 326*: 194-197
46 Laird CD. Proposed mechanism of inheritance and expression of the human fragile-X syndrome of mental retardation. *Genetics 1987; 177*: 587-599
47 Cavenee WK, Dryja TP, Phillips RA et al. Expression of recessive alleles by chromosomal mechanisms in retinoblastoma. *Nature 1983; 305*: 779-784
48 Orkin SH, Goldman DS, Sallan SE. Development of homozygosity for chromosome 11p markers in Wilms' tumour. *Nature 1984; 309*: 172-174
49 Toguchida J, Ishizaki K, Sasaki MS et al. Preferential mutation of paternally derived RB gene as the initial event in sporadic osteosarcoma. *Nature 1989; 338*: 156-158
50 Schroeder WT, Chao LY, Dao DD et al. Nonrandom loss of maternal chromosome 11 alleles in Wilms' tumour. *Am J Hum Genet 1987; 40*: 413-420
51 Van der Mey AGL, Maaswinkel-Mooy PD, Cornelisse CJ et al. Genomic imprinting in hereditary glomus tumours: evidence for new genetic theory. *Lancet 1989; ii*: 1291-1294
52 Julier C, Hyer RN, Davies J et al. Insulin-IGF2 region on chromosome 11p encodes a gene implicated in HLA-DR4-dependent diabetes susceptibility. *Nature 1991; 354*: 155-159
53 Barr E, Leiden JM. Systemic delivery of recombinant proteins by genetically modified myoblasts. *Science 1991; 254*: 1507-1509

GENETICS AND THE HEART

Paul JR Barton
National Heart and Lung Institute, London

MOLECULAR BIOLOGY AND THE HEART

Advances in molecular biology have resulted in rapid progress in the identification and cloning of genes involved in a wide variety of biological processes. In cardiology this has made a significant contribution to our understanding of the occurrence and distribution of many of the molecular constituents of the mycocardium, and in particular of the proteins of the contractile apparatus [1]. Moreover it has provided insight into the molecular mechanisms underlying cardiac disease, particularly that of cardiac hypertrophy. Some have heralded the advent of molecular biology as a new paradigm in cardiology of comparable importance to those marked by Starling's law and the principle of excitation-contraction coupling [2]. Several aspects of molecular biology can be identified, each of relevance to biomedical research in this field. These include molecular biology as a basic science and the application of molecular biology to questions of medical genetics.

Molecular biology as a basic science

The process of gene expression is the transmission of genetic information (coded in the DNA sequence contained in the nucleus of the cell) into the form of a cellular protein (Figure 1). The steps involved in this process start by transcription of the gene to form an RNA transcript (an RNA copy of the complete gene sequence), splicing (which involves the molecular editing of the primary RNA transcript often occurring in alternative ways) to produce one or more messenger RNA (mRNA) molecules and translation of the mRNA into a polypeptide chain. Nascent polypeptides are often subject to subsequent modification by, for example, glycosylation, phosphorylation or assembly into a multimeric unit before forming a functionally active protein.

Any one of these steps may be regulated in order to control the overall expression of a given gene, and it is the endeavour of basic molecular biology to determine how this is achieved. Three general questions are addressed in basic molecular biology: What signals control gene expression? At which step

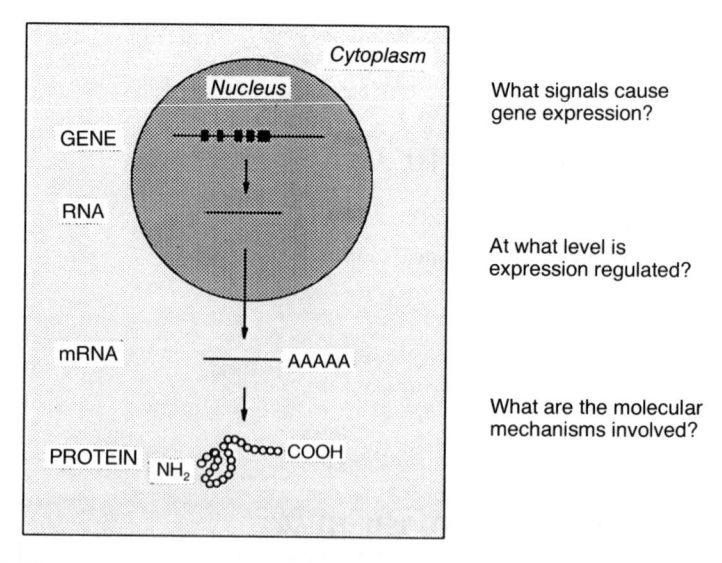

Figure 1. The process of gene expression and the principal questions addressed by basic molecular biology.

in the overall process of expression is regulation imposed? What are the molecular mechanisms involved in this regulation? Considerable effort is currently centred on these questions, much of which is concerned with transcription and the protein molecules (transcription factors) which regulate this process.

The impact of molecular biology in cardiology

A clear understanding of basic molecular biology is of considerable importance to questions of cardiac development and disease. It is now known, for example, that the heart responds to increased workload, as in the case of pressure overload hypertrophy, by regulating gene expression so as to alter the protein constituents of the contractile apparatus [3]. Most of the contractile protein genes have been cloned and the molecular regulation of their expression is a field of active research. Such studies are aimed at understanding normal patterns of regulation and how alterations in expression resulting from pressure overload are achieved. Several key elements of the hypertrophic response have been identified. Firstly, it is now well established that the altered pattern of expression seen in pressure overload hypertrophy is reminiscent of that seen during normal foetal growth [4]. Thus foetal isoforms of myosin and actin, as well as regulatory proteins including the Na, K-ATPase, are re-expressed in hypertrophy. This effect has been largely attributed to changes in gene expression due to altered transcriptional activity of the genes concerned. These changes can be reproduced in isolated cardiomyocytes in culture using a variety of stimuli including stimulation by catecholamines, phorbol esters and by direct physical stretch achieved by growing cells on the surface of deformable dishes [5]. Alterations in gene expression are also apparent in a wide variety of other disorders including dilated cardiomyopathy and end-stage heart failure, and are observed in many of the congenital malformations of the heart.

Concerning cardiac development two principal aspects are of interest [1]. Firstly, it is of importance to characterize the normal pattern of gene expression during cardiac development, both during embryonic life where cells become fixed to particular lineages, and during foetal growth where alterations in gene expression give rise to the changing characteristics of the developing myocardium [6, 7]. Secondly, it is of importance to identify those genes which play a direct role in regulating development. A rapidly increasing number of such genes have been identified and many of these play a significant role in cardiac development [8, 9]. These include growth factors such as the transforming growth factors (TGFβs), receptor molecules including the retinoic acid and growth hormone receptor families, and genes encoding transcription factors known to play a direct role in determining cell fate such as the so-called homeobox genes.

GENETIC DISEASES OF THE HEART

An increasing number of cardiac diseases are now suspected to be the direct result of genetic defects. Considerable progress has been made in our understanding of lipid metabolism and of the genes involved. For an account of the state of the art concerning genetics and lipid metabolism in relation to coronary heart disease the reader is referred to recent reviews on this subject [10, 11]. In most cases of genetic disease of the myocardium the exact lesion has yet to be defined and current interest is therefore centred on identifying families with clear modes of inheritance. Using such families it should be possible to use the techniques of gene cloning in order to locate, isolate and characterize the underlying genetic defects.

The case of familial hypertrophic cardiomyopathy (FHC)

One of the recent surprises in hypertrophic cardiomyopathy was the identification of genetic defects in myosin genes which can cause familial cases of this disease. The work leading to the definition of the myosin gene mutation is used here to illustrate the principles of this methodology of genetic analysis.

The discovery came about through a detailed genetic analysis of a large Canadian kindred with a documented history of FHC [12]. Having carried out accurate diagnosis on all existing members of the family it was possible to construct a picture of the mode of inheritance of the defective gene. Subsequent analysis concentrated on locating the position of the gene using restriction fragment length polymorphism (RFLP) markers covering the genome. This approach makes use of the fact that the DNA sequence of the genome varies between individuals, and these differences often result in the creation of sites susceptible to digestion by restriction enzymes (Figure 2). If such a site shows frequent variation in a population it is considered as being polymorphic and can be used to follow the pattern of segregation of that chromosomal region through family pedigrees (Figure 3). This is known as RFLP analysis and, by

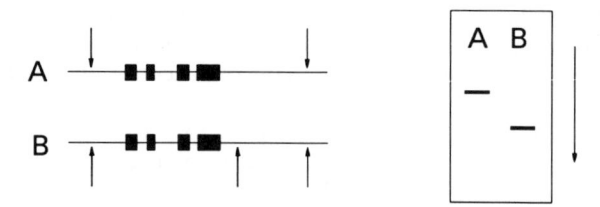

Figure 2. Detection of restriction fragment length polymorphism.
Left: the presence of an additional restriction site (vertical arrows) in the genomic DNA in B results in a change in the length of restriction fragment containing the gene (right) as detected by Southern blot analysis.

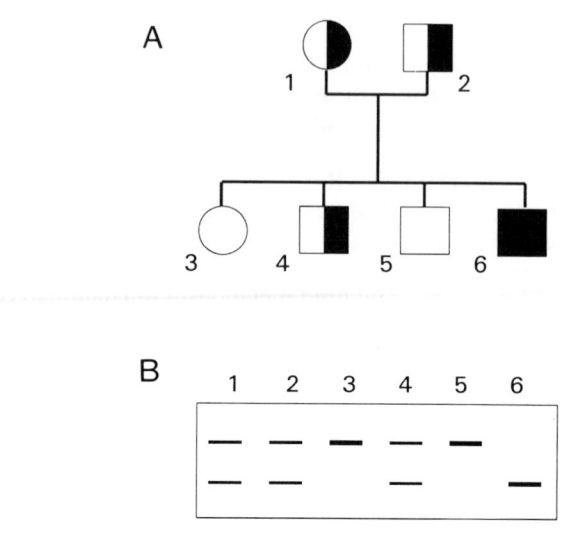

Figure 3. Analysis of a hypothetical family pedigree with a recessive gene defect (such as cystic fibrosis).
A: The family pedigree; circles denote females and squares males. Open symbols are normal individuals, part shaded symbols denote carriers and filled symbol denotes an affected child.
B: Restriction fragment length polymorphism analysis of the above pedigree. Note that in this case the mutant allele is defined by the presence of a shorter restriction fragment. Siblings 3 and 5 are therefore normal while 4 is a carrier for the disease.

using a large number of RFLP markers spread over the genome, it is usually possible to locate the position of an unknown gene by comparing its pattern of segregation relative to the RFLP markers: a gene located close to an RFLP marker will tend to co-segregate with high frequency whereas unlinked RFLP markers will show independent segregation.

In the case of the FHC pedigree, an extensive genetic analysis was carried out resulting in the identification of an RFLP marker located on chromosome 14 which shows close linkage to the FHC gene. This region of chromosome 14 contains several known genes including the cardiac isoforms of myosin heavy chain which therefore became candidates for the site of the mutation. Detailed analysis of the myosin genes in affected individuals identified a single nucleotide difference compared with unaffected individuals [13]. This difference results in an amino acid substitution in the resulting myosin protein, in a region which is otherwise highly conserved both between different myosin types and between species. This therefore defines the genetic mutation responsible for the hypertrophic cardiomyopathy in this family. The exact molecular mechanism of the resulting pathology remains obscure, however. The site of the mutation is in a region of the myosin molecule which is highly conserved but which is of unknown functional significance. The mode of inheritance of the disease is dominant (that is, affected individuals are heterozygotes and have both a normal and an abnormal allele) implying that the mutant myosin probably interferes with the function of the normal counterpart. This contrasts with recessive traits where the mutations most commonly cause loss-of-function, and where heterozygotes are usually phenotypically normal. One possibility is that the mutant myosin interferes with normal assembly of the thick filament, a suggestion which is consistent with the myofibre disarray characteristic of the disease.

Other candidates for gene defects
Idiopathic dilated cardiomyopathy
Dilated cardiomyopathy (DCM) is a disease of unknown aetiology which is characterized by dilation and impaired function of one or both ventricles, and has an estimated prevalence of 36 per 100,000 [14]. Several contributory factors have been implicated in DCM including viral infection, alcohol abuse and mitochondrial abnormalities. Moreover, the immune hypothesis of idiopathic DCM proposes an association with particular HLA (human leucocyte antigent) haplotyes [15]. Recent data now suggest that genetic factors may make a significant contribution to the disease with as many as 1 in 5 patients showing evidence of a familial trait [16]. In this report 59 index patients with idiopathic dilated cardiomyopathy were studied along with all available relatives (315 in total). Eighteen relatives from 12 families were found to have DCM suggesting that 12/59 (20.3%) of index patients had a familial form of the disease. This is considerably higher than previously suggested and raises the question as to the nature of the genetic lesion(s) involved.

The long QT syndrome
The long QT syndrome is characterized by a prolonged QT interval on electrocardiograms. Affected individuals show predisposition to recurrent fainting and sudden death at an early age resulting from ventricular tachycardia and fibrillation. The incidence of long QT syndrome in the population is uncertain but several cases of familial inheritance have been identified. Using one such family Keating et al [17] have recently localized the gene defect responsible for the disorder to chromosome 11 by linkage to the Harvey ras-1 (H-ras-1) gene locus. A total of 245 genetic markers, effectively covering over 60% of the

genome including the HLA locus, were tested in a five generation pedigree including 40 affected individuals before tight linkage to the H-ras-1 locus was found. The results suggest that the genetic lesion in this pedigree lies in extremely close proximity to the H-ras-1 gene, raising the intriguing possibility that the mutation may lie in the H-ras-1 gene itself. This is an attractive hypothesis as the H-ras-1 gene product is known to be a key player in many cell signalling pathways. Ras proteins are located on the inner surface of the cell membrane and are similar to G proteins which regulate myocardial and pacemaker ion channels. Structural analysis of the H-ras-1 gene in affected individuals in these families should, in the near future, determine whether mutations in this gene are indeed directly involved.

Congenital malformations of the heart
Congenital heart disease constitutes the largest category of birth defects. There is therefore considerable interest in defining in which cases the underlying cause can be attributed to specific genetic lesions. Molecular biology has provided significant advances in our understanding of the regulation of early development and numerous genes involved in regulating cell differentiation and growth have now been identified. Many of these constitute candidates for genetic lesions causing congenital heart defects. Those malformations suspected to have a genetic cause include atrioventricular septal defect, hypoplastic left heart syndrome and isomerism.

In some cases a genetic contribution is evident due to the presence of chromosomal abnormalities which are visible at the cytological level. The most obvious case is that of Down's syndrome where trisomy of chromosome 21 results in the developmental abnormalities associated with this syndrome, including atrioventricular defects. Identification of the gene(s) involved in this disorder is an intense area of research, and this is assisted by a mouse model resulting from trisomy of mouse chromosome 16. This model displays many of the characteristics of Down's syndrome including developmental abnormalities of the atrioventricular septum. In the case of DiGeorge's syndrome chromosomal deletions of chromosome 22 are believed to be responsible for multiple developmental abnormalities [18] which include interrupted aortic arch type B and truncus arteriosus.

CLINICAL RELEVANCE
The most immediate benefit of defining genetic lesions which underlie familial disease is in the field of genetic counselling. DNA analysis of family members can provide both accurate diagnosis (including prenatal diagnosis) and carrier detection. This can be of particular value in providing diagnosis prior to onset of symptoms thereby offering the potential for preventative treatment. In severe diseases it offers the option of early termination of pregnancy. It should be stressed, however, that the application of genetic information to clinical practice requires a clear understanding of the molecular mechanism of the pathology, particularly if the disease has a late onset or where differing degrees of severity are observed due to variable expression or incomplete penetrance. For an in-depth discussion of these questions and of the future

prospects of techniques in gene therapy the reader is referred to the excellent account given by Weatherall [19].

REFERENCES

1. Barton PJR. Molecular biology and the heart. In Yacoub MH, Pepper JR, eds. *Annual of Cardiac Surgery 1990-1991*. London: Current Science. 1991: 3-12
2. Molecular biology in cardiology, a paradigmatic shift (editorial). *J Mol Cell Cardiol 1988; 20*: 355-366
3. Nadal-Ginard B, Mahdavi V. Molecular basis of cardiac performance. *J Clin Invest 1989; 84*: 1693-1700
4. Izumo S, Nadal-Ginard B, Mahdavi V. Protooncogene induction and reprogramming of cardiac gene expression produced by pressure overload. *Proc Natl Acad Sci USA 1988; 84*: 339-343
5. Komuro I, Kaida T, Shibazaki Y et al. Stretching cardiac myocytes stimulates protooncogene expression. *J Biol Chem 1990; 265*: 3595-3598
6. Lyons GE, Schiaffino S, Sassoon D et al. Developmental regulation of myosin gene expression in mouse cardiac muscle. *J Cell Biol 1990; 111*: 2427-2436
7. Barton PJR, Moscoso G, Thompson RP. Detection of myosin gene expression in the developing heart using probes derived by polymerase chain reaction. *Int J Cardiol 1991; 30*: 116-118
8. Parker TG, Schneider MD. Growth factors, proto-oncogenes, and plasticity of the cardiac phenotype. *Ann Rev Physiol 1991; 53*: 179-200
9. Litvin J, Montgomery M, Gonzalez-Sanchez A et al. Commitment and differentiation of cardiac myocytes. *Trends in Cardiovascular Research 1991; 2*: 27-32
10. Assmann G. Genes and dyslipoproteinaemias. *Heart J 1990; 11 (Suppl H)*: 4-8
11. Breslow JL. Lipoprotein transport gene abnormalities underlying coronary heart disease susceptibility. *Ann Rev Med 1991; 42*: 357-371
12. Jarcho JA, McKenna W, Pare JAP et al. Mapping a gene for familial hypertrophic cardiomyopathy to chromosome 14q1. *N Engl J Med 1989; 321*: 1372-1378
13. Geisterfer-Lowrance AAT, Kass S, Tanigawa G et al. A molecular basis for familial hypertrophic cardiomyopathy: a β cardiac myosin heavy chain gene missense mutation. *Cell 1990; 62*: 999-1006
14. Codd MB, Sugrue DD, Gersh BJ, Melton LJ III. Epidemiology of idiopathic dilated and hypertrophic cardiomyopathy: a population-based study in Olmsted County, Minnesota 1975-1984. *Circulation 1989; 80*: 564-572
15. Bender JR. Idiopathic dilated cardiomyopathy. An immunologic, genetic, or infectious disease, or all of the above? *Circulation 1991; 83*: 704-706
16. Michels VV, Moll PP, Miller FA et al. The frequency of familial dilated cardiomyopathy in a series of patients with idiopathic dilated cardiomyopathy. *N Engl J Med 1992; 326*: 77-82
17. Keating M, Atkinson D, Dunn C, et al. Linkage of a cardiac arrhythmia, the long QT syndrome, and the Harvey *ras*-1 gene. *Science 1991; 252*: 704-706
18. Wilson DI, Cross IE, Goodship JA et al. DiGeorge syndrome with isolated aortic coarctation and isolated ventricular septal defect in three sibs with a 22q11 deletion of maternal origin. *Br Heart J 1991; 66*: 308-312
19. Weatherall DJ. *The New Genetics and Clinical Practice*. Oxford: Oxford University Press. 1991: 376 pp

CLINICAL GENETICS APPLIED TO ASTHMA

Julian Hopkin
Osler Chest Unit, Oxford

Asthma is characterized, clinically, by episodic breathlessness with chest tightness and, physiologically, by a state of labile airflow obstruction [1]. Airway calibre shows variability of at least 15% but in many individuals may amount to 30-40% reversible decline in expiratory flow measurements, such as peak flow rate, during a 24 hour spell [2]. Ten per cent of the population may suffer from asthma of some degree during their lives which causes 2000 deaths per year in Britain.

Asthma is a syndrome rather than a disease and has distinct underlying causes. Foremost amongst these is atopy [3, 4], the state of allergic responsiveness to common inhaled dusts that include pollens and the house dust mite. Atopic individuals suffer from asthma, rhinitis and eczema in variable combination; 95% of asthmatics between the ages of 5 and 40 are atopic [5].

In any form of established asthma, there is an increased responsiveness of the airways to a variety of non-specific insults (triggers) that can include cold air, exercise, emotion and irritant fumes. Histological studies on post-mortem material and biopsies taken at fibreoptic bronchoscopy demonstrates that bronchial inflammation is characteristic of asthma [6-8]. In atopy, inflammation is based on allergic reaction to a broad array of common, otherwise innocuous, inhaled antigens that include different plant pollens, house dust mite faecal particles, respirable moulds and danders from a variety of animals, e.g. the cat in the home environment or rat or mouse in the research laboratory. In experiments on bronchial challenge with antigen, an immediate response occurs with swift development of airflow obstruction but also, after recovery, the development of prolonged bronchial hyper-responsiveness, the late reaction [9]. One characteristic feature of atopic responsiveness is exuberant production of immunoglobulin E (IgE) to such common inhaled antigens [10]. IgE is produced by all individuals in response to helminth infection when it again mediates intense local inflammation which plays a protective role in the killing of parasites [11] and is unique amongst the immunoglobulins in having a site at its Fc region with very high affinity for mast cells but also lesser affinity for T- and B-lymphocytes, monocytes and eosinophils [12, 13]. Allergen specific IgE, bound to mast cells in the bronchial epithelium, reacts with its target antigen resulting in activation and degranulation of the mast cell with the release of a number of molecular mediators that cause the immediate inflammatory response and by interaction with CD4 T-lymphocytes and eosinophils, the late bronchial inflammatory response [14–16].

GENETICS

The cellular and molecular mechanisms that underlie the production of IgE, its binding to various cells but especially the mast cell, and the events that follow its interaction with antigens and subsequent degranulation of the mast cell, have been the focus of direct, intense study. Recognition of the key molecules that control these processes will offer the hope for new strategies of more effective prevention and treatment of disease. A complementary approach to the recognition of primary controlling elements in this complex process is genetic investigation. If there is a major genetic effect determining the development of asthma, mediated at one or two gene loci, then molecular genetic methods now offer the power of localizing and subsequently identifying such gene loci and their protein products [17, 18]. In cystic fibrosis (CF), genetic segregation and linkage analyses laid the foundation for identifying the genetic locus on chromosome 7 at which mutations cause CF [19].

One fundamental question therefore is how strong is any genetic influence on the development of asthma or perhaps underlying *atopy* or allergic response. Familial aggregation suggests that genetic factors may play a significant role; the interpretation of the results of the many genetic studies conducted is, however, hampered by the variety of disease or immunological phenotypes used.

Clinical disease

Studies confining their methods to questionnaire ascertainment of an established diagnosis of asthma show an incidence as low as 15% in the first degree relatives of asthmatics, whereas the community prevalence of asthma using the same methods may be 5% or more [20]. Therefore, with the rare exception of apparent dominant inheritance of asthma in certain kindreds [21], there is no evidence that clinical asthma is due to a single gene effect. In a study of histamine bronchial responsiveness in healthy infants, a positive family history as well as cigarette smoking both contributed significantly to the risk of bronchial responsiveness [22]. In a Finnish study of adult twin pairs [23] concordance for asthma was higher amongst monozygotic than dizygotic twins and has led to an estimate of *heritability* (that proportion of aetiology attributable to genetic factors) of 36% for asthma.

Extension of the clinical phenotype to include rhinitis and eczema, in similar studies, leads to an impression of a more important genetic effect on the development of atopy than asthma per se (one of its manifestations).

The early reports of Cooke and Van der Veer [3] emphasized familial clustering of atopy and they suggested a dominant mode of inheritance, based on the recognition of clinical disease (one or more of asthma, rhinitis or hay fever and eczema), though this conclusion was disputed by others. A recent genetic study, basing the recognition of atopy on clinical symptoms alone, found no pattern of simple Mendelian inheritance in a large sample of Finnish families; 50% of atopic children were born into families with no family history of disease [24].

However, the atopic state does seem to be an idiosyncratic one. Thus most atopics (70% or more) are reactive to more than one allergen [4, 25] suggesting their sensitization is not simply the result of chance allergen exposure; their risk of becoming sensitized to other antigens, e.g. certain occupational agents such as small mammal antigens in laboratory workers, is clearly different from non-atopics. Ninety-five per cent of animal laboratory workers developing symptoms within the first year of work were atopic; 40% of atopics entering such work became sensitized within the year but only 3% of non-atopics, judged by negative skin tests to common inhaled antigens [26].

In a twin study documenting asthma, seasonal rhinitis, skin test response, total serum IgE levels and specific RAST IgE, maximum likelihood tests of genetic and environmental components, based on concordance for these characters in mono- and dizygous twins, suggested a predominant genetic effect on the development of atopy with a lesser contribution from common environmental effects [27].

Total IgE levels

Much investigation of the genetics of atopy has focused on direct assay of IgE responsiveness. Measurement of total serum IgE, by solid phase immunoassay, offers one method of phenotype analysis, though its skewed continuous distribution and influences by age and smoking make perfect discrimination of atopic from non-atopic impossible [28, 29]. Despite this a decisive genetic effect on this continuous measurement was demonstrated in a study of over 7000 adult and childhood twins; the intra-pair variance of IgE levels was found to be smaller in monozygotic (identical) than dizygotic twins and the estimate of *heritability* for total serum IgE was 59% for adults and 79% for children [30]. Family studies of total serum IgE levels have led to conflicting conclusions on mode of inheritance. Some investigators found that segregation favoured autosomal recessive inheritance [31]; later supported by complex path and segregation analysis [32], but this was disputed by others whose findings supported dominant inheritance [33] or no consistent pattern [34]. It is likely that the arbitrariness of assigning atopy by this continuous variable accounts for the variable findings and conclusions; it is also common clinical experience that many symptomatic atopic individuals with clear IgE response to specific allergens may have levels of total IgE within the designated normal range [35].

Atopic IgE responsiveness

Because a significant proportion of atopic individuals, with specific allergen sensitization and typical bronchial or nasal symptoms, show low total IgE levels we have conducted in Oxford [36] a re-evaluation of the inheritance of generalized IgE responsiveness, identifying this state by either elevated total serum IgE or positive skin test or IgE specific (RAST) to any one or more common antigens including house dust mite, grass and tree pollens, respirable moulds and animal danders. Individuals were therefore designated IgE responsive or atopic if they satisfied any one of three tests (Table I). Using these criteria, 87% of designated atopics were found to have some symptoms in keeping with asthma or rhinitis of some degree although only 30% had an established clinical diagnosis of asthma or hay fever; in the adult population, only 40% of the designated atopics had an elevated total IgE level. A series of nuclear and extended families were examined, encompassing 1000 individuals.

TABLE I. Criteria for designation of atopic IgE responsiveness

Response to *any* one or more common allergens: house dust mite, pollens, moulds, danders	Skin prick test wheal 2mm>control IgE RAST>0.35 RAST units/ml
or Raised total IgE	>1SD above age-related geometric mean (children) >100kU/l (non-smoking adults)

Firstly, in a comparative study of the parents of asthmatic children and control subjects it was found that 90% of the atopic asthmatic children had one or both parents who could be identified themselves as IgE responsive [36, 37]. This evidence of vertical transmission, suggestive of autosomal dominant inheritance, was observed repeatedly in extended families, though the frequency of atopy complicates the pattern by introducing doubly affected marriage pairs and the likelihood of homozygosity for atopy. Sixty-two per cent of children from marriages between one atopic and one non-atopic parent were atopic, in keeping with dominant inheritance of a frequent disorder.

Interactive effects

A notable observation in these families demonstrating dominant inheritance of atopic or generalized IgE responsiveness was that the patterns of allergen specific IgE responses and clinical disease were quite variable within families [38]. This indicates that dominantly inherited atopic IgE responsiveness must interact with other factors to determine the pattern of specific response in any particular individual and hence clinical disease. Current evidence suggests that the predominant interactive factors are HLA variation in determining pollen sensitivity [39, 40] and hence rhinitis (since pollen grains are 20–40µm diameter and impact in the nose), but allergen exposure dosage in determining house dust mite sensitization [41] and hence asthma (respirable house dust mite pellets are generally 10µm in diameter and deposit in the bronchi).

Marsh [39, 40] has shown that correlation between particular HLA-D types (or immune response genes) and sensitization to particular allergens became stronger with more precise definition, by fractionation, of the test antigenic fragment; 95% of individuals sensitized to a 5000 molecular weight antigen from short ragweed (*Ambrosia artemisiifolia*, Amb a V) were found to be Dw2 positive. No linkage was found between general IgE responsiveness, assayed by total IgE level, and the HLA locus. The observed strong association between an HLA Class II variant and specific responsiveness to a low molecular weight antigenic fragment is in keeping with the now well-delineated function of these molecules in the co-presentation of processed foreign antigen by macrophages and other antigen presenting cells to CD4 helper T-lymphocytes as a central part of the development of specific immunity. Thus HLA Class II molecules mediate this process, but it remains to be determined how important the genetic variants at HLA loci are in determining overall risk of sensitization to varying doses of complex allergens, with many epitopes, in atopic individuals.

In an analysis of atopic sibling pairs discordant for house dust mite sensitization [41], those sensitized to the mite were found to have significantly greater levels of major mite allergens in their bed mattresses than their atopic but non-mite sensitized siblings.

ATOPY AND CHROMOSOME 11q

To test the model that atopic IgE responsiveness is determined by mutations at a single gene locus with a pattern of dominant inheritance, molecular genetic linkage studies were conducted. One of the fundamental laws of genetics (Mendel's second law) states that different gene loci are independently assorted at meiosis and the formation of gametes, except when genes are very closely aligned on any chromosome. This exception to the law of independent assortment, the co-transmission of alleles at proximate gene loci, is called *genetic linkage*. With the advent of techniques that have allowed the recognition of structural variants of DNA (particularly variation in lengths over certain non-coding sequences, termed restriction fragment length polymorphisms, RFLPs) there is the opportunity to test models of inheritance stringently and to assign loci conferring disease to chromosomal regions efficiently [17]. The probability that *genetic linkage* exists, and therefore that a disease locus is close to a particular test DNA marker, is generally expressed as a lod score (the log of the odds) and may be positive (favouring linkage) or negative (opposing linkage).

The segregation of atopy in our families was therefore compared with segregation of alleles from various loci demonstrating restriction fragment length polymorphisms. Negative lod scores were obtained with all but one of the first 17 probes tested; the exception was co-segregation of atopy with alleles from a polymorphic segment of DNA (MS.51) [42] which had previously been assigned by in situ hybridization to chromosome 11q13. A lod score of 5.6 was obtained in seven extended families providing a conservative probability of $p<0.0002$ favouring linkage in this data set [43]. To test the presence of genetic linkage further, analysis was conducted on over 60 young nuclear families; youth is associated with a clearer atopy phenotype; and clinical and total IgE data are not as frequently marred by cigarette smoking as in some older British families. An aggregate lod score of 3.8 was obtained from these nuclear families, supporting genetic linkage of atopy to the chromosome 11q locus [44]. A test for *genetic heterogeneity* (the possibility that atopy might be inherited at loci other than the 11q locus in some of the families) was performed; an estimate was obtained that atopy was inherited at the 11q locus in some 60% (95% confidence interval) of these young British families who demonstrated the typical clinical and immunological features of atopy [44].

Since then, a group from Osaka in Japan have shown a lod score of 4.9 for linkage between atopy and the same genetic marker MS.51, on chromosome 11q [45].

CONCLUSIONS

A more coherent picture of the genetics of asthma is emerging. The immunological phenotype of generalized IgE responsiveness (characteristic of atopy and which is the principal cause of asthma in older children and young adults) can be inherited as a dominant character at an, as yet unidentified, locus on chromosome 11q and which is within 10cM of the DNA test marker, MS.51. It is also clear that inherited generalized IgE responsiveness must interact with other factors to determine the pattern of allergen specific response and of clinical disease in any particular individual; genetic variation HLA Class II molecules and allergen exposure dosage are relevant (Figure 1).

Currently, the function of the chromosome 11q locus protein product remains speculative. The high prevalence of alleles conferring atopy (30–40% of any population are usually atopic) suggests that the mutations may have conferred advantage in some populations and it is possible that the character of ready response to a small amount of antigen, incorporating the production

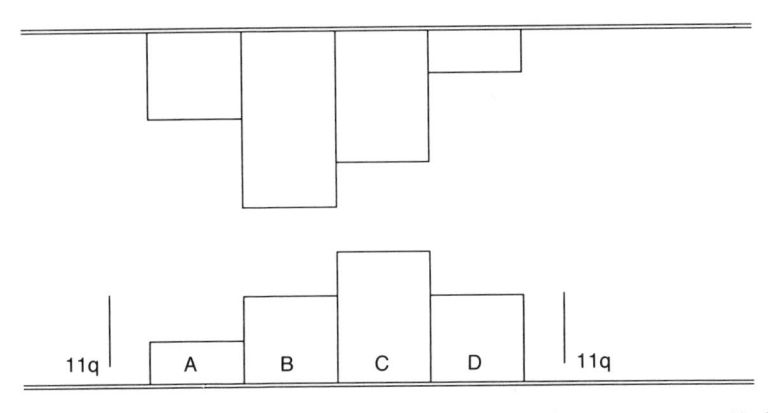

Figure 1. Representation of the possible pattern of interaction of the chromosome 11q locus with HLA locus action and allergen dosage in determining allergen specific sensitization in an individual. Avidity of HLA molecules for specific allergens is shown at the roof of the cage and dosage of the same allergens (A–D) is shown at the floor of the cage with increasing depth and increasing height representing, respectively, increasing avidity and increasing allergen exposure. Allergic response to any allergen is predicted to result when vertical overlapping occurs. The action of the 11q locus is to symmetrically lift the floor of the cage making overlap for any allergen more likely but without producing sufficient elevation to cause universal sensitization.

of IgE, might have offered significant protection against helminthic gut infestation. If the process of *reverse genetics* (in which the identification of a disease locus is based on the preliminary step of genetic linkage) can be applied successfully to the 11q locus, as in the case of cystic fibrosis on chromosome 7, then our understanding of allergic response and possibilities for new modes of prevention and treatment of asthma should be significantly enhanced.

REFERENCES

1. Clark TJH, Godfrey S. In *Asthma* 2nd edn. London: Chapman & Hall. 1983: 457–489
2. Holgate ST. Cellular and mediator mechanisms in asthma. In Borysiewicz LK, ed. *Horizons in Medicine No 2.* Cambridge: University Press. 1990: 1–15
3. Cooke RA, Van der Veer AJn. Human sensitization. *J Immunol 1916; 1*: 201–305
4. Stenius B, Wide L, Seymour W et al. Clinical significance of specific IgE to common allergens. *Clin Allergy 1971; 1*: 37–55
5. Dolovich J, Hargreave FE. The asthma syndrome: Inciters, inducers and host characters. *Thorax 1981; 36*: 641–644
6. Dunnill MS, Massarell GR, Anderson JA. A comparison of the quantitative anatomy of the bronchi in normal subjects in status asthmaticus in chronic bronchitis and in emphysema *Thorax 1969; 24*: 176–179
7. Beasley R, Roche WR, Roberts JA, Holgate ST. Cellular events in the bronchi in mild asthma and after bronchial provocation. *Am Rev Respir Dis 1989; 139*: 806–817
8. Djukanovic R, Roche WR, Wilson JW et al. Mucosal inflammation in asthma. *Am Rev Respir Dis 1990; 142*: 434–457
9. Pepys, J, Hutchcroft BJ. Bronchial provocation tests in the etiologic diagnosis and analysis of asthma. *Am Rev Respir Dis 1975; 112*: 829–859
10. Ishizaka K. Mechanisms of reaginic hypersensitivity. *Clin Allergy 1971; 1*: 9–24
11. Ogilvie BM. Reagin-like antibodies in animals immune to helminth parasites. *Nature 1964; 204*: 91–92
12. Metzger H, Alcaraz G, Hohman R et al. The receptor with high affinity for immunoglobulin E. *Ann Rev Immunol 1986; 4*: 419–470
13. Yodoi J, Hosoda M, Maeda Y et al. Low affinity IgE receptors: regulation and functional roles in cell activation. In *IgE, Mast Cells and the Allergic Response* (Ciba Foundation Symposium 147). Chichester: John Wiley & Sons. 1989: 133–152
14. Azzawi M, Bradley B, Jeffrey PK et al. Identification of activated T lymphocytes and eosinophils in bronchial biopsies in stable atopic asthma. *Am Rev Respir Dis 1990; 142*: 1407–1413
15. Kay AB, Ying S, Varney V et al. Messenger RNA expression of the cytokine gene cluster, IL-3, IL-5 and GM-CSF in allergen-induced late phase cutaneous reactions in atopic subjects. *J Exp Med 1991; 173*: 775–778
16. Venge P. What is the role of the eosinophil. *Thorax 1990; 45*: 161–163
17. Botstein D, White RL, Sholnik M, Davis RW. Construction of a genetic linkage map in man using restriction fragment length polymorphisms. *Am J Hum Genet 1980; 32*: 314–331
18. Little P. Finding the defective gene. *Nature 1986; 321*: 558–559
19. Rommens JM, Iannuzzi MC, Kerem B-S et al. Identification of the cystic fibrosis gene; chromosome walking and jumping. *Science 1989; 245*: 1059–1065
20. Sibbald B, Turner-Warwick M. Factors influencing the prevalence of asthma in first degree relatives of extrinsic and intrinsic asthmatics. *Thorax 1979; 34*: 332–337
21. Zhang DQ. An extensive pedigree of autosomal dominant inheritance of bronchial asthma. *Chung Hua Chieh Ho Ho Hu Hsi Tsa Chih 1989; 12*: 280–281
22. Young S, Le-Soeuf PN, Geelhoed GC et al. The influence of a family history of asthma and parental smoking on airway responsiveness in early infancy. *N Engl J Med 1991; 324*: 1168–1173
23. Nieminen MM, Kaprio J, Koskenvuo M. A population-based study of bronchial asthma in adult twin pairs. *Chest 1991; 100*: 70–75

24 Luoma R, Koivikko A. Occurrence of atopic disease in three generations. *Scand J Soc Med 1982; 10*: 49-56
25 Young RP. *House Dust Mite Sensitization: Genetic and Environmental Factors*. DPhil Thesis, University of Oxford. 1991
26 Botham PA, Davies GE, Teasdale EL. Allergy to laboratory animals: a prospective study of its incidence and of the influence of atopy on its development. *Br J Int Med 1987; 44*: 627-632
27 Hanson B, McGue M, Roitman-Johnson B et al. Atopic disease and immunoglobulin E in twins reared apart and together. *Am J Hum Genet 1991; 48*: 873-879
28 Holford-Strevens V, Warren P, Wong C, Manfreda J. Dystrophin: the protein product of the Duchenne muscular dystrophy locus. *Cell 1984; 51*: 919-928
29 Kjellman N-I, Johansson GO, Roth A. Serum IgE levels in healthy children quantified by a sandwich technique (PRIST). *Clin Allergy 1976; 6*: 51-59
30 Bazarel M, Orgel HA, Hamburger RN. Genetics of IgE and allergy: serum IgE levels in twins. *J Allergy Clin Immunol 1974; 54*: 288-304
31 Marsh DG, Bias W, Ishizaka K. Genetic control of basal serum immunoglobulin E level and its effect on specific reaginic sensitivity. *Proc Natl Acad Sci 1974; 71*: 3588-3592
32 Gerrard J, Rao D, Morton N. A genetic study of immunoglobulin E. *Am J Hum Genet 1978; 30*: 46-58
33 Blumenthal MN, Namboodiri N, Mendell N et al. Genetic transmission of serum IgE levels. *Am J Med Genet 1981; 10*: 219-228
34 Kuno-Saki H. Total serum IgE and specific IgE antibodies in children with bronchial asthma. *Ann Allergy 1986; 56*: 488-491
35 Meyers DA, Hasstedt SJ, Marsh DG et al. The inheritance of immunoglobulin E. *Am J Med Genet 1983; 16*: 575-581
36 Cookson WOCM, Hopkin JM. Dominant inheritance of atopic immunoglobulin-E responsiveness. *Lancet 1988; i*: 86-88
37 Hopkin JM. The genetics of atopy. *Clin Exp Allergy 1989; 19*: 1
38 Hopkin JM, Cookson WOCM, Young RP. Asthma, atopy and genetic linkage. In Piper PJ, Krell RD, eds. *Advances in the understanding and treatment of asthma*. *Ann New York Acad Sci 1991; 629*: 26-30
39 Marsh DG, Meyers DA, Friedhoff LR. HLA-Dw2: a genetic marker for human immune response to short ragweed pollen allergen Ra5 II. Response after ragweed immunotherapy. *J Exp Med 1982; 155*: 1452-1463
40 Ansari AA, Shinomiya N, Zwollo P, Marsh DG. HLA-D gene studies in relation to immune responsiveness to a grass allergen Lol p III. *Immunogenetics 1991; 33*: 24-32
41 Young RP, Hart BJ, Merret TG et al. House dust mite allergy: interaction of genetic factors and dosage of allergen exposure. *Clin Exp Allergy 1992; 22*: 205-211
42 Royle NJ, Clarkson R, Wong Z, Jeffreys AJ. Preferential localisation of hypervariable minisatellites near human telomeres. *HCGM9* (Proceedings of the 9th International Workshop on Human Gene Mapping). Basle: Karger. 1987: 685
43 Cookson WOCM, Sharp PA, Faux JA, Hopkin JM. Linkage between immunoglobulin E responses underlying asthma and rhinitis and chromosome 11q. *Lancet 1989; i*: 1292-1295
44 Young RP, Sharp PA, Faux JA et al. Confirmation of genetic linkage between atopic IgE responsiveness and chromosome 11q. *J Med Genet 1992; 29*: 236-238
45 Shirakawa T, Morimoto K, Hashimoto T et al. Linkage between IgE responses underlying asthma and rhinitis (atopy) and chromosome 11q in Japanese families. *XIth International Workshop on Human Gene Mapping*. London: ICRF. 1991

GENETIC MARKERS FOR POLYPOSIS COLI

MG Dunlop
Western General Hospital, Edinburgh

INTRODUCTION
Familial adenomatous polyposis (FAP) has an incidence rate of around 1:8000 and is the most common autosomal dominant heritable syndrome predisposing to cancer in which the gene defect has been characterized. Around 30% of all cases are new mutations, suggesting the presence of a large target gene, or perhaps a mutational 'hotspot'. The phenotypic characteristics of the disease include colorectal adenomatosis (typically greater than 100 polyps), duodenal, periampullary and small bowel adenomas, gastric hyperplastic polyps as well as adenomas, craniofacial osteomas, focal retinal pigmentation, desmoid tumours, epidermoid cysts and an excess incidence of brain tumours and of thyroid carcinoma in females. This paper reviews briefly the use of some of the clinical and molecular genetic markers in the context of their value in preclinical diagnosis of FAP.

CLINICAL MARKERS
Three clinical features of FAP are of practical value in preclinical diagnosis FAP, namely craniofacial osteomas, epidermoid cysts and focal pigmentation of the retina known as congenital hypertrophy of the retinal pigment epithelium (CHRPE). Although the presence of epidermoid cysts could never be used as a screening tool, it is mentioned here to emphasize the importance of the development of such lesions in childhood as a marker of FAP.

Craniofacial osteomas in association with FAP were first noted by Gardner [1] and have been demonstrated in up to 93% of cases [2, 3], such that it is now routine practice in some centres, particularly in Japan, to carry out bone surveys in family members at risk of FAP. The appearance of osteomas tends to precede the onset of polyps and so in at-risk individuals, the presence of osteomas can be taken to indicate that the patient is indeed affected, even if polyps have yet to become apparent. In individuals presenting to the dentist or oral surgeon with multiple osteomas but no family history of FAP, serious consideration should be given to the need for screening of the colon as the patient may be a sporadic case of FAP. Screening for osteomas by orthopantomogram is not particularly accurate, with a positive predictive value of 81% and a negative predictive value of 77%, due to the incidence of osteomas in the general population of between 4% and 16% [2, 3]. However, screening for FAP in such a manner can be used as an aid to conventional colonic screening and in genetic linkage analysis (see below). It is also vital that physicians, dentists and oral surgeons are aware of the association.

Multiple epidermoid cysts are also part of the FAP phenotype, originally thought to indicate the separate syndrome of Gardner's syndrome. However, as in the case of osteomas, when an active search is made, these lesions are common in all forms of familial adenomatous polyposis. The term sebaceous cyst has been used to describe these lesions but since this is a generic term including epidermoid and pilar cyst as well as steatocystoma multiplex, the lesions are best referred to as epidermoid cysts which are the only type associated with FAP [4]. In one study, they were detected by careful examination of the whole skin in 53% of all cases of FAP [5] and 33% have had one or more lesions removed in childhood [4]. An average of four cysts tend to occur on the face and scalp in FAP patients but in non-FAP cases the number of lesions is smaller, occurring in an older age group and more frequently on the back [5]. The appearance of an epidermoid cyst on the face or scalp of a prepubescent child should be regarded with some interest as these lesions are very uncommon in this age group when not associated with familial adenomatous polyposis.

Focal areas of retinal pigmentation known as CHRPE are now well described in association with polyposis coli [6–8]. Four types of lesions, usually affecting both eyes, can be detected: (1) multiple, small, black, flat, well-demarcated areas (as in Figure 1, individual II-1). (2) large areas of flat brownish-black pigmentation, usually fewer in number than in (1) (Figure 1, individual III-1); (3) large areas of pigmentation as in (2) but with patches of depigmentation (as in I-1); (4) areas of pigmentation intermediate between (1) and (2) with a surrounding depigmented halo. Few CHRPE lesions in FAP have been examined histologically but the smaller pigmented lesions (as in (1) above) exhibit hypertrophy of the pigment epithelial cells with increase in the size of the pigment granules within these cells and degeneration of the overlying photoreceptors. The CHRPE lesion with surrounding halo has been shown to consist of a hamartomatous growth of thinly myelinated axons and astrocytes in addition to hyperpigmentation of the pigment layer. The lesions have not been reported as causing symptoms or affecting visual fields or acuity.

CHRPE lesions are best visualized by indirect ophthalmoscopy as they are frequently peripheral. The CHRPE phenotype does allow presymptomatic diagnosis of the disease with some accuracy; 55–100% of gene carriers exhibit the feature when three or more lesions are considered positive [7–9]. Clearly CHRPE is a useful tool for demonstrating the presence of FAP but it is of lesser value in excluding inheritance of the mutant gene. It is also important to note that CHRPE lesions also occur in normal controls but whereas some patients with FAP have less than three CHRPE lesions, no normal controls

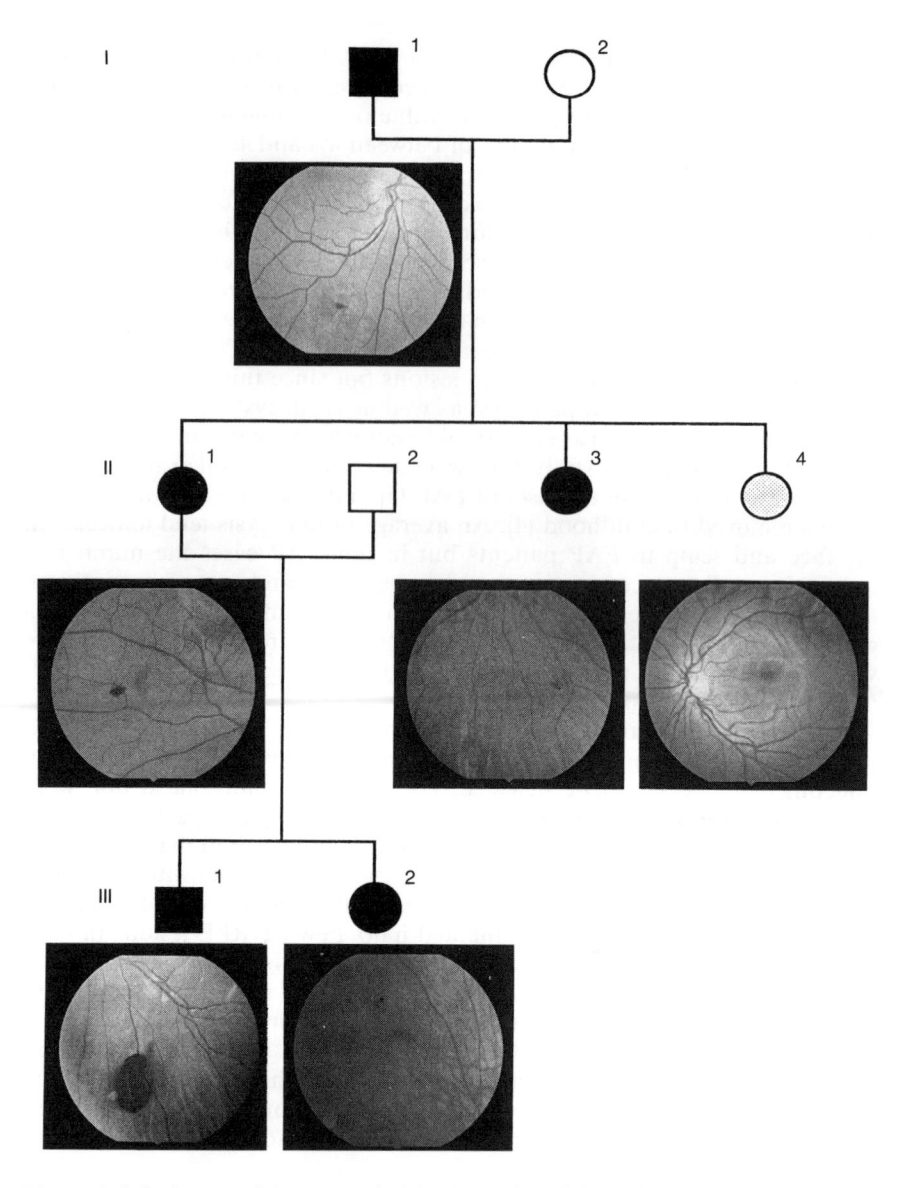

Figure 1. Inheritance of the congenital hypertrophy of the retinal pigment epithelium phenotype in a three generation FAP kindred. A normal fundal photograph is shown for individual II-4 for comparison.

were shown to have more than three in one study [7]. The presence of multiple typical CHRPE lesions in an at-risk individual must be considered to indicate the presence of the disease. Conversely, in some FAP families none of the gene carriers have CHRPE lesions [8]. By combining the detection rate of CHRPE in the above studies, it is possible to calculate that the presence of four or more CHRPE lesions in an at-risk individual has a positive predictive value of >99% but absence of the phenotype has a predictive value of non-gene carrier status of 90%, even in a family in which CHRPE is expressed as part of the trait. This level of risk is insufficiently accurate to influence current colonic screening but it can be combined with data from linked DNA markers to give highly accurate and complementary information [10, 11].

MOLECULAR GENETIC MARKERS

The offspring of patients affected by FAP have a 50% chance of inheriting the gene defect and so screening by regular endoscopy of the large bowel in such individuals is recommended from around the time of puberty until the age of 30 years. Some authors suggest screening should continue until 60 years of age. This burden could be radically altered by molecular genetic analysis of DNA purified from peripheral blood leucocytes. There are substantial numbers of individuals who could benefit from such genetic analysis since the incidence rate of FAP is around 1 in 8000 live births. This section discusses the methods of DNA analysis available.

Only two cytogenetic lesions in FAP have been reported to date [12, 13] and so chromosome analysis will never be of any value in the diagnosis of the disease. However, one of these reports was first to indicate the likely presence of the gene for FAP (known as *APC*) on the long arm of chromosome 5 [12]. This was followed up by the demonstration of genetic linkage to chromosome 5q markers [14, 15] and subsequent generation and linkage mapping of new markers from that region [16, 17]. In suitable families, these *linked markers* can be used in the clinical setting to provide a measure of the risk of having inherited the mutant gene from an affected parent. However, although the accuracy can approach 100%, it is not a definitive diagnosis [10, 11].

Following the fine linkage mapping studies, a massive effort on the part of two centres in the USA and one in Japan has resulted in the identification and sequencing of the gene responsible for FAP [18–21]. To date, mutations have been reported in nine FAP families. The potential value and drawbacks of direct mutation analysis as a preclinical marker for FAP are discussed below. Mutation analysis and risk assessment by linked DNA markers should not be considered in isolation and it is important that the two analyses are seen as complementary.

Linked DNA markers

Any of the markers which were originally generated and used in the process of identification of *APC* can be used to provide preclinical diagnosis of FAP. The problem with the use of such markers is that a number of affected and unaffected family members have to be sampled to provide data for even one at-risk family member. In addition, not all of the markers are informative in every family. However, a number of highly polymorphic linked markers which are very close to, and within, *APC* have recently been identified, which means that almost all families can benefit from the technique. Unfortunately, the offspring of cases due to new mutation will not benefit because there are insufficient relatives affected.

There is an inherent inaccuracy in the use of linked probes for diagnostic purposes. This inaccuracy is due to the occurrence of crossing-over to genetic material between homologous chromosomes at the time of meiosis and is a function of the genetic distance between the marker locus and the *APC* gene. The proportion of such crossing-over out of all meioses studied is known as the recombination fraction. If there is a recombination fraction of 5% between a probe and *APC*, then the probe will predict disease status correctly in 95% of tests carried out. The accuracy of the risk estimation can approach 100% when markers mapping to both sides of the *APC* gene are used. This is particularly so when clinical data are included in the estimation of risk [10]. A simple example of the use of linked markers is shown in Figure 2 and the family members correspond to those in Figure 1. YN5.48 and pi227 flank *APC* and have recombination fractions of 3% and 10% respectively. Therefore it can be calculated that since the boy inherited the A2, YN5.48 allele and the A2, pi227 allele from his mother, the risk is 99.7% that he is affected. III-1 was only 8 years of age but confirmation that he has inherited the mutant *APC* allele is indicated by the presence of multiple diagnostic CHRPE lesions (Figure 1). A more complex, though fundamentally similar, analysis is shown in Figure 3. The marker probes have been arranged into groups which are inherited together and are known as haplotypes. There has been a cross-over between the marker C11P11 and *APC*, serving to emphasize the importance of obtaining data from flanking probes. The stippled haplotype is associated

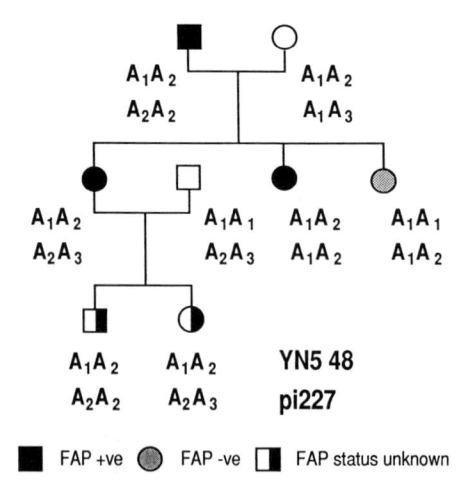

Figure 2. Preclinical diagnosis of individuals III-1 and III-2 using linked DNA probes YN5.48 and pi227. The family members correspond to those shown in Figure 1.

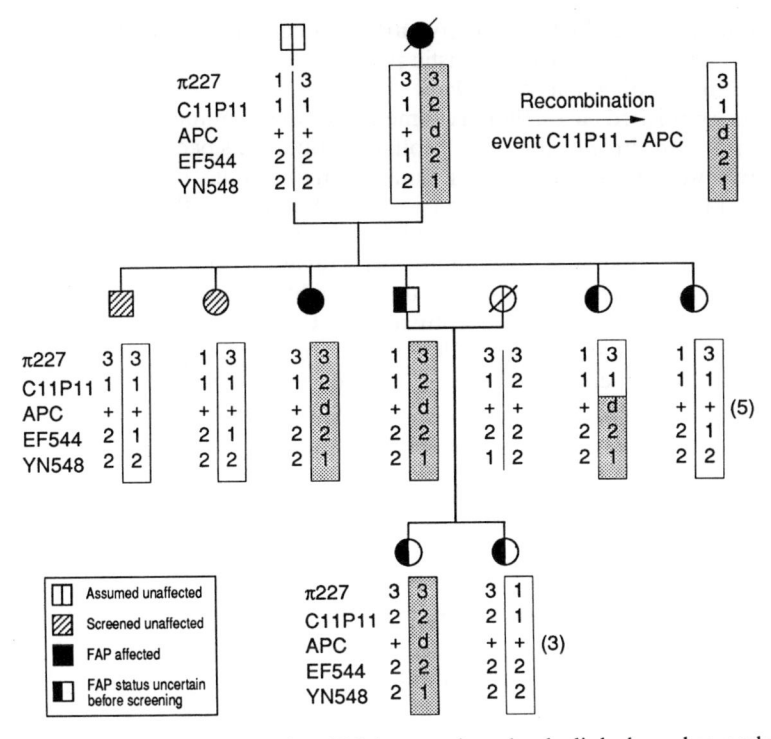

Figure 3. 5-locus haplotypes at the *APC* locus using closely linked marker probes. A recombination has occurred in one individual, stressing the importance of analysing each family with probes which map to both sides of *APC*.

with the mutant *APC* allele and each of those inheriting it was subsequently shown to have colonic polyposis.

Genotype data from linked markers could allow a substantial reduction in the frequency of screening procedures required for those with low risk although clinical screening could not be abandoned altogether. Conversely, those shown to be affected could be informed that they had inherited the mutant gene and followed up closely until polyps appeared when surgical intervention could be planned. Following the recent characterization of the *APC* gene, it seems even more likely that closely linked markers will still be required. There appears to be no 'hotspot' for mutation within the gene and so the task of searching the whole gene for a mutation in each family may prove too onerous for all but a few families (see below). Even when a mutation is identified in a family, it would be advisable to have independent confirmation from linked marker data.

Identification of mutations

The gene responsible for familial adenomatous polyposis is large, with 15 exons containing a coding sequence of around 8.5 kilobases of DNA with a predicted amino acid sequence 2843 residues long [18, 19]. There are no signs that mutations are clustered in any particular codon, or even exon, of the *APC* gene [20, 21]. This may cause logistic problems in the use of mutation analysis for preclinical diagnosis of FAP.

In the published cases, there is some clustering of mutations at position 302 in exon 8 with three of the nine published mutations occurring at that point. However, we have only found this mutation in one family out of 43 in a Scottish population. The techniques used in identification of the mutation in this patient are shown in Figure 4. Details of the principles and methodology of these techniques are not given in this brief review as they are widely available in the literature. The initial screen used was by the identification of a single strand conformational polymorphism (SSCP) change in DNA amplified by the polymerase chain reaction (PCR). The position of the mutation was then confirmed by a chemical cleavage mismatch technique using hydroxylamine and osmium tetroxide (HOT). The complete exon 8 was then sequenced from PCR amplified DNA and a heterozygous G to A (C to T in the reverse, transcribed direction) mutation can be seen. Clearly such analysis is time consuming and expensive but if the mutations were clustered in only a few exons, it may be practical to use mutation analysis for preclinical diagnosis of FAP. However, the mutations reported in the literature to date were identified in nine different families and eight of these resulted in the generation of a stop codon either directly or downstream of the mutation by frameshift. Due to

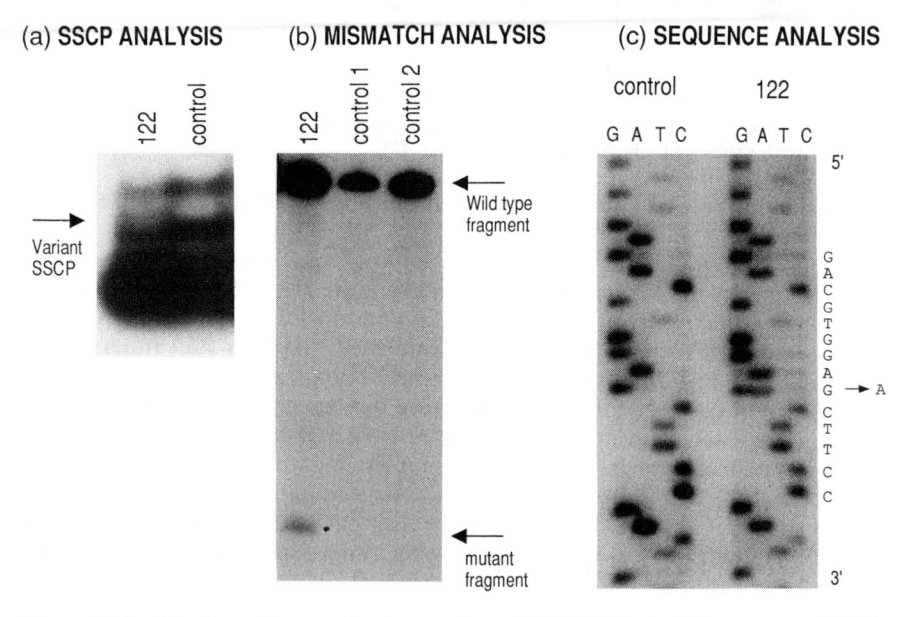

Figure 4. Identification of a mutation in a patient with FAP. The initial screen was SSCP analysis (a) followed by a chemical cleavage technique (b) and final confirmation by sequencing of PCR amplified DNA (c). The heterozygous mutation is a G to A change, or C to T in the opposite direction which is the direction of transcription, and results in an in-frame CGA(Arg) to TGA(stop codon).

the dramatic effect of a stop codon on expression of the gene, there is no tendency for mutational 'hotspots' to occur as might be expected in regions of functional importance were the mutations to result in amino acid changes. Hence it is likely that mutations will be scattered throughout the gene and so mutation analysis may only be possible for a minority of FAP families. Until the full characterization of all the different types of mutations involving *ACP* and their relative frequency has been established, most preclinical diagnosis will continue to be carried out by use of linked markers.

CONCLUSIONS

Genetic markers for familial adenomatous polyposis are not merely of academic interest. Cancer can be prevented by appropriate screening and prophylactic surgery. It is vital for the astute physician, ophthalmologist and dentist to be aware of the association of epidermoid cysts, craniofacial osteomas and CHRPE lesions with FAP since patients present with these conditions outside the confines of a screening programme. Several sad, preventable deaths have arisen in our own series. One patient presented with troublesome mandibular osteomas 10 years before returning with an inoperable colonic cancer at the age of 40. Clinical awareness is all the more important since 30% of all cases are new mutations which can never be identified by DNA analysis and will continue to rely on clinical means for their detection. DNA analysis holds much for the future. New highly informative markers are now available and so most families will benefit. Definitive diagnosis of at-risk individuals by mutation analysis may be available to some centres with an academic interest but until the epidemiology of *APC* mutations within the FAP patient population has been established, it will not be widely accessible.

ACKNOWLEDGEMENTS

Thanks to Dr J Prosser for the example of the HOT technique used in *APC* mutation analysis.

REFERENCES

1 Gardner EJ. A genetic and clinical study of intestinal polyposis, a predisposing factor for carcinoma of the colon and rectum. *Am J Hum Genet 1951; 3*: 167–176
2 Utsonomiya J, Nakamura T. The occult osteomatous changes in the mandible in patients with familial polyposis coli. *Br J Surg 1975; 62*: 45–51
3 Bulow S, Sondergaard JO, Witt IN et al. Mandibular osteomas in familial polyposis coli. *Dis Colon Rectum 1984; 27*: 105–108
4 Leppard BJ, Bussey HJR. Epidermoid cysts, polyposis coli and Gardner's syndrome. *Br J Surg 1975; 62*: 387–393
5 Leppard BJ. Epidermoid cysts and polyposis coli. *Proc Roy Soc Med 1974; 67*: 1036–1037
6 Blair NP, Trempe CL. Hypertrophy of the retinal pigment epithelium associated with Gardner's syndrome. *Am J Ophthalmol 1980; 90*: 661–667
7 Chapman PD, Church W, Burn J, Gunn A. The detection of congenital hypertrophy of the retinal pigment epithelium (CHRPE) by indirect ophthalmoscopy; a reliable clinical feature of familial adenomatous polyposis. *Br Med J 1989; 298*: 353–354
8 Polkinghorne PJ, Ritchie S, Neale K et al. Pigmental lesions of the retinal pigment epithelium and familial adenomatous polyposis. *Eye 1990; 4*: 216–221
9 Iwama T, Mishima Y, Okomato N, Inoue J. Association of congenital hypertrophy of the

retinal pigment epithelium with familial adenomatous polyposis. *Br J Surg 1990; 77*: 273-276

10 Dunlop MG, Wyllie AH, Steel CM et al. Linked DNA markers for presymptomatic diagnosis of familial adenomatous polyposis. *Lancet 1991; 337*: 313-316

11 Burn J, Chapman P, Delhanty J et al. The Northern region genetic register for familial adenomatous polyposis coli; use of age of onset, CHRPE and DNA markers in risk calculations. *J Med Genet 1991; 28*: 289-296

12 Herrera L, Kakati S, Gibas L et al. Gardner Syndrome in a man with an interstitial deletion of 5q. *Am J Med Genet 1986; 25*: 473-476

13 Hockey KA, Mulcahy MT, Montgomery P, Levitt S. Deletion of chromosome 5q and familial adenomatous polyposis. *J Med Genet 1989; 26*: 61-68

14 Bodmer WF, Bailey CJ, Bodmer J et al. Localisation of the gene for familial polyposis coli on chromosome 5. *Nature 1987; 328*: 614-616

15 Leppert M, Dobbs M, Scambler P et al. The gene for familial polyposis maps to the long arm of chromosome 5. *Science 1987; 238*: 1411-1413

16 Nakamura Y, Lathrop M, Leppert M et al. Localization of the genetic defect in familial adenomatous polyposis within a small region of chromosome 5. *Am J Hum Genet 1988; 43*: 638-644

17 Dunlop MG, Wyllie AH, Nakamura Y et al. Genetic linkage map of 6 polymorphic DNA markers around the gene for Familial Adenomatous Polyposis on chromosome 5. *Am J Hum Genet 1990; 47*: 982-987

18 Joslyn G, Carlson M, Thliveris A et al. Identification of deletion mutations and three new genes at the Familial Polyposis locus. *Cell 1991; 66*: 601-613

19 Kinzler KW, Nilbert MC, Su L-K et al. Identification of FAP locus genes from chromosome 5q21. *Science 1991; 253*: 661-665

20 Groden J, Thliveris A, Samowitz W et al. Identification and characterization of the Familial Adenomatous Polyposis Coli gene. *Cell 1991; 66*: 589-600

21 Nishisho I, Nakamura Y, Miyoshi Y et al. Mutations of chromosome 5q21 genes in FAP and colorectal cancer patients. *Science 1991; 253*: 665-669

DIABETES: ARE WE DOING BETTER THAN 10 YEARS AGO?

Stephen Tomlinson
The Manchester Diabetes Centre, Manchester

INTRODUCTION

Diabetes affects 1-2% of the population in the UK but its prevalence is much higher in some ethnic groups such as Asians and Afro-Caribbeans. The prevalence of diabetes amongst people from the Asian sub-continent is three- to fourfold higher than it is amongst whites, and in people of Afro-Caribbean origin it is two to three times higher than it is amongst whites. Moreover, the prevalence of diabetes in Asians over the age of 60 may be as high as 25%. The incidence of both type I and type II diabetes is increasing. Mortality has been shown to be increased in diabetes largely as a result of heart disease and renal failure; the risk of blindness is increased tenfold compared with non-diabetics and there is at least a 15-fold increase in the risk of amputation. There are important problems associated with diabetes in pregnancy, especially an increased risk of congenital malformations in the infants of diabetic mothers. Some 50% of men under the age of 40 with insulin-dependent diabetes are said to be impotent. Both diabetic ketoacidosis and hypoglycaemia are acute complications which sometimes need hospital admission and diabetes causes prolonged stays in hospital as a result of foot problems. There can be major social problems associated with employment, eligibility for driving licences and insurance, as well as the psychological consequences of chronic illness. In Central Manchester it has been calculated that the inpatient costs per annum for diabetes are at least £2 million per year and extending this to the North Western Region as a whole this comes to around £40 million per year. Nationally, this figure would reach almost £600,000,000 and if other costs are added such as outpatient costs, benefits, etc., the total is nearer £1,000,000,000 [1-3].

The importance of diabetes as a health problem has been recognized both nationally and internationally: the St Vincent Declaration of 1989 established both general goals for people with diabetes and 5-year targets [4] and the problem of diabetes has been highlighted in the recent publication *The Health of the Nation*. There has been major investment in diabetes care in the last 10–20 years, especially in relationship to management of chronic complications: because of the availability of chronic ambulatory peritoneal dialysis and renal transplantation people with diabetes need no longer die of chronic renal failure; blindness is largely preventable with appropriate use of laser treatment; furthermore, patient education, more effective use of antibiotics and improved surgical management have reduced the need for major amputations, and a teamwork approach has changed the outlook in diabetic pregnancy.

Large sums of money have been invested in a new approach to diabetes care which makes much more effective use of health care professionals as well as doctors; diabetes specialist nurses have an increasing role as educators and both dietitians and chiropodists figure much more prominently in care plans than they used to. There has been major capital investment in diabetes centres which provide open access for patients and which are aimed at prevention of problems through education and self-care. The Health Service reforms have encouraged GPs to become much more involved in diabetes and many GPs now run their own diabetes mini-clinics. Has all this investment in new technology, manpower, buildings and changed approaches to management shown any signs of benefit?

MORTALITY AMD MACROVASCULAR COMPLICATIONS OF DIABETES

Between 1914 and 1922 the life expectancy of somebody with newly-diagnosed insulin-dependent diabetes (IDDM) was not more than 3 years. Following the discovery and widespread availability of insulin, this increased to 26 years in 1930 and to around 60 years in 1960. By the 1970s there had been a 40% reduction in mortality over a period of about 50 years but this was still associated with a marked increase in relative mortality. Recent evidence suggests that this relative mortality is largely associated with proteinuria, with a twofold increase in people with IDDM without proteinuria and a 100-fold increase in mortality in people with proteinuria [5]. From the onset of proteinuria to death in IDDM is of the order of 8 years and mortality is 15% per annum. Thus proteinuria appears to be a key prognostic indicator in diabetes. The main cause of death in these patients is coronary artery disease – in patients with type I diabetes associated with proteinuria up to 40% of deaths before the age of 50 are due to cardiovoascular disease. Undoubtedly, therefore, there is a link between mortality caused by type I diabetes and proteinuria and the mortality is not simply a consequence of renal failure but mainly of coronary artery disease. The reduction in mortality due to IDDM over the last 50 years or so may be partly a consequence of the reduction in the incidence of nephropathy; for example, it has been shown that the incidence of nephropathy in people with IDDM of 15 years' duration fell from 24% in 1957 to 11% in 1987 [6]. It is clear, therefore, that mortality from IDDM has declined, that life expectancy is still reduced and that proteinuria is a sign of poor prognosis. The relationship between proteinuria and coronary artery disease is not clear; it may be related to associated dyslipidaemia and changes in mechanisms of blood coagulation or thrombolysis.

Recent studies using death certification did not show a decline in mortality from diabetes in men over 45, but did show a small reduction (11.5%) in women. However, in people aged less than 45 there has been an overall decline in mortality between 1975 and 1985 of 31% in men and 24% in women. This is partly a result of a reduction in mortality due to ischaemic heart disease of 18% in men and 23% in women, a relatively modest improvement in mortality compared with non-diabetics where mortality due to ischaemic heart disease has fallen by 31% in men and 40% in women [7]. It can be inferred from these data, therefore, that any overall decline in mortality due to diabetes, especially that related to ischaemic heart disease, has occurred in younger people and that this may reflect the decline in mortality in insulin-dependent diabetes, as described above, rather than non-insulin-dependent diabetes (NIDDM). This is confirmed by no improvement in the average reduction in life expectancy in NIDDM, which has remained at 7–8 years for people diagnosed between the ages of 40–59 and 3–6 years for those diagnosed over the age of 60 between the years 1975 and 1988 [8]. As with IDDM, the causes of coronary artery disease in NIDDM have not yet been defined but they may be multifactorial and include obesity, dyslipidaemia and hypertension as well as the diabetes itself [9].

MICROVASCULAR COMPLICATIONS OF DIABETES
Renal disease
A reduction in cumulative incidence of nephropathy has been reported in successive cohorts of people with insulin-dependent diabetes in the last 20–40 years (see above). A recent study from Leicester confirms this impression of a declining incidence in diabetic nephropathy [10]. This may be a result of increased emphasis on metabolic control and management of hypertension. Hypertension in particular is now recognized to play a major role in accelerating deterioration of renal function once proteinuria develops; furthermore, reduction in blood pressure has been shown to slow the rate of progression and decrease proteinuria. Before the widespread use of chronic ambulatory peritoneal dialysis (CAPD) people with established renal failure died; indeed in the early 1980s it was reported that 25% of deaths in people less than 31 years old were secondary to diabetic nephropathy [11]. A joint British Diabetic Association, Renal Association and Royal College of Physicians working party on diabetic renal failure in 1988 reported that in the UK, 273 people with diabetes had started renal replacement treatment in 1985 compared with 199 in 1984, 160 in 1983 and 106 in 1982 [12]. At the Manchester Royal Infirmary there are currently about 20 people with diabetes on CAPD, representing 15% of the total number on this form of renal replacement treatment, and over 100 patients have been managed on CAPD in the last 5 years: about 50% have NIDDM and the proportion is increasing. Between the years 1985 and 1987, 10 people with diabetes underwent renal transplantation, representing 3.5% of the total number of renal transplants, whereas between 1988 and 1990, 31 people with diabetes were treated in this way, 7% of the total. This trend towards more active management of renal failure in diabetes, with CAPD being seen as a prelude to renal transplantation, will continue.

Diabetic retinopathy
Sight-threatening diabetic retinopathy is unfortunately still relatively common. After excluding all people with known retinopathy a survey at the Manchester Royal Infirmary Diabetic Clinic in 1986 revealed 5% of approximately 700 patients with sight-threatening retinopathy. In Nabarro's personal series of almost 7000 patients betwen 1954 and 1988, the number of people with sight-threatening retinopathy remained constant at about 8 patients per year but there was a striking reduction in blindness after 1970 [13]. This reduction in blindness coincided with the advent of photocoagulation and he was able to observe in people with insulin-dependent diabetes a reduction in blindness from 2.84 to 1.21 patients per year. Similarly, there was a reduction in blindness in people with non-insulin-dependent diabetes from 1.74 to 0.63 patients per year. With improvements in glycaemic control, and increasing awareness of the importance of screening for diabetic eye disease, as well as effective treatment, up to 80% of blindness due to diabetes might be preventable. The relevant importance of maculopathy in people with type II diabetes will increase.

Foot problems of diabetes
Diabetes may now account for the majority of non-traumatic lower limb amputations. Foot problems due to diabetes are the commonest cause for diabetes-related hospital admissions; at the Manchester Royal Infirmary an average length of stay of 42 days has been recorded for patients with diabetes proceeding to lower limb amputation. There is evidence that many amputations are preventable. Prevention depends upon the identification of the foot at risk which means determining whether there is neuropathy and/or impaired vascular supply; the establishment of multi-professional foot clinics which include chiropodists, nurses, orthotists, physicians and surgeons, with the implementation of educational programmes, has been shown to reduce amputations by up to 50% [14, 15].

Data on the prevalence of risk factors such as impaired sensation and vascular occlusion are difficult to interpret because of differences in populations studied and methods of detection.

Outcome of pregnancy [16–18]
One of the main achievements in the management of diabetes over the last 50 years has been the steady decline in foetal mortality from almost 30% in the 1940s to 15% in the 1950s, 10% in the 1960s and just over 2% in the 1980s; however, this is still more than twice that of the non-diabetic. Several studies have shown that this improvement seems to be related to better glycaemic control throughout pregnancy. There is now good evidence that optimal glycaemic control in the first trimester of pregnancy can reduce the incidence of congenital anomalies in the infants of mothers with diabetes.

The obstetric/diabetes team at the Diabetes Centre and St Mary's Hospital, Manchester, have been able to increase vaginal deliveries from 23% to 50% of of babies per annum, reduce elective caesarean sections from 55% to 20% and reduce the need for prolonged stays in intensive care (longer than 24 hours) from 38% to 13% of all babies delivered. These successes largely relate to a team of highly motivated, committed and enthusiastic health care professionals working in partnership with the mothers through education and intensive monitoring and management.

DIABETES CENTRES AND DELIVERY OF CARE [19-21]

Diabetes Centres mean different things to different people; it may be a room or rooms within the hospital environment set aside for the provision of education of people with diabetes usually by diabetes specialist nurses and dietitians; at the other extreme, it might be a conversion or a purpose-built centre on or off the hospital site which provides a focus for all outpatient diabetes activities. In most circumstances it provides a location for enthusiastic health professionals to come together for the common purpose of providing first-class care for people with diabetes. It is the diabetes team which is essential not a Diabetes Centre. The key element in the provision of care from a Centre is ease of access; ease of access to the traditional once- or twice-weekly diabetic clinic was impossible and direct comparison between the two kinds of health care delivery is considered by some to be unfair. With the advent of the new GP contract and the health service reforms a more valid approach would be comparison (both in terms of cost and effectiveness) between care provided exclusively in GP diabetes mini-clinics or in Diabetes Centres with shared care.

The Diabetes Centre in Manchester is on the Manchester Royal Infirmary, Royal Manchester Eye Hospital and St Mary's Hospital site. It is a conversion from two semi-detached houses with a Portakabin addition, the total capital cost being £190,000 in 1988. The traditional diabetic clinic was abandoned when the Diabetes Centre was opened in 1988. The Centre is open 5 days a week from 9.00 to 5.00 and there is a drop-in and telephone advice facility, as well as an out-of-hours facility via a British Telecom radio pager. There are medical, nursing, dietetic and chiropody sessions and specialist renal, ophthalmological and psychosexual clinics. The joint obstetric service is partly based in the Centre and partly in St Mary's Hospital next door. A foot clinic attended by a physician, chiropodist, orthotist and specialist foot nurse is held in the Foot Hospital, 5 minutes from the Centre.

When the Centre first opened there were 2300 patients on the register and there are now 3400. Each patient attends an average of 1.5 medical sessions per year, 3 nursing sessions per year and a dietetic and chiropody session every couple of years. Recently the dietetic input has been increased and we anticipate that we should be able now to fulfil the objective of one dietetic contact per annum for each patient. Interestingly this increased dietetic input has been followed by a 10% reduction in people with NIDDM on oral hypoglycaemic agents representing a saving of almost £12,000 on the drugs bill.

The Centre is a focus for education not only for patients but also for health care professionals. There are regular sessions held for nurses locally and nationally, and a newly established weekend course for practice nurses. A distance learning package is being developed which will be associated with a structured course, including continuing education for all kinds of nurses.

Focusing attention upon the educational needs of practice nurses is a reflection of the increasing involvement of general practice in the delivery of health care for people with diabetes. The diabetes team has been much involved in helping GPs to establish mini-clinics and in providing access to advice for GPs and practice nurses which has helped to establish good working relationships. These working relationships have been further enhanced by the appointment of a GP nurse facilitator whose responsibility it is to ascertain the needs of the local GPs which will be important in defining contracts. Built into the contracts will be a major element of quality assessment which will depend very much upon the established computerized database that includes the patients' demographic details, and comprehensive clinical and biochemical information, as well as data which will provide the basis for activity analysis; the clinical information system in the Centre is to be linked into the hospital patient administration system (PAS) so that the impact of the outpatient service on inpatient episodes can be evaluated. The information accumulated in this way not only has major service implications but provides opportunities for developing our clinical research programmes.

Of course the delivery of care and its evaluation has to be linked to the costing of the service. Detailed costing of the revenue consequences of the Centre has been undertaken by our Finance Department and the grand total in terms of cost per patient per year comes to about £150. The mean cost per contact, irrespective of type is, therefore, approximately £30 per patient. The grant total revenue consequence for the Centre is just over £400,000 but this applies only to the diabetes service based in the Centre and does not include onward tertiary referrals for evaluation and treatment of retinopathy, nephropathy (e.g. dialysis, transplantation, etc.), macrovascular disease (e.g. cardiac, peripheral vascular) or pregnancy. The costing, therefore, is for the core service and tertiary and inpatient costs would have to be added on as appropriate. Furthermore, there is no element built into the costs above for further development of the service.

GLYCAEMIC CONTROL, PATIENT KNOWLEDGE AND PATIENT SATISFACTION

With the increasing recognition that microvascular complications are associated with hyperglycaemia, major efforts have been made to help the patients improve glycaemic control. Many studies have shown that this is possible in the short to medium term. At the Manchester Diabetes Centre over the last 5 years there has been a highly significant fall in glycated haemoglobin from 10.9% to 10.3%; the fall in people with insulin-dependent diabetes has been relatively modest from 10.8% to 10.5% whereas people with non-insulin-dependent diabetes have shown an improvement from 10.9% to 10.2%. With an increasing emphasis on education, attempts have been made to analyse whether knowledge of diabetes has improved amongst patients. From our own studies it is very clear that knowledge scores amongst people with non-insulin-dependent diabetes are much worse than those with insulin-dependent diabetes. This is partly related to a decline in knowledge with age which occurs irrespective of the type of treatment used. Improvements in knowledge have been observed in relationship to the significance of different levels of blood sugar, the link between blood sugar and complications and some aspects of diet; nevertheless on the whole results have been disappointing and it may be that attitudes, beliefs and behaviours are more important than factual knowledge.

With the opening of the Diabetes Centre in Manchester there have been major improvements in patient satisfaction which have been sustained over a period of 3 years [22]. For example, 91% of patients reported that opening times in the Diabetes Centre were better than in the old clinic, 97% thought that the environment was better, 79% that waiting times were better, 79% that the information and education they received was better, and 83% that the clinical care they were receiving was better. Perceptions of clinical care have also improved: only 86% of patients recognized that their diabetes was being checked in the old clinic but in the Diabetes Centre 98% recognized that this is one of the purposes of their visit; the number of people who reported that their feet were checked increased from 29% in the clinic to 77% in the Centre, that their eyes were checked from 54% to 85%, that their kidneys were checked from 18% to 56% and that their heart and circulation were checked from 49% to 91% of patients.

CONCLUSIONS

There is no doubt, therefore, that there have been improvements in mortality due to diabetes but this is mainly in people with insulin-dependent diabetes and is probably attributable to reductions in death, especially from heart disease but also from chronic renal failure. Mortality amongst people with non-insulin-dependent diabetes remains high and is largely attributable to coronary artery disease. Some aspects of morbidity have improved including blindness from retinopathy and amputations as a consequence of peripheral neuropathy and occlusive vascular disease. There is now a great deal of evidence that spectacular improvements in outcome of pregnancy are possible in women with diabetes.

Finally, following reorganization of a diabetes service with the emphasis on a multiprofessional approach, patient education and self-care, it is possible to demonstrate improvements in glycaemic control, patient knowledge of diabetes, and satisfaction with the service being provided. Although it remains to be established what the long-term significance of these improvements will be in terms of outcome, the teamwork approach to diabetes care and Diabetes Centres are here to stay.

REFERENCES

1. Borch-Johnsen K, Kreiner S, Deckert T. Mortality of Type 1 (insulin-dependent) diabetes mellitus in Denmark. A study of relative mortality in 2,930 Danish type I diabetic patients diagnosed from 1933 to 1972. *Diabetologia* 1986; 29: 767–772
2. Gries FA. NIDDM – prevalence, incidence, complications, prevention. The impact of arteriosclerotic complications. *Giornale Italiano di Diabetalogia* 1990; 10 (suppl): 21–25
3. Gerard K, Donaldson C, Maynard A. The cost of diabetes. *Diabet Med* 1989; 6: 164–170
4. Diabetes Care and Research in Europe – the St Vincent Declaration. *Giornale Italiano di Diabetologia* 1990; 10 (suppl): 143–144

5 Borch-Johnsen K, Anderson AR, Deckert T. Effect of proteinuria on relative mortality in Type I (insulin-dependent) diabetes mellitus. *Diabetologia 1985; 28*: 590–596
6 Cofoed-Enevoldsen A, Borch-Johnsen K, Kreiner S et al. Declining incidence of persistent proteinuria in Type I (insulin-dependent) diabetic patients in Denmark. *Diabetes 1987; 36*: 205–209
7 Stephenson J, Swerdlo AJ, Devis T, Fuller JH. Recent trends in diabetes mortality in England and Wales. *Diabet Med 1992; 9*: 417–421
8 Panzram G, Zabel-Langhennine R. Prognosis of diabetes mellitus in a geographically defined population. *Diabetologia 1981; 20*: 587–591
9 De Fronzo RA, Ferrannini E. Insulin resistance: a multifaceted syndrome responsible for NIDDM, obesity, hypertension, dyslipidaemia and atherosclerotic cardiovascular disease. *Diabetes Care 1991; 14; 3*: 173–194
10 McNally PG, Burden AC, Swift PGF et al. The prevalence and risk factors associated with the onset of diabetic nephropathy in juvenile onset (insulin-dependent) diabetics diagnosed under the age of 17 years in Leicestershire 1930–1985. *Q J Med 1990; 280*: 831–844
11 Moloney A, Tunbridge WMG, Ireland JP, Watkins PJ. Mortality from diabetic nephropathy in the United Kingdom. *Diabetologia 1983; 25*: 26–33
12 Joint Working Party on diabetic renal failure of the British Diabetic Association, the Renal Association and the Research Unit of the Royal College of Physicians. *Diabet Med 1988; 5*: 79–84
13 Nabarro JDN. Diabetes in the United Kingdom: a personal series. *Diabet Med 1991; 8*: 59–68
14 Thompson FJ, Veves A, Ashe H et al. A team approach to diabetic footcare – the Manchester experience. *Foot 1991; 2*: 75–82
15 Edmonds ME, Blundell MP, Morris ME et al. Improved survival of the diabetic foot: the role of a specialised foot clinic. *Q J Med 1986; 60*: 763–771
16 Steel JM, Johnsen FD, Hepburn DA, Smith AF. Can prepregnancy care of diabetic women reduce the risk of abnormal babies? *Br Med J 1990; 301*: 1070–1074
17 Mountain KR. The infant of the diabetic mother. In Oats JN ed. *Baillière's Clinical Obstetrics and Gynaecology. Diabetes in Practice*. London: Baillière Tindall, 1991: 413–442
18 Rosenn B, Miodovinik N, Mimouni F et al. Patient experience in a diabetic programme project improves subsequent pregnancy outcome. *Obstet Gynecol 1991; 77*: 87–91
19 Knight AH, Redmond S. District diabetes centre in the United Kingdom and Eire. *Diabet Med 1989; 7*: 639–641
20 Gill GV, McFarlane IA. Defending the diabetic clinic. *Practical Diabetes 1989; 6*: 23
21 Tomlinson S. Should diabetes centres have a research/education function? The experience of the Manchester Diabetes Centre. *Practical Diabetes 1991; 8*: 183–186
22 Harrison CJ, Roaf E, Boulton AJM, Tomlinson S. An audit of patient satisfaction following the establishment of the Manchester Diabetes Centre. *Practical Diabetes* 1992 (in press)

NEUTRAL ENDOPEPTIDASE - THERAPEUTIC POSSIBILITIES OF ATRIAL NATRIURETIC FACTOR

John MC Connell, Alan G Jardine
Western Infirmary, Glasgow

INTRODUCTION
Atrial natriuretic factor (ANF) is a cardiac hormone which is natriuretic, diuretic and venodilator and suppresses the renin-angiotensin system [1]. Given at near physiological concentrations it lowers blood pressure in normal [2] and hypertensive man [3], and has effects on central cardiac haemodynamics [4] which would be beneficial in long-term treatment of cardiac failure. However, these potential therapeutic benefits are frustrated by the lack of bioavailability of ANF by other than intravenous administration. Because of this, interest has centred on utilizing ANF by raising endogenous levels through inhibition of its breakdown.

NEUTRAL ENDOPEPTIDASE
ANF is inactivated by a zinc-containing metallo-endopeptidase (EC3.4.24.11), neutral endopeptidase (NEP), which cleaves the peptide at the CYS_{105}-PHE_{106} bond, disrupting its ring structure [5-7]. The enzyme is widely distributed in tissues, being present in lung, brain, gut, placenta and in high concentrations in the brush border of the proximal tubule of the kidney [8-10].

A range of peptides are substrates for NEP in vitro. In addition to ANF, brain natriuretic peptide, bradykinin, endothelin, angiotensin II, luteinizing hormone releasing hormone (LHRH) and enkephalins can all be metabolized by the enzyme [9]. Indeed, initial studies of NEP were based on its ability to metabolize opioid peptides in the central nervous system [11]. Compounds which inhibited metabolism of enkephalins by NEP (such as phosphoramidon or thiorphan) were shown to be effective antinociceptive agents [11]. However, since the discovery that NEP in the peripheral circulation was a major route of metabolism for ANF, interest has centred on the therapeutic implications of inhibition of the enzyme to modulate levels of this cardiac hormone. Inhibition of ANF breakdown should allow increased availability of the hormone to its biologically active guanylate-cyclase linked receptors, thereby increasing its renal, endocrine and haemodynamic actions.

PHARMACOLOGICAL INHIBITION OF NEP
Initial assessment of pharmacological inhibition of NEP in vitro confirmed that the breakdown of ANF could be delayed (using renal tissue homogenates [7]). When given to intact experimental animals, inhibitors of NEP delayed the elimination of exogenous ANF, and this was associated with the predicted increase in natriuresis and diuresis [12]. In a number of studies, administration of NEP inhibitors also raised endogenous ANF levels, resulting in similar changes in renal function [13–15]. These studies demonstrated, therefore, that inhibition of NEP could have significant effects on ANF metabolism in vivo resulting in actions which were of potential therapeutic benefit.

In rat models of hypertension the effects of these compounds have been less consistent. Blood pressure has been reported to fall after 5 days' administration of the NEP inhibitor SCH34,826 to spontaneously hypertensive rats [16], while in other studies blood pressure in deoxycorticosterone acetate (DOCA)-salt hypertensive rats has also been reduced [17]. Our own studies with SCH34,826 have been carried out in rats made hypertensive by administration of DOCA-salt. The DOCA-salt hypertensive rats were compared with untreated rats and each group divided into two sub-groups of six animals 3 weeks after commencement of DOCA treatment/placebo. The sub-groups then either received incremental doses of SCH34,826 at 0, 10, 30, or 100mg/kg twice daily. The doses were administered in ascending order, for 3 days each, with the exception of the 100mg/kg which was continued for 5 days. At the end of each treatment phase blood pressure was measured indirectly by the tail cuff method and exchangeable sodium determined isotopically.

The NEP inhibition had no effect on blood pressure in the normal rat, but prevented the development of hypertension in the DOCA-salt group (Figure 1). Plasma ANF levels, measured on the last day of the study, revealed a 10-fold increase in ANF in the DOCA-salt treated rats as expected, with a 50% increase in plasma level in both the placebo and DOCA-salt treated groups following treatment with SCH34,826. It is of interest (Figure 1, lower part) that the fall in blood pressure and increase in ANF was not associated with natriuresis nor significant change in body exchangeable sodium content. It may be that in this model of hypertension the effects of NEP inhibition on blood pressure reflect vasodilatation, possibly as a consequence of altered ANF metabolism. It does appear, however, from these studies that NEP inhibition might have some therapeutic potential in hypertension.

NEP INHIBITION IN MAN
The first studies of NEP inhibition in man used an intravenous preparation (UK69,578, Candoxatrilat, Pfizer Central Research, UK)[18]. In single doses given to normal man we showed that this drug raised endogenous levels of ANF, with no apparent dose–response relationship [19]. Associated with this rise in ANF was natriuresis and diuresis without concomitant potassium loss. No change in blood pressure or heart rate was noted in these single dose studies. Plasma active renin concentration was, however, suppressed, consistent with the fall in renin noted during administration of ANF [1].

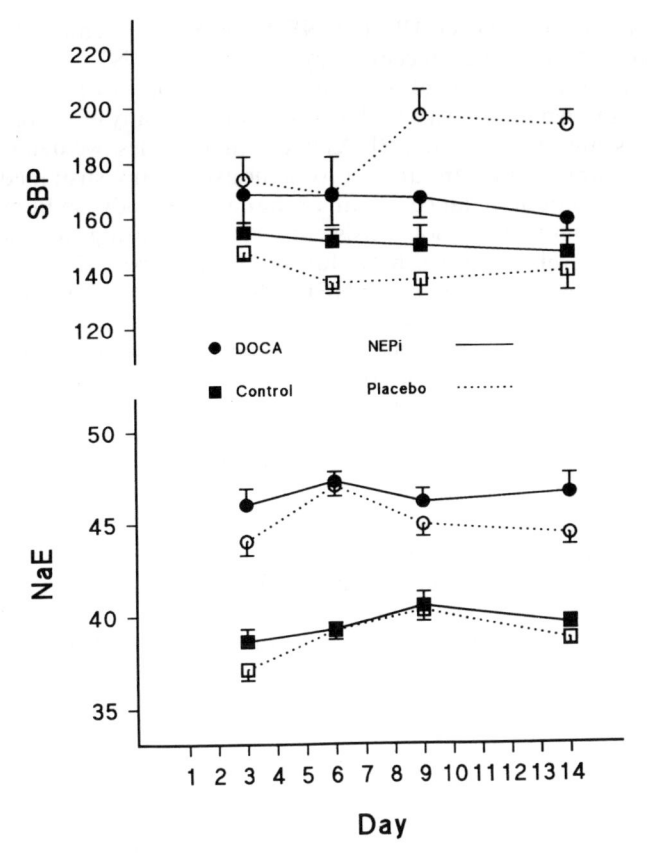

Figure 1. Effect of SCH34,826 (for details of dosing see text) on systolic blood pressure (SBP) and exchangeable body sodium (NaE) in rats given DOCA (25 mg + 1% NaCl in drinking water) or control (1% NaCl in drinking water). n=6 in each group.

Subsequent studies with this compound have used an oral preparation (UK79,300, Candoxatril) which yields the active enantiomer of UK69,578. In normal human subjects Richards and colleagues showed that this agent raised ANF levels and caused a modest natriuresis and diuresis over a 4 day period [20]: at the end of this time subjects remained in negative sodium balance. The drug did not lower blood pressure significantly, and there was a trend for renin levels to be lower in the actively treated group. At the end of the study Richards and colleagues showed that the elimination half-life of endogenous ANF was still reduced [21] indicating dependence of the peptide on NEP for elimination during repeated dosing.

These authors also reported that urinary levels of cyclic guanosine monophosphate (GMP) remained elevated throughout the dosing period: urinary cyclic GMP levels rise after intravenous administration of ANF and reflect activation of renal guanylate cyclase receptors by the peptide [22]. This sustained rise in cyclic GMP after NEP inhibition is consistent with prolonged activation of such receptors by endogenous ANF.

After 10 days of treatment with UK79,300 (200mg twice a day) in normal subjects, our own group was unable to demonstrate any effect of the drug on blood pressure or heart rate [23]. As with other studies, we demonstrated an initial natriuresis but were unable to demonstrate any sustained change in cumulative sodium balance or in exchangeable body sodium. Although plasma ANF levels were not consistently elevated during treatment, urinary cyclic GMP levels remained high during the study period.

These studies have shown that NEP inhibition can raise plasma levels of ANF and cause sustained activation of renal guanylate cyclase receptors. In some studies a modest natriuretic effect has been seen, and it seems reasonable to ask if these changes can be translated into clinically relevant actions in subjects with cardiovascular disease.

STUDIES IN ESSENTIAL HYPERTENSION

Infusion of ANF in hypertensive subjects lowers blood pressure acutely and when given over a 5 day period [24]. Initial uncontrolled studies in hypertensive patients with an NEP inhibitor (sinorphan) reported a fall in both systolic and diastolic blood pressure [25]. Our own more rigorous studies with UK79,300 have shown that after single dosing in subjects with hypertension ANF levels rise, and that this is associated with natriuresis at high dose administration (200mg) [26]. However, after 30 days of treatment with UK79,300 in a placebo-controlled, parallel group study of 40 subjects we could demonstrate only a small fall in standing systolic blood pressure [27]. Other haemodynamic measurements were unaffected. In this study plasma ANF levels remained increased by chronic NEP inhibition.

These initial studies, therefore, do not show major changes in blood pressure in hypertensive patients treated either acutely or chronically with an effective inhibitor of NEP. In view of the promising initial animal and normal human subject studies, the results are a little disappointing and the reasons for the failure to lower blood pressure with chronic therapy are unclear. There may be, however, a number of possible contributory factors. There are a number of other potential vasoactive substrates for NEP in addition to ANF, and inhibition of breakdown of these may well offset any potential benefit from chronic prolongation of the elimination of ANF. For example, angiotensin II is broken down by NEP. We have shown that angiotensin II levels in plasma during infusion of synthetic angiotensin II are increased by NEP inhibition, although basal levels of the peptide appear to be unaffected [19]. More detailed studies of angiotensin II kinetics in subjects during treatment with NEP inhibitors need to be carried out. Furthermore, generation and metabolism of endothelin are also affected by NEP inhibition and it is possible that a change in the breakdown of this peptide could contribute to the lack of antihypertensive effect.

CHRONIC HEART FAILURE

In subjects with chronic heart failure endogenous levels of ANF are increased [28]. The profile of action of the hormone, with venodilatation, natriuresis and diuresis would be expected to be of benefit in subjects with heart failure and initial studies of ANF administration in this syndrome showed potentially beneficial haemodynamic changes [4, 29]. In an animal model of heart failure (dog) NEP inhibition resulted in natriuresis and diuresis [30]; in an uncontrolled open study of sinorphan in subjects with severe heart failue beneficial haemodynamic changes were noted [31]. We reported, in initial studies with UK69,578, that intravenous administration of the drug to subjects with mild heart failure resulted in a rise in plasma levels of ANF (from an already elevated baseline), with associated natriuresis and diuresis [32]. These changes coincided with a fall in cardiac filling pressures. If sustained, such effects would be clinically advantageous in heart failure. More recently, Lang and colleagues have reported that single dose administration of UK79,300 in mild chronic heart failure raises levels of both ANF and the related hormone brain natriuretic peptide (BNP) [28]. The significance of the change in BNP is unclear, and longer-term studies with NEP inhibitors are still to report on this syndrome.

SUMMARY

In summary, inhibition of NEP provides a novel method of influencing the action of ANF. The currently available drugs do cause an increased action of ANF at guanylate cyclase receptors, but this has yet to be shown to translate into therapeutically useful effects. The role of such agents in the management of heart failure syndrome remains to be defined.

REFERENCES

1 Kenyon CJ, Jardine AG. Atrial natriuretic peptide: water and electrolyte homeostasis. *Clin Endocrinol Metab 1989; 3*: 431–450
2 Richards AM, Nicholls MG, Ikram H et al. Renal, haemodynamic and hormonal effects of human alpha natriuretic peptide in healthy volunteers. *Lancet 1985; i*: 545–549
3 Tonolo G, Richards AM, Manunta P et al. Low-dose infusion of atrial natriuretic factor in mild essential hypertension. *Circulation 1986; 80*: 893–902
4 Northridge DB, McMurray J, Dargie HJ. Atrial natriuretic factor in chronic heart failure. *Herz 1991; 16*: 92–101
5 Sonnenberg JL, Sakane Y, Jeng AY et al. Identification of protease endopeptidase 24.11 as the major atrial natriuretic factor degrading enzyme in the rat kidney. *Peptides 1987; 9*: 173–180
6 Stephenson SL, Kenny AJ. The hydrolysis of α-human natriuretic peptide by pig kidney microvillar membranes is initiated by endopeptidase 24.11. *Biochem J 1987; 243*: 183–187
7 Olins GM, Krieter PA, Trapani AJ et al. Specific inhibitors of endopeptidase 24.11 inhibit the metabolism of atrial natriuretic peptides in vitro and in vivo. *Mol Cell Endocrinol 1989; 61*: 201–208
8 Kerr MA, Kenny AJ. The molecular weight and properties of a neutral metallopeptidase from rabbit kidney brush border. *Biochem J 1974; 137*: 489–495
9 Erdos EG, Skidgell RA. Neutral endopeptidase 24.11 (enkephalinase) and related regulators of peptide hormones. *FASEB J 1989; 3*: 145–151

10 Kenny AJ, Stephenson SL. Role of endopeptidase 24.11 in the inactivation of atrial natriuretic peptide. *FEBS Lett 1988; 232*: 1-8
11 Llorens C, Gacel G, Swertz J et al. Rational design of enkephalinase inhibitors: substrate specificity of enkephalinase studied from inhibitory potencies of various dipeptides. *Biochem Biophys Res Comm 1980; 96*: 1710-1716
12 Seymour AA, Fennell SA, Swerdel JN. Potentiation of renal effects of atrial natriuretic factor by SQ 29,072. *Hypertension 1989; 14*: 87-97
13 Danielwicz JC, Barclay PL, Barnish IT et al. UK 69,578, a novel inhibitor of EC 3.4.24.11 which increases endogenous ANF levels and is natriuretic and diuretic. *Biochem Biophys Res Comm 1989; 164*: 58-65
14 Lafferty HM, Gunning M, Silva P et al. Enkephalinase inhibition increases plasma atrial natriuretic peptide levels, glomerular filtration rate, and urinary sodium excretion in rats with reduced renal rate. *Circulation Res 1989; 65*: 640-646
15 Shepperson NB, Barclay PL, Bennett JA, Samuels GMR. Inhibition of neutral endopeptidase leads to an atrial natriuretic factor mediated natriuretic, diuretic and antihypertensive response in rodents. *Clin Sci 1991; 80*: 265-269
16 Sybertz EF, Chiu PJS, Vemulapaali S et al. Atrial natriuretic factor potentiating and antihypertensive effects of SCH 34826. *Hypertension 1990; 15*: 152-161
17 Sybertz EJ, Chiu PJS, Vemulapaali S et al. SCH 39370, a neutral endopeptidase inhibitor potentiates the biological responses to atrial natriuretic factor and lowers blood pressure in deoxycorticosterone acetate-sodium hypertensive rats. *J Pharmacol Exp Ther 1989; 250*: 624-631
18 Northridge DB, Jardine AG, Alabaster CT et al. Effects of UK 69,578: a novel atriopeptidase inhibitor. *Lancet 1989; ii*: 591-594
19 Jardine AG, Connell JMC, Northridge DB et al. The atriopeptidase inhibitor UK 68,578 increases plasma atrial natriuretic factor and causes a natriuresis in normal man. *Am J Hypertension 1990; 3*: 661-667
20 Richards M, Espiner E, Ikram H et al. Inhibition of endopeptidase EC 24.11 in humans: renal and endocrine effects. *Hypertension 1990; 16*: 269-276
21 Richards AM, Wittert G, Espiner EA et al. EC 24.11 inhibitor in man alters clearance of atrial natriuretic peptide. *J Clin Endocrinol Metab 1991; 72*: 1317-1322
22 Chinkers M, Garbers DL, Chang MS et al. A membrane form of guanylate cyclase in an atrial natriuretic peptide receptor. *Nature 1989; 338*: 78-83
23 O'Connell JE, Jardine AG, Davidson G et al. A ten day study of UK 79,300, an orally acting neutral endopeptidase inhibitor in man. *Ottawa Symposium on Atrial Natriuretic Factor.* University of Ottawa Heart Institute 1990, p 98
24 Janssen WMT, de Zeeuw D, Gdalt K, de Jong PE. Antihypertensive effect of a five day infusion of atrial natriuretic factor in humans. *Hypertension 1989; 13*: 640-646
25 LeFrancois P, Clerk G, Duchier J et al. Antihypertensive activity of sinorphan. *Lancet 1990; 336*: 307-308
26 O'Connell J, Jardine AG, Davidson G, Connell JMC. Candoxatril, an orally active neutral endopeptidase inhibitor, raises plasma atrial natriuretic factor and is natriuretic in essential hypertension. *J Hypertension 1992; 10*: 271-278
27 Bevan BG, McInnes GT, Lorimer AR et al. Efficacy and tolerability of an atriopeptidase inhibitor, Candoxatril, in essential hypertension. *Eur Soc Hypertension, 1991*; Abstract 6
28 Lang CC, Motwani J, Coutie WJ, Struthers AD. Influence of Candoxatril on plasma brain natriuretic peptide in heart failure. *Lancet 1991; 338*: 255
29 Cody RJ, Atlas SA, Laragh JH et al. Atrial natriuretic factor in normal subjects and heart failure patients. *J Clin Invest 1986; 78*: 1362-1374
30 Cavero PG, Marguiles KB, Winaver J et al. Cardiorenal actions of neutral endopeptidase inhibition in experimental congestive heart failure. *Circulation 1990; 82*: 196-201
31 Khan JC, Patey M, Dubois-Rande JL et al. Effect of sinorphan on plasma atrial natriuretic factor in congestive cardiac failure. *Lancet 1990; 36*: 118-119
32 Northridge D, Jardine AG, Dilly SD et al. Inhibition of the metabolism of atrial natriuretic factor causes diuresis and natriuresis in chronic heart failure. *Am J Hypertension 1990; 3*: 682-687

OSTEOPOROSIS: ADVANCES AND CONTROVERSIES

Roger Smith
Nuffield Orthopaedic Centre, Oxford

INTRODUCTION
Osteoporosis was last dealt with in the Advanced Medicine series in 1988 [1]. Since then it has been indexed in 2500 indexed papers and numerous conferences and reviews (see for instance references 2 and 3). This frenzied activity is based on the supposition that bone loss causes fracture; on the possibility that skeletal failure may be predicted and prevented; and on the undoubted medical, socio-economic and financial advantages which would follow. Clarity has not followed from quantity but it is possible to extract some apparently significant advances from the intellectual quagmire of osteoporosis research. Examples include the importance of heritability and mechanical factors to skeletal mass, the development of accurate biochemical measurements of bone turnover, the prediction of fracture risk and the effectiveness and safety of hormone replacement therapy. Amongst the equal number of controversies population screening for osteoporosis is an outstanding current example. To understand osteoporosis it is necessary to summarize the ways in which bone mass is controlled and the potential for influencing them.

BONE MASS
This is determined by the interaction of genetic and mechanical factors modulated by hormonal status and calcium intake (Figure 1) [4]. Recent investigations have filled in some details of this scheme. Thus (clockwise left to right) collagen gene mutations have been described in a family considered to have osteoporosis (but most likely mild osteogenesis imperfecta) [5]. The cause of the greater bone mass in blacks remains mysterious, but appears only in adolescence [6]. Bone mass is influenced by dietary calcium, particularly during growth [7] and in men [8] as well as women, and bone mineral density is reduced by episodes of adolescent and early adult ovulatory disturbances [9]. Anorexia nervosa shows the deleterious skeletal effects of combined nutritional and oestrogen deficiency [10]. The mass of bone is undoubtedly related to the mechanical forces through it, both in animals and

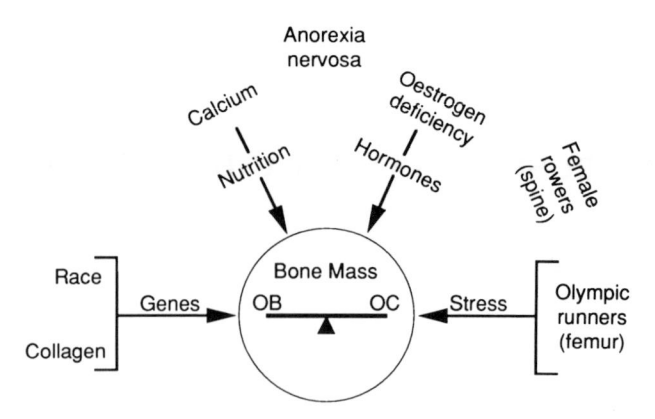

Figure 1. The major effects of genetics and mechanical influences on bone mass and the modulating effect of calcium intake and hormones. OB = osteoblast; OC = osteoclast.

man. Female rowers have a greater spinal bone mass density (BMD) (measured by quantitative computed tomography – QCT) than normal non-rowers, but this increase is less in the amenorrhoeic group; likewise Olympic runners show an increase in femoral shaft cortical bone density in comparison to rowers, dancers and sedentary subjects [11, 12].

All these effects are mediated through the bone cells, particularly the osteoblast (Figure 2). This cell comes from the stromal cell line (which includes adipocytes and fibroblasts [13]), and is the precursor of the osteocyte. It controls the activity of the osteoclast, which is haemopoietic in origin. Its osteoblasts are influenced by calciotrophic and other hormones, by many short acting chemical messengers or cytokines, and possibly by the effect of non-collagen proteins liberated from bone matrix; these include the newly characterized bone morphogenetic proteins [14]. Bone cells work in multicellular units (BMUs) in which activation of osteoclast precursors is followed by resorption of bone and its subsequent replacement by osteoblasts and a period of quiescence.

Bone mass increases during childhood and adolescence and young adult life to a peak at about 30 years and decreases in both sexes from then on with a temporary rapid postmenopausal phase in women. It depends on the balance between resorption and formation; and it is by manipulation of this balance that osteoporosis can be prevented and treated.

BONE MASS AND FRACTURE

The main determinants of the amount of bone in later life are the previous maximum amount (peak bone mass) and the subsequent rate of loss. In women peak bone mass adjusted for lean body mass is near to that of men but subsequent bone loss is more rapid, and life span is greater. Thus women spend many more years with a bone density below the fracture 'threshold' than men. Low bone density is a major risk factor for fracture, with a direct but not close association between the two [15]. When combined with pre-

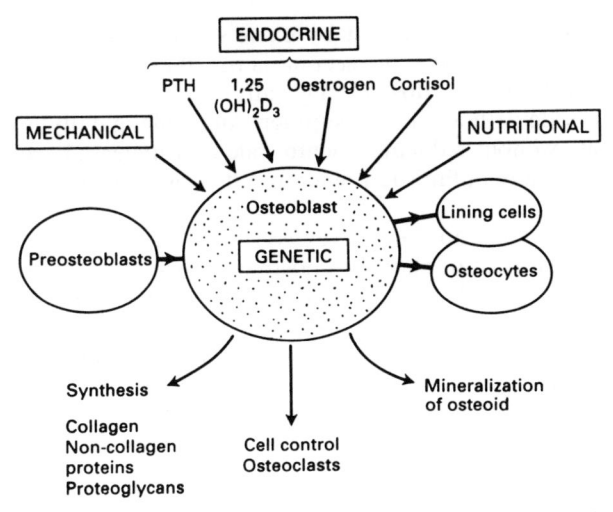

Figure 2. The central position of the osteoblast. PTH = parathyroid hormone; $1,25(OH)_2D_3$ = 1,25-dihydroxyvitamin D_3.

existing fractures, bone mass is a powerful predictor of subsequent fracture [16]. Current measurements of bone density give no information about structure, which may be equally important [17]. The rate of falling increases with age probably more so in women, to become the main cause of fractures [18]. Measurement of bone density (in the opposite hip) of those subjects who have had a proximal femoral fracture shows that there is considerable overlap with age-matched non-fracture controls. Such observations reduce the rationale and enthusiasm for bone density population screening to prevent hip fracture (see below [19]).

PREVENTION OF OSTEOPOROSIS

Despite the relatively poor correlation between bone density and fracture virtually all current recommendations to prevent skeletal failure depend on preserving the skeleton rather than preventing injury. This preservation may be achieved by increasing peak bone mass and reducing subsequent loss. Since it is not possible to alter the genetic contribution to bone mass, optimal peak bone density depends on using the skeleton, on sufficient intake of calcium [20] and on the avoidance of risk factors (excessive alcohol, smoking, immobility, excessive thinness). Likewise subsequent bone loss depends on avoiding the same risk factors, continued exercise and sufficient calcium (although this last recommendation is still controversial [21]). Some feel strongly that smoking is deleterious to the skeleton [19].

Methods to prevent bone loss divide by their predicted effect on bone cells, either by increasing osteoblastic bone formation, or decreasing osteoclastic bone resorption, or doing both. Since bone cells talk to each other, it is very difficult to separately influence their activities in the long-term scale, though temporary dissociation can be achieved, and may be effective [22, 23].

Bone formation is increased by exercise and also by sodium fluoride; whilst the first is harmless, the second is not, though the effects may depend on dose. On the higher dose (75mg daily) used in the USA study [24] oral sodium fluoride with a calcium supplement (1500mg daily) increased spinal bone density without reducing fracture rate and increased appendicular fractures. Despite more optimistic French results [25] fluoride therapy is currently under a cloud.

Bone resorption can be prevented by hormone replacement therapy (HRT), the treatment of choice in postmenopausal women, by oral calcium, by cyclical Didronel (etidronate) and by calcitonin (by injection or intranasally). The first three require further discussion (see below). Calcitonin is rarely given to prevent or treat osteoporosis in the UK although it is used in continental Europe and elsewhere.

RECOMMENDATIONS

Against this background the management of osteoporosis should be simple, but in practice this is not always so. The following recommendations will need to be modified for each individual.

1. At all ages exclude obvious causes for osteoporosis. Most osteoporotic subjects are postmenopausal women, but osteoporosis can occur without identifiable cause in growing children, pregnancy and young adults. Known causes of secondary accelerated osteoporosis are hormonal (corticosteroid excess), Cushing's syndrome, thyrotoxicosis, hypogonadism, immobility, gastrointestinal disease, mastocytosis and mild osteogenesis imperfecta.
2. In peri- and postmenopausal women measure bone density to aid in therapeutic decisions and to assess the risk of fracture in relation to other risk factors.
3. In those with low bone density recommend HRT (oestrogen with or without progestogen according to presence of the uterus or not). Consider HRT also for those with normal bone density because of cardiovascular and other advantages.
4. Make sure that the calcium intake is adequate (up to 1500mg daily), preferably by increasing the amount in the diet.
5. Maintain and where possible increased weight-bearing exercise.
6. Avoid known risk factors for further bone loss; stop smoking, excessive alcohol or excessive weight loss.
7. For those subjects where HRT is inappropriate or contraindicated consider alternatives, possibly cyclical etidronate, for established vertebral osteoporosis.

Surprisingly only 1, 5 and 6 are non-controversial; opinions differ on the usefulness of bone densitometry, on the effectiveness of HRT (particularly with progestogen), on the justification for additional calcium and on the role of etidronate in osteoporosis.

BONE DENSITY MEASUREMENT
Instruments which can measure the amount of bone accurately and rapidly at the site of interest such as the spine or femoral neck have been a great help in research. They have established that the risk of subsequent fracture is directly related to the amount of bone, and provide a quantitative assessment both of the degree of bone loss and the effectiveness of methods of intervention.

Apart from its use in research there are two different situations in which the measurement of bone density can be considered as appropriate. The first is to provide a measure of the amount of bone present to confirm (or disprove) a diagnosis of osteoporosis (a reduction of bone by more than 2SD from the mean), to give some idea of skeletal prognosis and provide information for a therapeutic decision, and where necessary to follow the effect of treatment. Such measurements (by single photon absorptiometry – SPA, dual photon absorptiometry – DPA, QCT or dual energy X-ray absorptiometry – DEXA) should be part of the clinical care of a patient referred for a skeletal opinion, in the same way that patients with anaemia have full blood counts and those with cardiovascular disease have plasma cholesterol measurements.

It is in the second situation, population screening, that bone density measurements are controversial and questions are asked. Is it economical (or medically appropriate) to measure the bone density in all perimenopausal women within the population, in order to identify those with a low bone density and presumably an increased risk of fracture [19]? The issue is a complicated one and the necessary studies have not been done. So far as femoral neck fractures are concerned it seems that the bone density of the unfractured opposite femur may often be within the normal range for the age of the patient [26]; and the overlap in bone densities between those who fracture and those who do not is too great to justify the use of population screening [19]. On the whole the recommendations for bone density measurement expressed by Melton et al [27] and at the last osteoporosis conference in Copenhagen [28] still stand.

HORMONE REPLACEMENT THERAPY
Most long-term studies are concerned with the effect of oestrogen alone and have established that oestrogen prevents postmenopausal bone loss and reduces hip fracture rate [29]. Additionally, and quantitatively more importantly, oestrogens appear to halve mortality due to cardiovascular disease but not stroke [30]. However, oestrogen given alone considerably increases the prevalence of endometrial carcinoma, a risk which is abolished by giving progestogen for 10 or more days per month [31]. In postmenopausal women who have had a hysterectomy unopposed oestrogen can be given to full advantage on the skeleton and cardiovascular system, with the very slightly increased risk of breast cancer after prolonged treatment [32]. Where a hysterectomy has not been done there are unanswered questions posed by giving progestogen as well, since it is not known whether this abolishes the cardiovascular advantage of oestrogen alone. There are unsettled questions about HRT. For instance, it is not established whether bone loss occurs at an accelerated early postmenopausal rate when replacement therapy is stopped, and

if so to what extent the skeletal advantage of HRT is lost in older women [33]. There is also the suggestion that those few who take HRT and continue with it are self-selected and change their life style in other ways compared with those not on HRT [34].

It is for these and other reasons that a randomized trial of the use of HRT in osteoporosis is necessary and proposed [35, 36]. Even if such a trial confirms the apparently beneficial effects of HRT extending into those with established osteoporosis [37] it is currently prescribed by few doctors and acceptable to few women [38].

EFFECT OF CALCIUM

Despite lengthy and continuing controversy [39, 40] recent studies suggest that dietary calcium is an important contributor to peak bone mass in the young and an increase may slow bone loss in the adult [41]. Thus in an American study of healthy women whose menopause had occurred at least 6 years previously and who had a daily calcium intake of less than 400mg, an increase up to 800mg daily reduced bone loss at axial and appendicular sites [42]; and from Perth, Australia Prince et al [43] compared the effect of exercise, calcium supplementation and hormone replacement therapy on forearm bone density of postmenopausal women of mean age 56 years, finding that exercise plus calcium (1000mg daily) but not exercise alone significantly slowed bone loss.

ETIDRONATE IN OSTEOPOROSIS

Disodium etidronate (EHDP, Didronel) was first used to treat Paget's disease 20 years ago. In doses of 10–20mg/kg body weight daily for 3–6 months bone cell suppression (resorption before formation) was predictable and sustained. It has now been used for osteoporosis in a cyclical manner and smaller doses, i.e. 400mg daily for 2 weeks in every 15 with a continuous calcium supplement. Two detailed studies, from Denmark [22] and the USA [23], showed that spinal bone density increased and the rate of spinal fractures (assessed radiologically and by change in height) decreased.

The early studies covered less than 3 years of treatment and further information is awaited. This is essential because any agent which suppresses bone resorption (such as calcitonin) will cause an apparent increase in bone mineral density within the first year or so, supposedly because osteoblastic activity continues unabated. However, continued increase in bone mineral density would be unexpected and would represent a significant advance in the management of osteoporosis. Importantly the beneficial effects of etidronate have been shown only for vertebral osteoporosis.

CONCLUSION

Current research in osteoporosis is finally beginning to provide scientific evidence for what many doctors would regard as common sense, namely that genetically determined bone mass is maintained and fracture rate reduced by a tripartite combination of exercise, calcium and HRT where appropriate [44]. Economists wonder which of these we can afford and propose population strategies which exclude most of them [19]. Meanwhile epidemiologists come up with tantalizing findings. For example, in a follow-up of 9704 American women aged 65 and older, low initial proximal forearm bone density was associated with subsequently increased mortality; but this increase was not due to fractures; and the most significant relationship was between low bone density and stroke [45]. What then is the significance of low bone density; is it merely one indicator of biological age; and is the relationship between low bone density and fracture in other studies more apparent than real; and where does this leave bone density screening programmes?

Finally, lest we forget it, a recent study has redirected our attention to the likely effects on bone mass of changes in vitamin D status within the physiological range. At latitude 42 (Boston, Massachusetts) healthy postmenopausal women with daily vitamin D intakes of 100iu (2.5µg) can apparently significantly reduce late wintertime bone loss and improve net spinal bone density over one year by increasing their daily intake to 12.5µg [46]. We must wait to see if this has any long-term significance for osteoporosis prevention. Meanwhile there are many problems for the future (Table I): the last of these returns us to the osteoblast.

TABLE I. Osteoporosis: questions for the future

How effective is HRT; is the population selected?
Is population screening worthwhile; what does low bone density indicate?
What determines fracture; how can we measure bone strength?
Can we selectively stimulate osteogenesis?

REFERENCES

1 Smith R. Osteoporosis. Causes, consequences and control. *Adv Med 1988; 24*: 31–38
2 Smith R. *Osteoporosis 1990*. London: RCP Publications
3 Drife JO, Studd WW. *HRT and Osteoporosis*. London: Springer-Verlag. 1990
4 Heaney RP. Calcium, bone health and osteoporosis. *Bone Min Res 1986; 4*: 255–301
5 Spotila LD, Constantinou CD, Sereda L et al. Mutation in a gene for Type I procollagen (COL1A2) in a woman with postmenopausal osteoporosis: evidence for phenotypic and genotypic overlap with mild osteogenesis imperfecta. *Proc Natl Acad Sci USA 1991; 88*: 5423–5427
6 Gilsanz V, Roe TF, Mora S et al. Changes in vertebral bone density in black girls and white girls during childhood and puberty. *N Engl J Med 1991; 325*: 1597–1600
7 Miller JL, Slemenda CW, Johnston CC. Positive relationship between calcium intake and bone mass – co-twin control study. *3rd International Symposium on Osteoporosis*. Copenhagen 1990 (Abstract)
8 Kelly PJ, Pocock NA, Sambrook PN et al. Dietary calcium, sex hormones, and bone mineral density in men. *Br Med J 1990; 300*: 1361–1364
9 Prior J, Vigna YM, Schechter MT. Spinal bone loss and ovulatory disturbances. *N Engl J Med 1990; 323*: 1221–1227
10 Rigotti NA, Nussbaum SR, Herzog DB et al. Osteoporosis in women with anorexia nervosa. *N Engl J Med 1984; 311*: 1601–1606
11 Wolman RL, Clark P, McNally E et al. Menstrual state and exercise as determinants of spinal trabecular bone density in female athletes. *Br Med J 1990; 301*: 516–518
12 Wolman RL, Faulmann L, Clark P et al. Different training patterns and bone mineral density of the femoral shaft in elite, female athletes. *Ann Rheum Dis 1991; 50*: 487–489

13. Martin TJ, Ng KW, Nicholson GC. Cell biology of bone. *Baillières Clinical Endocrinology and Metabolism* 1988; *2*: 1-29
14. Bentz H, Nathan RM, Rosen DM et al. Purification and characterisation of a unique osteoconductive factor from bovine bone. *J Biol Chem* 1989; *264*: 20805-20810
15. Ross P, Davis JW, Vogel JM et al. A critical review of bone mass and the risk of fractures in osteoporosis. *Calcif Tissue Int* 1990; *46*: 149-161
16. Ross PD, Davis JW, Epstein RS et al. Pre-existing fractures and bone mass predict vertebral fracture incidence in women. *Ann Intern Med* 1991; *114*: 919-923
17. Kanis JA, McCloskey EV, Eyres KS et al. Screening techniques in the evaluation of osteoporosis. In Drife JO, Studd WW, eds. *HRT and Osteoporosis*. London: Springer-Verlag. 1990: 135-147
18. Evans JG. Falls and fractures. *Age Ageing 1988*; *17*: 361-364
19. Law MR, Wald NJ, Meade TW. Strategies for prevention of osteoporosis and hip fracture. *Br Med J 1991*; *303*: 453-459
20. Picard D, Ste-Mg, Coutu D et al. Premenopausal bone mineral content related to height, weight and calcium intake during adulthood. *Bone and Mineral 1988*; *4*: 299-309
21. Avioli LV, Heaney RP. Calcium intake and bone health. *Calcif Tissue Int 1991*; *48*: 221-223
22. Storm T, Thamsborg G, Steiniche T et al. Effect of intermittent cyclical etidronate therapy on bone mass and fracture rate in women with postmenopausal osteoporosis. *N Engl J Med; 1990*; *322*: 1265-1271
23. Watts NG, Harris ST, Genant HK et al. Intermittent cyclical etidronate treatment of postmenopausal osteoporosis. *N Engl J Med 1990*; *323*: 73-79
24. Riggs BL, Hodgson SF, O'Fallon WN et al. Effect of fluoride treatment on the fracture rate in postmenopausal women with osteoporosis. *N Engl J Med 1990*; *322*: 802-809
25. Mamelle N, Meunier PJ, Dusan R et al. Risk benefit ratio of sodium fluoride treatment in primary vertebral osteoporosis. *Lancet 1988*; *ii*: 361-365
26. Riggs BL, Melton LJ. Involutional osteoporosis. *N Engl J Med 1986*; *314*: 1676-1686
27. Melton LJ, Eddy DM, Johnston CC. Screening for osteoporosis. *Ann Intern Med 1990*; *112*: 517-528
28. Consensus development conference: Prophylaxis and treatment of osteoporosis. *Am J Med 1991*; *90*: 107-110
29. Naessen T, Persson I, Adam H-O et al. Hormone replacement therapy and the risk of first-hip fracture. *Ann Intern Med 1990*; *113*: 95-103
30. Stampfer MJ, Colditz GA, Willett WC et al. Postmenopausal oestrogen therapy and cardiovascular disease. *N Engl J Med 1991*; *325*: 756-762
31. Voigt LF, Weiss NS, Chu J et al. Progestogen supplementation of exogenous oestrogens and risk of endometrial cancer. *Lancet 1991*; *338*: 274-277
32. Bergkvist L, Amadi H-O, Persson I et al. The risk of breast cancer after oestrogen and oestrogen-progestogen replacement. *N Engl J Med 1989*; *321*: 293-297
33. Compston JE. Preventing osteoporosis. *Br Med J 1991*; *303*: 920-922
34. Barrett-Connor E. Postmenopausal oestrogen and prevention bias. *Ann Intern Med 1991*; *115*: 455-456
35. Goldman L, Tosteson ANA. Uncertainty about postmenopausal oestrogen. *N Engl J Med 1991*; *325*: 800-802
36. Anonymous. More than hot flushes. *Lancet 1991*; *338*: 917-918
37. Lindsay R, Tohme JF. Oestrogen treatment of patients with established postmenopausal osteoporosis. *Obstet Gynecol 1990*; *76*: 290-295
38. Wallace WA, Price VH, Elliott CA. Hormone replacement therapy acceptability to Nottingham postmenopausal women with a risk factor for osteoporosis. *J Roy Soc Med 1990*; *83*: 699-701
39. Kanis JA, Passmore R. Calcium supplementation of the diet. Not justified by present evidence. *Br Med J 1989*; *298*: 137-140, 205-208
40. Nordin BEC, Heaney RP. Calcium supplementation of the diet. Justified by present evidence. *Br Med J 1990*; *300*: 1056-1060
41. Cumming RG. Calcium intake and bone mass: A quantitative review of the evidence. *Calcif Tissue Int 1990*; *47*: 194-201
42. Dawson-Hughes B, Dallal GE, Krall EA et al. A controlled trial of the effect of calcium

supplementation on bone density in postmenopausal women. *N Engl J Med 1990; 323*: 878–883

43 Prince RL, Smith M, Dick IM et al. Prevention of postmenopausal osteoporosis. *N Engl J Med 1991; 325*: 1189–1195

44 Kelly PJ, Eisman JA, Sambrook PN. Interaction of genetic and environmental influences on peak bone density. *Osteoporosis Int 1990; 1*: 56–60

45 Browner WS, Seeley DG, Vogt TM et al. Non trauma mortality in elderly women with low bone mineral density. *Lancet 1991; 338*: 355–358

46 Dawson-Hughes B, Dallal GE, Krall EA et al. Effect of vitamin D supplementation on wintertime and overall bone loss in healthy postmenopausal women. *Ann Intern Med 1991; 115*: 505–512

OCTREOTIDE: THE SOMATOSTATIN ANALOGUE WITH DIVERSE THERAPEUTIC POTENTIAL

RN Clayton
North Staffordshire Royal Infirmary, Stoke-on-Trent

HISTORICAL PERSPECTIVE

In 1968 McCann's group [1], during attempts to discover growth hormone (GH) releasing factor, first discovered that hypothalamic extracts contained separable GH releasing and inhibiting activities each controlled by the central nervous system. Independently, workers using avian pancreatic islet extracts found that these inhibited islet cell insulin release in vitro [2]. Both groups had discovered somatostatin, which became the first of the hypothalamic releasing/inhibiting factors to be identified and subsequently characterized [3].

The initial concept that the 14 amino acid peptide, initially purified, and subsequently synthesized, had as its main function the regulation of GH secretion proved to be a gross oversimplification. Firstly, there is a large family of somatostatin-related peptides with several molecular forms [4] whose proportion not only differs between tissues of the same species but also exhibits wide species variation. Nevertheless, it appears that in mammals at least there is a single somatostatin gene [4] and the multiplicity of forms arises from (a) alternative splicing of the primary gene transcript and (b) alternative processing of the preprosomatostatin peptide. Such mechanism(s) for generating tissue and species protein diversity from a single gene is now widely recognized. Notwithstanding the more phylogenetically recent cellular mechanisms for generating such diversity, it appears that this neuropeptide gene is evolutionarily ancient being found in primitive invertebrates [5] and a protozoan [6].

As alluded to above the name somatostatin has turned out to be a misnomer since it inhibits many other hormones (Table I). Moreover, its almost global organ distribution suggests that function is likely to be selective depending upon anatomical location. Although widely distributed throughout the body (Table II) it should not be concluded that somatostatin inhibits everything and anything since some experimental evidence indicates increased electrical excitability of neurones in many central nervous system sites upon local exposure to the peptide, and stimulation of gut motility [7] (see references 8 and 9 for review).

TABLE I. Major hormones inhibited by somatostatin

Pituitary	Pancreas	Gut
Growth hormone	Insulin	Gastrin
TSH	Glucagon	VIP
	Gastrin	Secretin
	VIP	Cholecystokinin
	Pancreatic polypeptide	GIP
		Motilin
		Substance P
		Neurotensin
	Pancreatic	5HT
	exocrine function	Serotonin
		Tachykinins

TSH: thyroid stimulating hormone; VIP: vasoactive intestinal polypeptide; GIP: gastric inhibitory polypeptide; 5HT: 5-hydroxytryptamine.

TABLE II. Organ distribution of somatostatin

Nervous system	Gastrointestinal	Endocrine	Other
Central nervous system	Pancreatic islets (D cells)	Anterior pituitary	Renal collecting tubules
Hypothalamus	Gastric antrum	Parafollicular C cells of thyroid	
Limbic system	Neurones of sub-		
Brain stem	mucosa and		
Spinal cord	myenteric plexus		
Cerebral cortex	Salivary gland		
Peripheral nervous system			
Spinal sensory ganglia			
Retina/optic nerve			
Sympathetic neurones			

Consistent with the widespread tissue distribution and multiple actions of somatostatin is the demonstration of specific high affinity binding sites for the peptide in target sites. It is probable that there are several subtypes of somatostatin receptors as with other neurotransmitters/neuropeptides. Although in the pituitary somatotroph, somatostatin inhibited GH secretion is accompanied by reduced cyclic AMP production, this is probably not the major mechanism of action since somatostatin also inhibits cAMP induced GH secretion. Recent evidence links the somatostatin receptor to inhibition of membrane calcium channels and calcium permeability. Much remains to be learned about somatostatin receptors, their coupling to, and the nature of, their inhibitory effectors. This information could well be resolved when the gene for this receptor has been cloned (still awaited 20 years after the discovery of somatostatin).

PHARMACOLOGY OF SOMATOSTATIN AND OCTREOTIDE

Most of this work has been performed using suppression of GH secretion as the model. Thus, early human studies showed inhibition of GH secretion after intravenous injection to be extremely rapid and the duration of the effect extremely short (minutes), consistent with the 3–4 minute plasma half-life. Continuous intravenous or subcutaneous infusion of native somatostatin is required to maintain GH suppression.

Moreover, cessation of short-term somatostatin infusion is associated with rebound GH hypersecretion with GH levels exceeding pre-infusion values. These features, although demonstrating the potential therapeutic value for controlling GH hypersecretion, clearly made the native peptide impracticable for long-term treatment. Modification of the structure produced an octapeptide (octreotide) (Figure 1) which retained full biological activity for GH suppression with a plasma half-life of about 2 hours and which maintained suppression of GH hypersecretion for 6–8 hours after a single subcutaneous injection. Availability of this active analogue opened the way for long-term clinical trials for several indications which had been predicted from the extensive animal studies and short-term human studies.

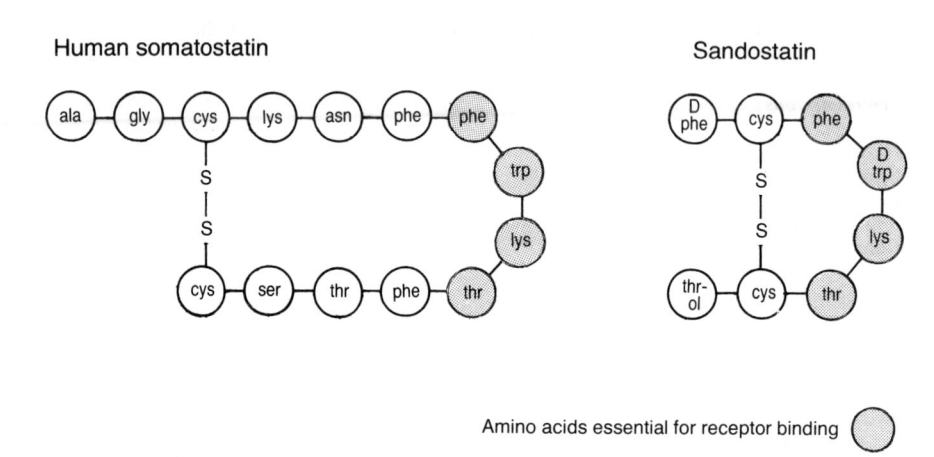

Figure 1. Amino acid sequence of natural somatostatin (left) and octreotide (Sandostatin) (right).

PHYSIOLOGY OF GH SECRETION

Unlike all other anterior pituitary hormones, growth hormone secretion is regulated by two hypothalamic releasing factors, one inhibitory (somatostatin), the other stimulatory (growth hormone releasing factor – GRF). There is a classical negative feedback loop whereby circulating insulin-like growth factor-1 (IGF-1, previously known as somatomedin C) produced predominantly, though not exclusively, by the liver inhibits somatotrophs, at both the pituitary and hypothalamic level (Figure 2). GH secretion is pulsatile and, expressed simplistically, the pulse is generated by simultaneous inhibition of somato-

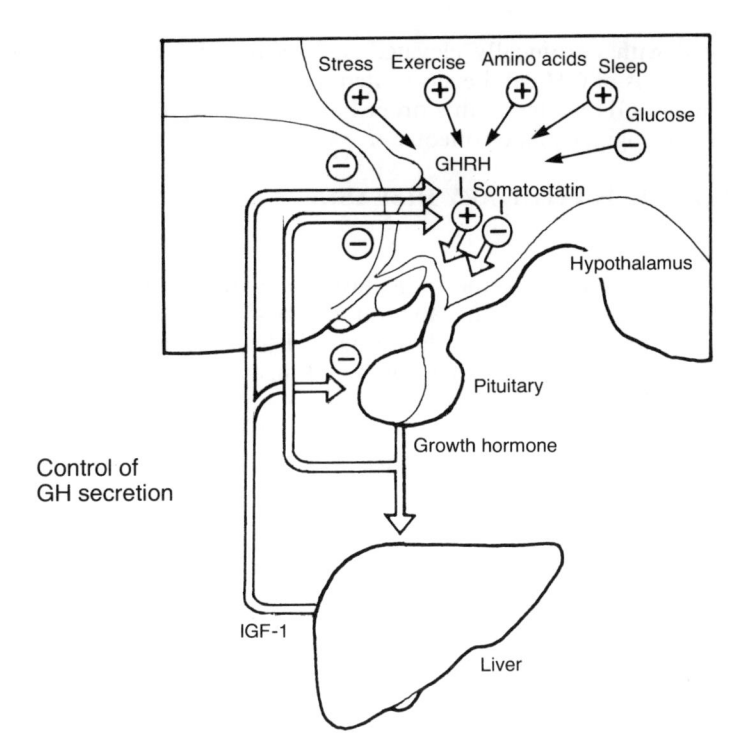

Figure 2. Control of GH secretion. IGF-1 = insulin-like growth factor 1 (somatomedin C).

statin release and stimulation of GRF release. The neuropharmacology of this *synchronized* inhibition/stimulation of two distinct sets of neurones has been extensively investigated, is extremely complicated, and is beyond the scope of this review. However, it is worth emphasizing that in the vast majority of acromegalics due to somatotroph adenomas this pulsatile nature of GH secretion is maintained, though the baseline about which the oscillations occur is elevated. Physiologically, most GH secretion occurs in childhood and adolescence when the largest bursts are synchronized with rapid eye movement (REM) sleep. In adulthood (>20 years) the amplitude of GH pulses gradually diminishes and there are long periods throughout the day (hours) when no GH secretion can be detected by currently available assays. It is, however, likely that small bursts of GH secretion are occurring but our ability to detect them is absent.

Many physiological factors control GH secretion including physical activity, nutrients and sleep. For example, in malnourished states, including malignant cachexia and anorexia nervosa, GH levels are elevated, probably due to the very low levels of IGF-1 produced by the liver. It is important to realize that IGF-1 can be measured reliably in serum, where it is bound to a variety of carrier proteins, and is a good long-term index of prevailing GH exposure. IGF-1 can be viewed as analogous to HbA_1C in diabetes, and the former may be elevated with chronically elevated low mean GH levels of 5–10mU/l. These low levels of GH can be associated with untreated acromegaly, and in the past mean GH values of this order have been designated as a 'cure' but this is now recognized as erroneous.

OCTREOTIDE IN PITUITARY DISEASE

Acromegaly

This is the primary endocrine indication for octreotide treatment both in terms of numbers of patients and on the basis of the pathophysiology. Octreotide is highly effective at lowering GH levels in acromegalics and a single subcutaneous dose of 100µg, with GH measurement 2, 4, 6 hours later is a good predictor of GH reduction with long-term treatment. Several studies [10, 14] have now reported results of long-term treatment (1–3 years) with octreotide and the following generalizations can be made:

1. 60–70% of patients have GH levels lowered by >50% and about 50% have levels suppressed to <10mU/l. This is a superior response to bromocriptine where only about 10% of patients achieve values of <10mU/l. IGF-1 levels show similar suppression.
2. There is concomitant improvement in clinical features of hyperhidrosis, soft tissue swelling (objectively measured as ring size or hand/foot volume), headache, carpal tunnel syndrome, and hypertension (see later).
3. Dose ranging studies indicate no advantage of increasing above 200µg three times daily, and the majority of patients respond maximally to 100µg three times daily. It is important to space the doses evenly at 8 hourly intervals. No evidence of diminishing response (i.e. tachyphylaxis) with up to 3 years' treatment is observed.
4. Significant tumour shrinkage occurs in 50–60% of patients, the extent of volume reduction being 40–50% [15]. This is a slow process taking 3–6 months to achieve. This contrasts with the much more rapid response of prolactinomas to bromocriptine where shrinkage can be observed within days. Consequently octreotide should not be used generally as an alternative to surgery where vision is impaired.
5. Side-effects – initial, usually transient 1–2 weeks, loose stool/diarrhoea and generalized abdominal discomfort. Generally, there is no need to discontinue treatment, and side-effects should be treated symptomatically. Longer term, there is good ultrasound evidence for an increase in biliary sludge and possibly gallstone formation in up to 40–50% of patients after 12–18 months' treatment [16]. However, the clinical significance remains to be determined. There is *no* impairment of glucose tolerance or deterioration in HbA_1C levels because the suppression of insulin levels is counterbalanced by lowering of the diabetogenic hormones, GH and glucagon.

Some additional observations, largely anecdotal and not thoroughly evaluated, deserve mention. There is preliminary evidence that resistant heart failure in a few acromegalics is improved as a consequence of increased stroke volume and reduced filling pressures [17]. Other studies document improvement in hypertension. However, it is likely that these cardiovascular benefits accrue whatever means is used to lower GH, rather than this being a specific effect of octreotide on the heart. Sleep apnoea is also improved with improvement in nocturnal oxygen saturation [18]; again this occurs with lowering of GH by other means.

It is self-evident that those adenomas responding to octreotide express somatostatin receptors on their somatotrophs. This may have potential value for targeting of high energy radionuclides to octreotide in very aggressive resistant tumours whose growth cannot be controlled by conventional means. Recent imaging studies using radio-labelled octreotide demonstrate significant pituitary specific uptake [19] which correlates with GH suppression.

Despite the obvious effectiveness of octreotide in treatment of GH hypersecretion, there are major obstacles to its prolonged use: (i) the inconvenience of thrice daily subcutaneous administration; (ii) the long-term side-effect profile, especially with respect to gallstones; (iii) the cost – currently about £6000/annum at 300µg/day (£12,000 at 600µg/day). It should be possible to develop a slow release depot preparation for once monthly injection as has been done with gonadotrophin releasing hormone (GnRH) analogues; or a nasal spray, which would enhance patient acceptability. The cost is a major consideration if years of treatment are envisaged.

Thus, it is appropriate to consider the objectives of treatment in acromegaly and where octreotide fits into this [20]. It is currently held that the objective should be to *eliminate* GH secretion if one is to achieve a *cure* in adults. As discussed earlier there is very little GH detected in adults and even mean levels of 5–10mU/l may be associated with high IGF-1 levels and long-term complications of which the most lethal are cardiovascular. For these reasons I believe every *reasonable* effort should be made, especially in the young/middle aged acromegalic (<60 years old). The problem we face is that there is no information available, nor is there likely to be for a number of years, on whether currently acceptable treatment objectives influence long-term morbidity or mortality. We, therefore, base our views on the unproven assumption that elimination of GH secretion is the gold standard. The main reason that this is probably naive is that patients have frequently had the disease for several years prior to the diagnosis being made, and damage to the cardiovascular system may be irreversible.

The widely acceptable approach which is most likely to achieve a hormonal cure is outlined in Figure 3. Based on currently available evidence my principle is to use octreotide if GH and IGF-1 levels remain elevated *after* radiotherapy and if bromocriptine in reasonable dosage fails to suppress levels further. My approach is pragmatic. I do not treat all patients in this category, treating each case on its merits depending upon symptoms and complications. There is the very rare patient with acromegaly caused by ectopic GH or GRF secretion, usually from a bronchial/gut carcinoid tumour. These respond well to octreotide if the primary source is unresectable.

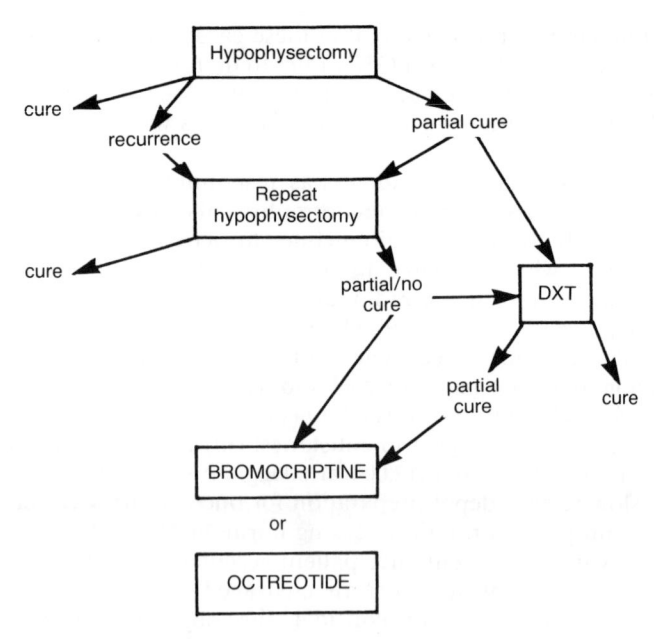

Figure 3. Modern management of somatotroph adenoma.

Other pituitary tumours
Octreotide successfully suppresses tumoral TSH secretion and corrects hyperthyroidism in rare TSH secreting adenomas [21]. However, octreotide is not generally of any therapeutic value in Cushing's syndrome whether caused by pituitary ACTH secreting adenomas or ectopic ACTH secretion, unless the latter is due to a carcinoid tumour, in which there have been anecdotal reports of benefit. Octreotide has no place in the treatment of prolactinomas or non-functional adenomas in which reduction of the tumour size is minimal if at all.

OCTREOTIDE IN GASTROENTEROPANCREATIC ENDOCRINE TUMOURS

These are rarer than acromegaly but may present with devastating and life-threatening symptoms due to high levels of hormone secretion (vasoactive intestinal polypeptide (VIP)/glucagon/gastrin/insulin) usually when liver metastases are already present. Because these tumours and their metastases are relatively slow growing and survival in, for example, carcinoid syndrome can be as high as 50% at 5 years [22], symptomatic relief is required for prolonged periods.

Carcinoid syndrome
The majority (80%) of primary tumours are in the gastrointestinal tract and 50–60% have liver metastases at presentation [23]. Adbominal pain, diarrhoea

and flushing are present in the majority of patients at some stage of the disease. Whilst these tumours produce a variety of biogenic amines (serotonin, 5HT) or vasoactive peptides (tachykinins), 5-hydroxyindole-acetic acid (5-HIAA) remains the most informative diagnostic and monitoring biochemical investigation. Treatment with octreotide may produce rapid (few days) and dramatic relief of abdominal pain, diarrhoea, flushing and wheezing in 60-70% of patients [24], and >50% reduction in 5-HIAA excretion occurs in similar proportion, though normalization of levels is rare. Doses of octreotide vary from 100 to 500μg three times daily. There is no evidence that octreotide reduces tumour bulk or prolongs survival. The role of octreotide is for symptomatic relief. It aborts hypotensive crises and prevents these if given before tumour debulking operations or hepatic embolization [22]. Eventually, resistance to the drug occurs as tumour bulk increases. The author has anecdotal experience of two patients with metastatic carcinoid in whom diarrhoea was abolished and flushing markedly reduced for 6-12 months of treatment.

VIPoma, glucagonomas, and AIDS-related diarrhoea
Less common than carcinoid syndrome these pancreatic neoplasms are associated with profound watery diarrhoea, dehydration, hypokalaemia, and achlorhydria. Although largely anecdotal, rapid and dramatic improvements in the fluid loss with weight gain (VIPoma) and rash (glucagonoma) have been documented [23-25]. Octreotide should be used prior to surgical resection in these patients. There are preliminary reports that octreotide will reduce stool volume in about 30% of patients with AIDS diarrhoea, refractory to other treatments though these studies need confirming.

Gastrinoma/Zollinger-Ellison syndrome
By suppression of gastrin secretion from benign and metastatic gastrinoma, patients' gastric acidity is diminished and healing of intractable ulcers can be obtained. Whilst in the former, surgery is the treatment of choice, octreotide has a place in symptomatic relief for patients with malignant gastrinoma.

Insulinoma and nesidioblastosis
Some patients with metastatic insulinoma respond to octreotide and it may reduce the frequency of and even prevent hypoglycaemic attacks [23-25]. In a patient treated by the author with octreotide 100μg, 100μg, 200μg at 8 hourly intervals for up to 9 months, from requiring a 10% dextrose drip to prevent hypoglycaemia, the patient is at home free of hypoglycaemia and not requiring glucose supplementation despite obvious clinical progression of hepatic metastases. Persistent hyperinsulinaemic hypoglycaemia of infancy due to nesidioblastosis may also respond to octreotide by reduction in glucose requirements and is worthy of trial prior to pancreatectomy [26]. An islet cell tumour causing hypercalcaemia due to high parathyroid hormone (PTH) related peptide production has been successfully treated with octreotide.

OCTREOTIDE IN ACUTE GASTROINESTINAL BLEEDING

Bleeding varices

Somatostatin reduces splanchnic blood flow in humans [27], particularly in the azygous and variceal vessels [28], and octreotide has the same actions. No clear reduction of portal pressure has been shown. Theoretically these actions might be expected to benefit patients with acute variceal bleeding and there have been several randomized trials comparing intravenous somatostatin or octreotide with vasopressin and balloon tamponade (reviewed in reference 29). The problem identified by Burroughs [29] is in the definition of end-points for comparison of the several treatment options in this condition. It would appear from the several studies reviewed that somatostatin was as effective as the more conventional treatments [30], though with fewer complications (e.g. ischaemic events with vasopressin or local gastro-oesophageal ulceration/perforation with balloon tamponade). There is conflicting evidence regarding whether somatostatin reduces transfusion requirements, and re-bleeding rates. There is no evidence that mortality is reduced. A comparison of somatostatin with emergency sclerotherapy showed equal control of bleeding in the first 5 days [31], and further studies are required to evaluate the place of octreotide prior to emergency sclerotherapy in the management of acute variceal bleeding. If these early results can be confirmed the simplicity of use and lack of side-effects may provide an important medical therapy in acute variceal bleeding. In the longer term we need to know whether octreotide given after sclerotherapy will reduce the frequency of re-bleeding and the long-term mortality from the complication of portal hypertension.

Acute gastrointestinal bleeding from other sites

Because of its beneficial effects on splanchnic blood flow and gastric acid secretion it was thought that octreotide may be beneficial in acute bleeding from peptic ulceration. This has not been demonstrated yet.

PANCREATITIS AND PANCREATIC FISTULAE

Inhibition of pancreatic enzymes, bicarbonate, and water secretion by octreotide suggest a beneficial role in acute pancreatitis and in pancreatic fistulae. Experimentally induced acute haemorrhagic pancreatitis in rats is attenuated by octreotide treatment [32]. No randomized placebo-controlled studies have been reported in humans with acute pancreatitis. It is possible that octreotide may be beneficial in patients undergoing pancreatic transplantation for end-stage diabetes where problems with pancreatic exocrine secretion can lead to failure of anastomosis healing. There are anecdotal reports that octreotide reduces secretions from external pancreatic fistulae and facilitates closure of both internal and external fistulae [33, 34].

OTHER GASTROINTESTINAL CONDITIONS

Octreotide reduces gastric emptying in post-gastrectomy patients and produces substantial symptomatic improvement in delayed dumping syndrome in which hyperinsulinaemia and hypoglycaemia are prevented [35]. Patients with short-bowel syndrome have high stool volume and excessive loss of water and electrolytes, all of which can be reduced by octreotide enhancement of gastrointestinal fluid absorption [36]. Patients with scleroderma have disordered gastrointestinal and oesophageal motility, pseudo-obstruction, and are prone to bacterial overgrowth and attendant malabsorption. A recent publication [7] showed that octreotide increased gastrointestinal motility in scleroderma patients and improved abdominal symptoms. Hydrogen breath excretion, reflecting gut bacterial overgrowth, was reduced. These effects of octreotide were independent of effects on motilin, whose plasma levels were reduced with treatment [7].

DIABETES MELLITUS
It was hoped that the suppressive effects of octreotide on GH and glucagon would improve glycaemic control and reduce insulin requirements in insulin-dependent diabetes (IDDM). However, this expectation has not been realized and instances of severe and unpredictable hypoglycaemia have been reported. No improvement in glycaemic control has been found in non-insulin-dependent diabetes (NIDDM) patients. There does not appear to be a place for octreotide management of hyperglycaemia of diabetes. Chronic octreotide treatment does not appear to alter either background or proliferative retinopathy. However, the increased renal blood flow, renal size, and higher glomerular filtration rate which are signs of early diabetic nephropathy were reduced after 3 months' treatment [37] opening the way for further studies to determine whether this drug has a place in preventing or delaying progression of nephropathy in IDDM.

ONCOLOGY
Somatostatin receptors have been identified on a wide variety of neuro-endocrine derived cells in vitro, and the availability of an iodinated analogue of octreotide has enabled in vivo scintigraphy to show good correlation with in vitro autoradiography. This subject is extensively reviewed in Lamberts [19]. Besides their usefulness for detection of primary tumours and metastatic deposits it is possible that analogues can be used to target high dose radionuclides or antimitotic prodrugs.

Various animal models of in vivo tumorigenesis and in vitro studies with several cell lines appear to show an antitumour effect of octreotide/ somatostatin. Whether the mechanism for this is indirect via lowering of GH/ IGF-1 and other growth factors including angiogenic factors, or is direct via effects on the tumour cells, is debatable and there is evidence for both of these possibilities [19]. Irrespective of the mechanism proposed for the antitumour activity of octreotide in animals it remains to be seen whether any similar activity will be found in humans.

Intrathecal octreotide by continuous infusion can be a potent analgesic in patients with intractable cancer pain [38]. Moreover, headache associated with pituitary tumours can be relieved irrespective of tumour shrinkage [39].

PSORIASIS
Improvement in plaque thickness and erythema has been reported in a double-blind placebo-controlled study lasting 12 weeks [40]. How octreotide achieves this is unknown.

POLYCYSTIC OVARY SYNDROME
Octreotide, 100μg twice daily for 7 days, significantly reduced luteinizing hormone (LH) pulse amplitude, mean LH, and LH response to a GnRH analogue in 10 amenorrhoeic women with polycystic ovary syndrome (PCOS) [41]. Accompanying this was a significant reduction in mean (over 4 hours) testosterone and androstenedione levels. Insulin responses to oral glucose were also suppressed. Because insulin levels (basal and carbohydrate stimulated) are elevated in PCOS and hyperinsulinaemia can directly stimulate ovarian androgen production, the observed results may partly be explained by the effects of octreotide on insulin secretion. This study (Prelevic et al [41]) merits further longer-term investigations in a double-blind placebo-controlled trial.

CONCLUSION
It is evident that somatostatin has a host of functions many of which have been known for some time. However, exploitation of these for therapeutic benefit was delayed until a long acting analogue became available. Now its potential has been realized in relatively uncommon endocrine tumours in some of which the symptomatic benefits are dramatic. However, the use of the drug for many other indications has led to promising possibilities, some of which may have wider implications in medicine (Table III). The issue of the clinical importance of disturbance in gallbladder function with long-term treatment will have to be addressed. Other side-effects appear to be transient and disappear with continued treatment. More controlled longer-term clinical trials are, however, needed. These should be paralleled by pharmacological developments to produce a more patient-acceptable depot formulation, and a reduction in the cost.

TABLE III. Therapeutic uses of octreotide

Definitive value	Potential value	Possible value
Acromegaly	Bleeding varices	Diabetic nephropathy
Gastrointestinal tumours carcinoids	Pancreatic fistulae	Pain relief (in cancer)
VIPomas glucagonomas	Post-gastrectomy dumping	Polycystic ovary syndrome
gatrinomas	Systemic sclerosis	Psoriasis
(Imaging endocrine tumours)	Autonomic neuropathy diarrhoea postural hypotension Headache associated with pituitary tumours	

REFERENCES

1. Krulich L, Dhariwal APS, McCann SM. Stimulatory and inhibitory effects of purified hypothalamic extracts on growth hormone release from rat pituitary in vitro. *Endocrinology* 1968; *83*: 783–790
2. Hellman B, Lernmark A. Inhibition of the in vitro secretion of insulin by an extract of pancreatic cells. *Endocrinology* 1969; *84*: 1484–1487
3. Brazeau P, Vale W, Burgus R et al. Hypothalamic peptide that inhibits the secretion of immunoreactive pituitary growth hormone. *Science* 1973; *179*: 77–79
4. Goodman RH, Jacobs JW, Dee PC, Habener JF. Somatostatin-28 encoded in a cloned cDNA obtained from a rat medullary thyroid carcinoma. *J Biol Chem* 1982; *257*: 1156–1159
5. Jackson IMD. Phylogenetic distribution and function of the hypophysiotropic hormones of the hypothalamus. *Am Zoologist* 1978; *18*: 385–399
6. Berelowitz M, LeRoith D, von Schenk H et al. Somatostatin-like immunoreactivity is present in *Tetrahymena pyriformis*, a ciliated protozoan. *Endocrinology* 1982; *110*: 1939–1944
7. Soudah HC, Hasler WL, Owyang C. Effect of octreotide on intestinal motility and bacterial overgrowth in scleroderma. *N Engl J Med* 1991; *325*: 1461–1467
8. Reichlin S. Somatostatin. *N Engl J Med* 1983; *309*: 1495–1501
9. Reichlin S. Somatostatin. *N Engl J Med* 1983; *309*: 1556–1563
10. Harris AG, Prestele H, Herald K et al. Long-term efficacy of sandostatin (SMS 201-995, octreotide) in 178 acromegalic patients. Results from the International Multicentre Acromegaly Study Group. In Lamberts SWJ, ed. *Sandostatin in the Treatment of Acromegaly; consensus round table, Amsterdam 1987*. Berlin: Springer-Verlag 1988: 117–125
11. Page MD, Willward ME, Taylor A et al. Long-term treatment of acromegaly with a long-acting analogue of Somatostatin octreotide. *Q J Med* 1990; *74*: 189–201
12. McKnight JA, McCance DR, Sheridan B et al. A long-term dose response study of somatostatin analogue (SMS 201-995, octreotide) in resistant acromegaly. *Clin Endocrinol* 1991; *34*: 119–125
13. Lamberts SWJ. The role of somatostatin in the regulation of anterior pituitary hormone secretion and the use of its analogs in the treatment of human pituitary tumours. *Endocrine Reviews* 1988; *9*: 417–436
14. Sandler IM, Burrin JM, Williams G et al. Effective long-term treatment of acromegaly with a long-acting somatostatin analogue (SMS 201-995). *Clin Endocrinol* 1987; *26*: 89–95
15. Barkan AL, Lloyd RV, Chandler WF et al. Preoperative treatment of acromegaly with long-acting somatostatin analog SMS 201-995. Shrinkage of invasive pituitary macroadenomas and improved surgical remission rate. *J Clin Endocrinol Metab* 1988; *67*: 1040–1048
16. Wass JAH, Anderson JV, Besser GM, Dowling RH. Gallstones and treatment with octreotide for acromegaly. *Br Med J* 1989; *299*: 1162–1163
17. Chanson P, Timsit J, Masquet C, Warnet A et al. Cardiovascular effects of the somatostatin analog octreotide in acromegaly. *Ann Intern Med* 1990; *113*: 921–925
18. Sebastian JP, Allen M, Pearson SB, Belchetz PE. Lung function and sleep apnoea in acromegaly. *J Endocrinol* 1990; *127*: Suppl. Abs 32
19. Lamberts SWJ, Kreaning EP, Reubi J-C. The role of somatostatin and its analogs in the diagnosis and treatment of tumours. *Endocrine Reviews* 1991 *12*: 450–482
20. Frohman LA. Therapeutic options in acromegaly. *J Clin Endocrinol Metab* 1991; *72*: 1175–1181
21. Beck-Peccoz P, Roncoroni R, Mariotti S et al. Sex hormone-binding globulin measurement in patients with inappropriate secretion of thyrotropin (IST): evidence against selective pituitary thyroid hormone resistance in non-neoplastic IST. *J Clin Endocrinol Metab* 1990; *71*: 19–25
22. Wynick D, Bloom SR. The use of the long-acting somatostatin analog octreotide in the treatment of gut neuroendocrine tumours. *J Clin Endocrinol Metab* 1991; *73*: 1–3
23. Woods HF, Bax NDS, Ainsworth I. Abdominal carcinoid tumours in Sheffield. *Digestion* 1990; *45* (suppl 1): 17–22
24. Buchanan KD, Collins JSA, Varghese A et al. Sandostatin and the Belfast Experience. *Digestion* 1990; *45* (suppl 1): 11–16
25. Wynick D, Bloom SR. Sandostatin and the Hammersmith Experience. *Digestion 1990*:

45 (suppl 1); 5-10
26 Glaser B, Landaw H. Long-term treatment with the Somatostatin analogue SMS 201-995: alternative to pancreatectomy in persistent hyperinsulinaemic hypoglycaemia of infancy. *Digestion 1990; 145* (suppl 1): 27-35
27 Sonnenberg GE, Keller U, Perruchnd A et al. Effect of somatostatin on splanchnic haemodynamics in patients with cirrhosis of the liver and in normal subjects. *Gastroenterology 1981; 80*: 526-532
28 McCormick PA, Dick R, Siringo S et al. Octreotide reduces azygous blood flow in cirrhotic patients with portal hypertension. *Eur J Gastroenterol Hepatol 1990; 2*: 489-492
29 Burroughs AK. Somatostatin and octreotide for variceal bleeding. *J Hepatol 1991; 13*: 1-4
30 McKee RA. A study of octreotide in oesophageal varices. *Digestion 1990; 45* (suppl 1): 60-65
31 Jenkins SA, Baxter JN, Ellenbogen S, Sheilds R. A prospective randomised controlled clinical trial comparing sandostatin and injection sclerotherapy in the control of acute variceal haemorrhage: preliminary results. *Gut 1988; 29*: A1431
32 Toledano AE, Reis ED, Ribeiro MLB et al. The effect of secretion and somatostatin analog (SMS 201-995) on survival in taurocholate-induced acute pancreatitis in rats. *Pancreas 1988; 3*: 620-625
33 Lansden FT, Adams DB, Anderson MC. Treatment of external pancreatic fistula with somatostatin. *Am Surg 1989; 55*: 695-698
34 Scott NA, Finnegan S, Irving MH. Octreotide and gastrointestinal fistulae. *Digestion 1990; 45* (suppl 1): 66-71
35 Primrose JN. Octreotide in the treatment of dumping syndrome. *Digestion 1990; 45* (suppl 1): 49-59
36 Nightingale JMD, Walker ER, Burnham WR et al. Short bowel syndrome. *Digestion 1990;* (suppl 1): 77-83
37 Serri O, Beauregard H, Brazean P et al. Sandostatin reduces increased kidney function and size in type 1 diabetes. *Diabetologia 1990; 33* (suppl): A76
38 Penn RD, Paice JA, Kroin JS. Intrathecal octreotide for cancer pain. *Lancet 1990; i*: 738
39 Williams G, Ball JA, Lawson RA et al. Analgesic effect of somatostatin analogue (octreotide) in headache associated with pituitary tumours. *Br Med J 1987; 3295*: 247-248
40 Camisa C, O'Dorisio TM, Placeyko RF et al. Treatment of psoriasis with chronic subcutaneous administration of somatostatin analog 201-995 I, an open-label pilot study. *Cleveland Clinic J Med 1990; 57*: 1 71-76
41 Prelevic GM, Wurzburger MI, Balint-Perie L, Neric JS. Inhibitory effect of sandostatin on secretion of luteinising hormone and ovarian steroids in polycystic ovary syndrome. *Lancet 1990; ii*: 900-903

TRANSIENT ISCHAEMIC ATTACKS AND STROKE: PROGNOSIS AND MANAGEMENT

Martin Dennis
Western General Hospital, Edinburgh

INTRODUCTION

Each year in the UK over 100,000 people have a first stroke and almost 25,000 consult their doctor having had a transient ischaemic attack (TIA). Stroke is the third commonest cause of death in most developed countries, and a major cause of severe disability, accounting for more than 5% of all NHS resources. In such an important disease it is essential to know its prognosis and how management can affect this.

Stroke and TIA are both diagnoses which are defined primarily by their clinical features rather than by laboratory investigations. A TIA has been defined as an acute loss of focal cerebral monocular function with symptoms lasting less than 24 hours and which after adequate investigation are presumed to be caused by embolic or thrombotic vascular disease [1]. A stroke could be defined in the same way except that the symptoms last more than 24 hours or lead to death within that time. Unfortunately, and especially in the case of TIAs, these definitions are often not rigorously applied in everyday clinical practice. However, the data presented in this paper apply only to groups of patients with TIAs and stroke who fulfil these strict clinical definitions.

In this paper I refer to prognosis rather than natural history since most patients now receive some treatment even if it is only moderately effective. Published data on the prognosis of TIAs and strokes have varied widely and depend critically on the methodology used (which will not be discussed in detail in this paper) and the selection or mix of patients included in the studies. To overcome this, I will only present data from unselected cohorts of patients identified in a community-based study (Oxfordshire Community Stroke Project – OCSP [2–4]) which fulfil the criteria shown in Table I. The reader's perception of their patients' prognosis may differ from that presented here due to the selected nature of patients they are seeing. For example, a neurosurgeon will tend to see a large number of haemorrhagic strokes who have a much worse than average prognosis. For TIA and stroke patients we generally describe prognosis in terms of risk of death (subdivided into all deaths and vascular deaths), stroke (or recurrent stroke) and myocardial infarction. For stroke it is also useful to describe prognosis in terms of disability, and psychological and social outcome although these are more difficult to measure.

TABLE I. Important features of studies of prognosis

Unselected cohort of patients to ensure maximum generalizability of results
Large enough to give precise information
Identification of patients at an early and uniform time in the course of the disease
Prospective assessment using strict diagnostic criteria to ensure homogeneity
Prospective, complete and prolonged follow-up
Clearly defined outcomes
Appropriate analysis, e.g. life table

Prognostic data for groups of patients are valuable when planning randomized clinical trials and in health service planning, but the busy clinician is more often interested in predicting the prognosis in individual patients. An accurate prediction allows us to give reliable advice to patients and relatives, to balance the risks and benefits of different treatment options and to plan other aspects of management such as the timing of hospital discharge. For this reason I shall describe those variables, the prognostic variables, which indicate whether a particular patient is at high or low risk of having an unfavourable outcome.

THE PROGNOSIS OF TIAs

Following a patient's first presentation to a doctor with a TIA, his/her annual risk of death is about 6% although this is only slightly greater than would be expected for TIA free individuals of a similar age; the relative risk is about 1.4:1. The risk of stroke after a TIA is illustrated in Figure 1. The risk is highest early on and is about 12% (or about 13 times that of an unaffected individual) in the first year and about 4% per year (five times that of an unaffected individual) over the next few years. Patients who have had TIAs also have an increased risk of other vascular events such as myocardial infarction (2–3%/year); indeed this is a more common cause of death than stroke after a TIA. The overall annual risk of having a stroke or myocardial infarction or vascular death is about 8%.

Prognostic variables for TIAs

Several factors have been identified as being related to a greater or lesser than average risk of death, stroke or myocardial infarction after a TIA. These are shown in Table II (courtesy of Dr G Hankey). In patients with TIAs in the carotid distribution the degree of ipsilateral carotid stenosis appears to be related to the risk of ipsilateral stroke, the tighter the stenosis the higher the risk. By combining, and suitably weighting different variables, Hankey et al [5] have produced a prognostic equation but even this is relatively imprecise in predicting an individual's risk of a stroke, myocardial infarction or vascular

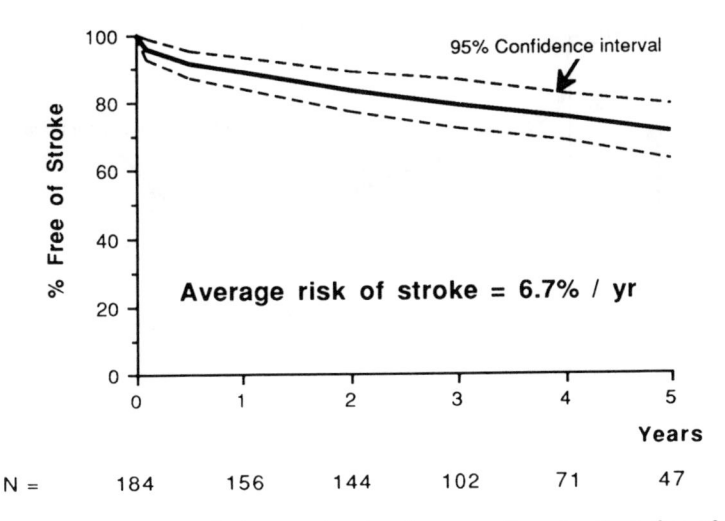

Figure 1. A Kaplan Meier survival curve showing the proportion of patients free of stroke after a TIA in the Oxfordshire Community Stroke Project.

death, although it is more reliable in dichotomizing patients into those at high and low risk.

TABLE II. Factors related to a poor outcome after a TIA

Increasing age
Male sex
Cerebral (rather than monocular) ischaemic attacks
Multiple TIAs during last 3 months
TIAs in both carotid and vertebrobasilar distributions
Residual neurological signs
Peripheral vascular disease
Left ventricular hypertrophy (on ECG)

THE PROGNOSIS OF STROKE

The survival following a first stroke is illustrated in Figure 2. Approximately 20% of patients die within the first 30 days, most dying within the first week from the direct neurological consequences of their stroke. Pneumonia, pulmonary emboli and secondary vascular events account for a few of these very early deaths but become an increasingly common cause over the next few weeks. By 1 year approximately 30% of patients will have died and about 20-30% are dependent on others for activities of daily living, but the remainder are able to live independently. After the first year patients continue to have about a 6% annual risk of death, about two or three times that of stroke free individuals. The risk of recurrent stroke and myocardial infarction in a stroke survivor is similar to that following a TIA and for practical purposes the approach to secondary prevention is similar for TIAs and minor

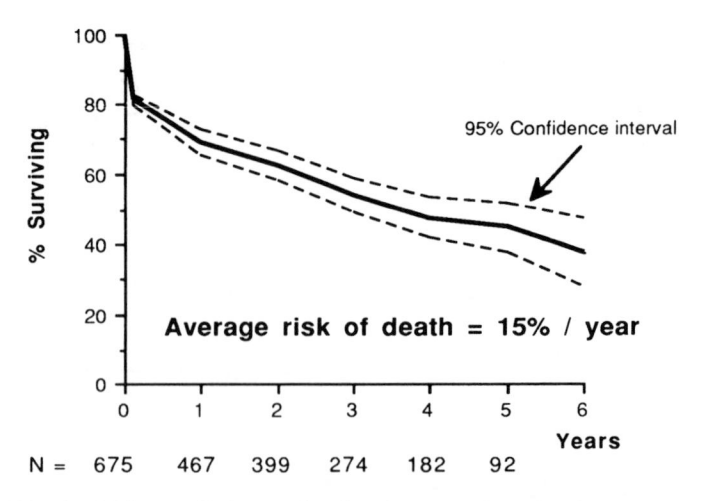

Figure 2. A Kaplan Meier survival curve showing the proportion of patients surviving after a first-ever stroke in the Oxfordshire Community Stroke project.

ischaemic strokes. Psychological problems are common in stroke survivors and include anxiety states, agoraphobia, apathy and self-neglect, irritability, pathological emotionalism and occasionally major depression [6, 7]. Social problems including isolation, marital disharmony, housing problems, poverty and unemployment are important but are difficult to quantify and have therefore been little studied. These psychological and social aspects of outcome are frequently ignored by clinicians although they may have a major bearing on the patients' and carers' quality of life and may respond to appropriate interventions.

Prognostic variables for stroke
Patients with either a primary intracerebral haemorrhage or subarachnoid haemorrhage have a much greater risk of early death compared with the patients with cerebral infarction. The 30 day case fatality rates are about 52%, 45% and 10% respectively [8]. However, having survived this early period, patients with intracranial haemorrhage are less likely than those with cerebral infarction to remain severely disabled or dependent on others. There is no convincing evidence that recurrence rates are different for different pathological types although in patients with subarachnoid haemorrhage in whom the primary cause is treated, e.g. the aneurysm is clipped or the AV malformation resected, recurrence is uncommon.

A number of clinical features indicate a high risk of early death. These comprise signs of severe brain stem dysfunction such as altered conscious level, gaze palsies, bilateral neurological signs and abnormal breathing patterns. These may result from direct involvement of the brain stem by the stroke or more commonly result from pressure effects from supratentorial strokes. Patients with these signs who survive, in addition to those with evidence of a large volume of cerebral damage (e.g. combination of hemiparesis, hemianopia with either dysphasia or neglect), are also likely to have a poor functional outcome. Urinary incontinence which persists for more than 3 days is probably the single most powerful prognostic factor to discriminate between patients with a good and bad outcome [9]. Several workers have combined factors into prognostic scores (e.g. Allen [10]) to improve predictive accuracy although most have not been validated in second cohorts of patients and cannot therefore be recommended for general use.

MANAGEMENT

The management of TIAs and strokes is complex and multifaceted. The major components are shown in Table III. In this paper discussion is limited to the medical (i.e. pharmacological) and surgical treatment of acute stroke and secondary prevention. Rehabilitation, that broad process which involves assessment and re-training of patients to make optimal use of their residual function, may have an important effect on functional, psychological and social outcome. However, a detailed discussion of this important subject is beyond the scope of this paper.

TABLE III. The management of stroke

Diagnosis
Assessment
Acute treatment (medical/surgical)
Rehabilitation
Terminal care
Placement and discharge planning
Follow-up
Secondary prevention

with education and counselling at all stages

Medical treatment of acute stroke

Over the last three decades many drugs have been tried in acute stroke. These include treatments which reduce cerebral oedema (e.g. steroids, glycerol), protect ischaemic neurones (e.g. calcium antagonists, naftidrofuryl) or improve blood flow (haemodilution, thrombolysis). Table IV shows the drugs which have been evaluated in randomized trials and the total number of patients randomized in each group of trials. A quantitative overview of these trials (unpublished data from H Willem and P Sandercock) demonstrates that no treatment appears to have a significant effect on mortality in acute stroke. Even where large numbers (>3000) of patients have been randomized (i.e. calcium entry blockers and haemodilution) the overview suggests little effect although the results are compatible (due to the wide confidence intervals) with them either preventing or causing 10 or 20 deaths per thousand patients treated. Further, much larger trials of the more promising treatments for acute stroke are urgently required to test their efficacy, since to demonstrate reliably that a drug reduces the risk of dying after an acute stroke by 20%

requires a trial of about 20,000 patients, which is more than 10 times larger than the largest acute stroke trial so far. If such a drug was simple and could be given to most stroke patients (cf. aspirin in acute myocardial infarction), then even if only moderately effective it could save many thousands of lives each year and may prevent many more patients being severely disabled. A major change in organization of stroke services, with the establishment of acute units, will be required to facilitate such trials.

TABLE IV. Randomized trials of medical therapies for acute stroke

Therapy	Number of trials	Total number of patients randomized
Anticoagulants	11	1079
Antiplatelet	1	30
Thrombolysis	7	573
Haemodilution	18	3313
Prostacyclin	4	168
Calcium entry blockers	15	3999
GM1-ganglioside	3	555
Naftidrofuryl	2	210
Naloxone	2	155
Steroids	11	684
Glycerol	10	830
Total	84	11596

Surgical treatment in acute stroke

The main indication for surgical treatment is in patients with haemorrhage and less often infarction of the cerebellum who deteriorate due to obstructive hydrocephalus. Insertion of a ventricular drainage device, decompression and/or aspiration of the haematoma may be lifesaving. The role of surgery in patients with supratentorial intracerebral haemorrhages is more controversial. Enthusiastic surgeons have experimented with a variety of operations for patients with major cerebral infarcts. These have included acute carotid endarterectomy and even decompression of the swollen hemisphere by a craniotomy but none have been properly evaluated and they are seldom performed.

Secondary prevention

In patients who have had a TIA or who have a reasonable quality of life following a first stroke the prevention of a further stroke, myocardial infarction or death is of great importance. All TIA and stroke patients should be thoroughly assessed to exclude uncommon but remediable causes of stroke such as temporal arteritis, syphilis and endocarditis. Treatment of these conditions will usually substantially reduce the risk of recurrence.

Epidemiological evidence and that from trials of primary prevention suggests that we can reduce the risk of secondary events by modifying risk factors such as smoking, hypertension and hypercholesterolaemia in TIA and stroke survivors. However, this has not been and may not be able to be confirmed by randomized clinical trials.

Antiplatelet drugs
An overview of all randomized trials of antiplatelet agents (APT [11]) demonstrated that drugs such as aspirin reduce the risk of further vascular events (including recurrent stroke and myocardial infarctions) by about 25% (e.g. 8%/year to 6%/year). Doses of aspirin as low as 75mg have been shown to be effective [12] and a recent trial comparing 30mg with 283mg showed no significant difference in outcome [13]. The APT has not demonstrated any differences in the effectiveness of aspirin in men and women, in different age groups and no other antiplatelet agent (e.g. ticlopidine, Persantin) is clearly more effective than aspirin.

Anticoagulation
The role of anticoagulation with warfarin in secondary prevention, especially in patients with a potential source of cardiac embolism, is still uncertain. The European Atrial Fibrillation Trial should yield some valuable information within the next year or two.

Carotid endarterectomy
During the past year, two large multicentre randomized trials [14, 15] of carotid endarterectomy have shown that for patients with TIAs and minor ischaemic strokes in the carotid distribution who have a stenosis of 70% or more in the ipsilateral carotid artery, carotid endarterectomy reduces the risk of subsequent stroke despite the not inconsiderable surgical morbidity and mortality. Patients with a less than 30% stenosis do not appear to benefit from treatment and the situation is still unclear for those with a stenosis of 30–69%. These studies are continuing to define further the role of carotid endarterectomy in the secondary prevention of stroke. Unlike antiplatelet agents, carotid endarterectomy only has an effect on the risk of ipsilateral stroke and is unlikely to prevent myocardial infarction and non-stroke vascular deaths.

THE FUTURE
During the next few years I believe that our ability to predict the likely outcome in individual patients will improve. Randomized trials, both current and planned, will define more precisely which patients are likely to benefit from anticoagulation and carotid endarterectomy. Even more exciting will be the evaluation of both existing and new drugs which may influence the outcome in acute stroke although their evaluation will depend upon us making major changes in the organization of health care for stroke patients. Perhaps, in the next few years the negative attitudes exhibited by many doctors towards stroke patients will be exchanged for more positive ones.

ACKNOWLEDGEMENTS

Dr M Dennis is supported by the Stroke Association and most of the data presented in this paper come from studies supported by the Medical Research Council and Stroke Association.

REFERENCES

1. Warlow CP, Morris PJ. Introduction. In Warlow CP, Morris PJ, eds. *Transient Ischaemic Attacks*. New York: Marcel Dekker. 1982: vii–xi
2. Bamford J, Sandercock P, Dennis M et al. A prospective study of acute cerebrovascular disease in the community: The Oxfordshire Community Stroke Project – 1981-1986: 1. Methodology, demography and incident cases of first stroke. *J Neurol Neurosurg Psychiatry 1988; 51*: 1373-1380
3. Bamford J, Sandercock P, Dennis M et al. A prospective study of acute cerebrovascular disease in the community: The Oxfordshire Community Stroke Project – 1981-1986. 2. Incidence, case fatality rates and overall outcome at one year of cerebral infarction, primary intracerebral and subarachnoid haemorrhage. *J Neurol Neurosurg Psychiatry 1990; 53*: 16-22
4. Dennis M, Bamford J, Sandercock P, Warlow C. Prognosis of transient ischaemic attacks in the Oxfordshire Community Stroke Project. *Stroke 1990; 21*: 848-853
5. Hankey GJ, Slattery JM, Warlow CP. Transient ischaemic attacks: which patients are at high (and low) risk of serious vascular events? *J Neurol Neurosurg Psychiatry* in press
6. House A, Dennis M, Mogridge L. Mood disorders in the year after first stroke. *Br J Psychiatry 1991; 158*: 83-92
7. House A, Dennis M, Molyneux A et al. Emotionalism after stroke. *Br Med J 1989; 298*: 991-994
8. Bamford J, Dennis M, Sandercock P et al. The frequency, causes and timing of death within 30 days of a first stroke: The Oxfordshire Community Stroke Project. *J Neurol Neurosurg Psychiatry 1990; 53*: 824-829
9. Wade DT, Hewer RL. Outlook after an acute stroke: urinary incontinence and loss of consciousness compared in 532 patients. *Q J Med 1985; 221*: 601-608
10. Allen CMC. Predicting the outcome of acute stroke: a prognostic score. *J Neurol Neurosurg Psychiatry 1984; 47*: 475-480
11. Antiplatelet Trialists' Collaboration. Secondary prevention of vascular disease by prolonged antiplatelet treatment. *Br Med J 1988; 296*: 320-331
12. The SALT Collaborative Group. Swedish Aspirin Low-dose Trial (SALT) of 75mg aspirin as secondary prophylaxis after cerebrovascular ischaemic events. *Lancet 1991; 338*: 1345-1349
13. The Dutch TIA Trial Study Group. A comparison of two doses of Aspirin (30mg vs. 283mg a day) in patients after a transient ischaemic attack or minor ischaemic stroke. *N Engl J Med 1991; 325*: 1261-1266
14. European Carotid Surgery Trialists' Collaborative Group. MRC European Carotid Surgery Trial: interim results for symptomatic patients with severe (70-99%) or with mild (0-29%) carotid stenosis. *Lancet 1991; 337*: 1235-1243
15. North American Symptomatic Carotid Endarterectomy Trial (NASCET) collaborators. Beneficial effect of carotid endarterectomy in symptomatic patients with high-grade stenosis. *N Engl J Med 1991; 325*: 445-453

PHARMACOLOGICAL MANAGEMENT OF EPILEPSY IN ADOLESCENTS AND ADULTS

Martin J Brodie
Western Infirmary, Glasgow

INTRODUCTION

Around 50 million people worldwide have epilepsy. The incidence is 20-70 individuals per 100,000 per year with a point prevalence of 4-10/1000 [1]. Incidence rates vary considerably with age. They are highest in childhood, plateau from 15 to 65 years and rise again in the elderly. It is estimated that 2-5% of the general population will have a fit at some time in their lives. Seizures represent the clinical expression of a number of diverse disorders, although a specific cause cannot be identified in around 70% of patients [2]. The diagnosis is made from the clinical description of the fits. Management consists largely of antiepileptic drugs, which are sometimes given for life [3]. A majority of patients remain seizure-free on taking prophylactic medication. Indeed, the condition will remit in a proportion of patients, and in these treatment can often be safely withdrawn [4]. Epilepsy becomes refractory in about 20% of patients, and particularly affects those with an anatomical basis for their seizure disorder [5].

Most neurologists in the UK do not initiate treatment following a single seizure, but await a second or occasionally further fits, if the situation remains unclear [2]. A witness to the seizure is an essential component for a correct diagnosis. A seizure is a symptom and not a pathological process. It is, therefore, important to determine whether epilepsy is primary (i.e. no underlying lesion; often a family history) or secondary (i.e. aura, cerebral damage, tumour, congenital malformation etc.) by appropriate investigations, such as electroencephalography and brain scanning. For a successful therapeutic outcome, the patient must understand the reason for taking an antiepileptic drug and be convinced about the benefits of continuing treatment for some years. Accordingly, if there is any doubt about the diagnosis or the patient's willingness to accept it, a wait-and-see policy is advisable. Poor compliance with medication, either as a consequence of lack of understanding of the prophylactic nature of the treatment or because of poor motivation, is a common reason for continuing seizures. Poor seizure control early in the course of the disorder may increase the patient's risk of developing refractory epilepsy [6].

CHOICE OF DRUG

The choice of drug to initiate therapy depends on seizure type, which is based on the classification (Table I) published by the International League against Epilepsy [7]. Consideration must be given to efficacy, side-effects, adverse reactions, and ease of use. In this paper, treatment of epilepsy in adolescents and adults only will be considered. The management of seizures in infancy and childhood presents different problems and has been reviewed recently elsewhere [8, 9].

TABLE I. International classification of seizure type

I. *Partial seizures*
    A Simple partial seizures
        (1) With motor signs
        (2) With somatosensory or special sensory hallucinations
        (3) With autonomic symptoms and signs
        (4) With psychic symptoms

    B Complex partial seizures
        (1) Simple partial onset followed by impairment of consciousness
        (2) With impaired consciousness at onset

    C Secondary generalization
        (1) Simple partial seizures evolving to generalized tonic–clonic seizures
        (2) Complex partial seizures evolving to generalized tonic–clonic seizures
        (3) Simple partial evolving to complex partial seizures and then to generalized tonic–clonic seizures

II *Generalized seizures*
    A (1) Absence seizures
        (2) Atypical absence
    B   Myoclonic seizures
    C   Clonic seizures
    D   Tonic seizures
    E   Tonic–clonic seizures
    F   Atonic seizures

III *Unclassifiable epileptic seizures*

For most adolescents or adults with newly diagnosed epilepsy, carbamazepine (CBZ) or sodium valproate (VPA) represents the drug of choice (Table II) [2]. CBZ should be chosen first for patients with partial seizures and VPA preferred for the primary generalized epilepsies [3]. CBZ is ineffective for the treatment of absence [10] and myoclonic epilepsies [11]. Phenytoin (PHT) is as effective as CBZ against partial and generalized tonic–clonic seizures, but can now be regarded as second-line therapy because of its potential to produce cosmetic and psychosocial side-effects, and the difficulty in determining the optimum dose due to the sudden change from first to zero order kinetics [3].

Ethosuximide (ETH) is still useful in the treatment of absence seizures. Phenobarbitone (PB) is out of favour, because of its propensity to produce sedation and tolerance. Nevertheless, it is an effective drug [12], which has an important role in the developing world as it is cheap and easy to use [13]. There is little place now for primidone (PRIM), which depends on metabolism to PB for its clinical action, but is more toxic [12]. Clonazepam (CLON), a sedative benzodiazepine, is of limited value. Few patients benefit greatly from long-term treatment with this drug and seizure control will worsen in around 50% when it is withdrawn [14]. Clobazam (CLB), a 1,5 benzodiazepine, less sedative than CLON and can be helpful in the treatment of refractory partial seizures [15], particularly when given as intermittent therapy to avoid tolerance [16]. Vigabatrin (VGB) and lamotrigine (LTG) have been licensed recently as additional therapeutic agents, when more established antiepileptic drugs have failed to provide adequate seizure control. VGB is particularly useful for partial seizures [17], while LTG is also promising for the primary generalized epilepsies [18].

TABLE II. Choice of drug for initiation of anticonvulsant therapy for the common seizure types in adolescents and adults

Seizure type	First line	Second line
Tonic–clonic	Sodium valproate Carbamazepine	Phenytoin
Absence	Sodium valproate	Ethosuximide
Myoclonic	Sodium valproate	Clonazepam
Partial	Carbamazepine	Phenytoin Sodium valproate
Unclassified	Carbamazepine Sodium valproate	Phenytoin

MONOTHERAPY

Treatment should be started in patients with newly diagnosed epilepsy using a single drug at low dosage (Table II). Subsequent titration should be undertaken on an individual basis over a period of months (Table III). This will help avoid concentration-dependent side-effects – in particular central nervous system toxicity, the presence of which is likely to discourage the patient from persevering with long-term therapy. An additional benefit of a cautious approach is to allow tolerance to develop to subjective cognitive impairment [19]. Such a policy will also detect early the emergence of idiosyncratic reactions, such as rash, hepatotoxicity and blood dyscrasias.

If the first drug chosen does not fully abolish seizures or produces unacceptable toxicity, a second should be substituted [3]. Again initial dosage should be low and titrated upwards as necessary at 4 weekly intervals. Until a therapeutic dose of the second drug is achieved, it is advisable not to change

TABLE III. Prescribing antiepileptic drugs in adolescents and adults

Drug	Indications	Starting dose	Maintenance dosing	Dosage schedule	Target range
Carbamazepine	Partial and generalized tonic–clonic seizures	100–200mg	400–2000mg	*Once or twice daily	4–12mg/l (17–50µmol/l)
Clobazam	Adjunctive therapy for refractory partial seizures	10mg	10–40mg	Once or twice daily	None
Clonazepam	Myoclonic and generalized tonic–clonic seizures	0.5–1mg	2–8mg	Once or twice daily	None
Ethosuximide	Absence seizures	500mg	500–2000mg	Once or twice daily	† 40–100mg/l (283–708µmol/l)
Lamotrigine	Adjuvant therapy for partial and generalized tonic–clonic seizures	25–50mg	100–400mg	Twice daily	‡ 2–4mg/l (7.8–15.6µmol/l)
Phenobarbitone	Partial and generalized tonic–clonic seizures	30–60mg	60–240mg	Once or twice daily	† 10–40mg/l (40–172µmol/l)
Phenytoin	Partial and generalized tonic–clonic seizures	200–300mg	100–700mg	Once or twice daily	10–20mg/l (40–80µmol/l)
Primidone	Partial and generalized tonic–clonic seizures	125–250mg	250–1500mg	Twice daily	† 6–12mg/l (25–55µmol/l)
Sodium valproate	Primary generalized epilepsies. Partial and secondary tonic–clonic seizures	500mg	500–3000mg	Once or twice daily	† 50–100mg/l (347–693µmol/l)
Vigabatrin	Adjunctive therapy for refractory partial seizures	500–1000mg	2–4g	Once or twice daily	None

* Using the controlled-release formulation. † Target range unhelpful. ‡ Target range not validated.

the dose of the first drug. Once seizure control has been established, the first drug can be withdrawn over a period of weeks or months. As pharmacokinetic interactions are almost inevitable between pairs of anticonvulsants, measuring the concentrations of both drugs can be helpful if problems arise. More rapid substitution is indicated if the first drug produces a rash or other unwanted effect.

A diary listing all the fits noted by the patient and his or her family is an essential aid to assessing control. This should include a description of each seizure. Careful supervision and support is essential at this stage to answer the patient's questions, allay fears and encourage compliance with medication. Time spent counselling the patient on the nature of the condition, the importance of perfect compliance and the likely repercussions of the diagnosis on his or her lifestyle, driving, employment, marriage, reproduction etc., will pay dividends in the long run in improved seizure control and better quality of life. Reassurance and encouragement will help build back the confidence lost by the shock of the diagnosis and the anticipation of further seizures.

Anticonvulsant monitoring
Monitoring circulating anticonvulsant concentrations may help to optimize the dose, particularly with PHT, and will certainly identify the poor compliers [20]. A drug level, however, can only be regarded as a guide, around which to alter the dose in line with the clinical situation [21]. The target range (Table III) applies only to a minority of patients. It is best defined for PHT and least useful for VPA, PB and PRIM. If complete seizure control proves elusive, the anticonvulsant dose should be increased monthly to the maximum tolerated by the patient without being too concerned about the circulating concentration.

Individual drugs

Carbamazepine
CBZ should be introduced at low dosage to offset the development of mild neurotoxic symptoms (nausea, headache, diplopia, dizziness, ataxia) [19]. A morbilliform rash will limit its usefulness in 5–10% of patients. At high concentrations, hyponatraemia may develop due to a vasopression-like action [10]. This is usually asymptomatic, but if the serum sodium falls below 120mm/l, the patient may present with confusion, peripheral oedema and increased seizure frequency. Due to induction of hepatic metabolic enzymes, CBZ concentrations tend to drift downwards over the first few weeks of therapy [22]. The dose may, thus, need to be increased shortly after starting treatment to take into account these changes (Figure 1). This pharmacokinetic oddity can produce a drop in elimination half-life from initial values of 24–36 hours in the naive patient to around 8–12 hours on chronic dosing. High peak concentrations often result in intermittent neurotoxic side-effects around 2 hours after a dose, necessitating dividing the dosage to three or four times daily in some individuals. The introduction of the modified-release formulation of CBZ will flatten the concentration–time profile [23], allowing twice daily dosing for all patients treated with this drug [24].

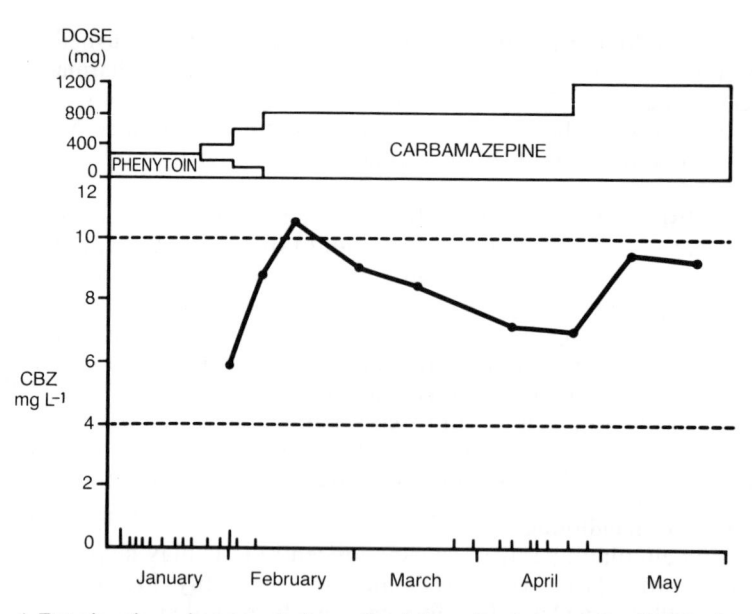

Figure 1. Deteriorating seizure control on a fixed dose of carbamazepine (CBZ) with falling plasma concentrations attributable to autoinduction of metabolism. Generalized tonic–clonic (longer lines) and partial (shorter lines) seizures are illustrated at the foot (from reference 22, with permission).

Sodium valproate
VPA is relatively free from sedative side-effects [25] and there is no need to give it more than twice daily to any patient (Table III). It is particularly effective in the treatment of the primary generalized epilepsies [26]. Common dose-related problems include tremor, weight gain due to appetite stimulation, thinning or loss of hair and peripheral oedema. Hepatotoxicity is rare above the age of 3 years [27]. As the drug can take some weeks to be fully effective [28], frequent adjustment of dose after initiating therapy is unjustified. There is no useful concentration–effect toxicity relationship; thus routine monitoring of VPA concentrations is unnecessary [20].

Phenytoin
There is a move away from using PHT as a first-line drug for two reasons [3]. Firstly, it produces an impressive array of side-effects, of which cosmetic changes (gum hyperplasia, acne, hirsutes, facial coarsening) and psychosocial disorders (aggression, sedation, impaired memory, depression) are the most troublesome. The second complicating factor is the sudden change in its elimination from first to zero order at concentrations around 15mg/l (60μmol/l) due to saturation of metabolism (Figure 2). Treatment should commence with an initial dose around 5mg/kg day. If urgent control is required, an oral loading dose of 15mg/kg can be given. Monitoring of PHT concentrations is often helpful in optimizing the dosage schedule. Without it, some patients

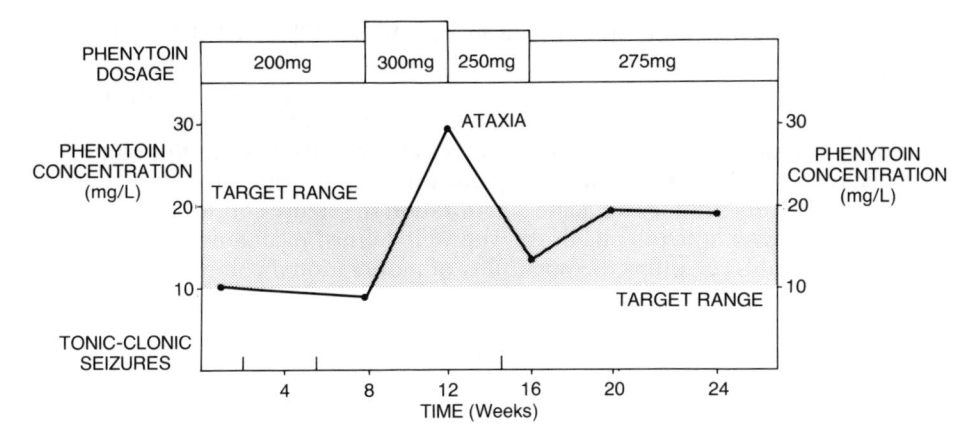

Figure 2. Effect of saturation of phenytoin metabolism on the relationship between dose and concentration. An increase from 200mg to 300mg daily trebled the circulating concentration, while subsequently dropping the dose to 250mg daily halved it (from reference 20, with permission).

will be undertreated, while others will develop neurotoxicity with mental slowing, depression and unsteadiness of gait. Examination will reveal nystagmus and ataxia (heel-toe walking is particularly sensitive). If the patient is not experiencing side-effects, PHT concentrations should be measured 4 weeks after starting treatment. Adjustment of dose can be undertaken in those still reporting seizures. If the PHT concentration is below 8mg/l (32μmol/l), an increment of 100mg should be made; patients with concentrations between 8 and 12 mg/l (32–48μmol/l) can be given an extra 50mg; above 12mg/l (48μmol/l) the dose should only be increased by 25mg at a time. Many patients remain seizure-free with concentrations of 5–10mg/l (20–40μmol/l) [29], while others will only respond optimally to circulating levels above 30mg/l (120μmol/l) without evidence of neurotoxicity [30].

POLYPHARMACY

Although seizures will be abolished in around 80% of patients with a single anticonvulsant, some patients require the addition of a second drug to obtain optimal control [31]. The proportion of patients with uncontrolled epilepsy who benefit from anticonvulsant polypharmacy is unknown; a figure as low as 10% has been suggested [12, 32]. Moreover, combinations of antiepileptic drugs can produce cognitive impairment [33] and complicated pharmacokinetic interactions [34].

There are no clear-cut guidelines on the choice of a second drug. Once all reasonable monotherapy options have been exhausted in patients with partial or generalized tonic–clonic seizures, most specialists combine two of the three most effective established drugs – namely CBZ, VPA and PHT – for no very good reason, as their mechanisms of action are complex and overlapping [35]. If an anatomical lesion is responsible for refractory complex partial seizures, it seems more appropriate to add VGB [17] or CLB [15]. If the patient reports predominantly generalized seizures, LTG is a better choice [18]. For myoclonic seizures, CLON should be added [2], while intractable absences may respond to a combination of VPA and ETH [36]. It seems illogical to introduce a sedative drug such as PB or PRIM, since this strategy is likely to be ineffective and subsequent withdrawal of the barbiturate will almost certainly produce an acute deterioration in seizure control. The development of novel antiepileptic drugs with well defined mechanisms of action, like VGB and LTG, offers the possibility of more rational combinations [34]. Controlled patient studies investigating additive or synergistic effects between pairs of anticonvulsants are currently lacking.

In some patients, who are truly refractory to pharmacotherapy, the law of diminishing returns will require patient and doctor to accept the persistence of some seizures. In such a situation it is important to balance adequacy of control with quality of life. If many seizures persist despite treatment with more than one anticonvulsant drug, little can be lost by gradually reducing the number of drugs and simplifying the dosage schedules. This manoeuvre will often reduce seizure frequency [37, 38]. Attempts to seek improvement by manipulating the drugs further should be resisted and the patient encouraged to accept a few seizures each month with as little cognitive impairment as can be achieved by pharmacological simplification. Producing less intrusive episodes, abolishing tonic–clonic fits and decreasing the likelihood of automatisms are all acceptable end-points. Alternatively, a surgical option can be explored [39] or the patient recruited for a clinical trial of a new antiepileptic drug.

Individual drugs

Vigabatrin
VGB is the newest antiepileptic drug to be licensed widely in Europe. It is a specific, irreversible inhibitor of gamma-aminobutyric acid (GABA) transaminase, the enzyme responsible for the breakdown of the inhibitory neurotransmitter, GABA [40]. It is particularly effective as adjunctive therapy in patients with refractory partial seizures [17]. Unfortunately, vigabatrin is sedative, although tolerance to this side-effect may occur. Around 5% of patients develop behavioural problems [41]. These consist of irritability, nervousness, confusion, aggression, and occasionally auditory and visual hallucinations leading in some individuals to frank psychosis. Rapid drug withdrawal can also precipitate psychosis. It is prudent to start with a low dose, usually 0.5–1g daily, and increase as necessary by a further 0.5g every 4 weeks (Table III). Some patients respond optimally to as little as 1g per day of VGB. The standard dose is around 2g daily and few patients benefit by taking more than 3g of the drug per day.

Clobazam
CLB is a useful adjunctive anticonvulsant in patients with refractory partial seizures [42]. Tolerance, however, is a particular problem. A few patients will achieve worthwhile improvement in seizure control with long-term dosing,

particularly those with an underlying intracerebral lesion [5]. Intermittent use reduces the likelihood of tolerance [16]. Short-term treatment can be effective prior to menstruation in women with catamenial exacerbations and as 'cover' for special events such as holidays, weddings and surgery. A single dose of 30mg may have a prophylactic action, if taken shortly after the first seizure in patients who have regular clusters. Sedation with CLB is less of a problem than with other benzodiazepines. Nevertheless, because deterioration in behaviour can occur in patients with mental retardation, this drug is probably best avoided in this patient population.

Lamotrigine
LTG has recently been marketed as 'add-on' therapy in refractory epilepsy in the UK and Ireland. Its principal actions are to stabilize neuronal membranes and inhibit release of excitatory amino acids, particularly glutamate, by blocking voltage sensitive sodium channels [43]. Treatment with other antiepileptic drugs substantially alters the metabolism of LTG. Enzyme inducers (CBZ, PHT, PB, PRIM) reduce its elimination half-life, while VPA inhibits its metabolism doubling the half-life from 30 to 60 hours [44]. Accordingly, in patients receiving VPA alone, the starting dose of LTG should be 25mg daily, while 50mg daily is usually given to patients receiving other antiepileptic drugs (Table III). Careful dosage titration can then be continued to the limit of tolerance. Side-effects may include headache, diplopia, dizziness, blurred vision and ataxia [45]. Rashes occur in about 3% of patients and other idiosyncratic drug reactions can be expected. Cognitive impairment seems not to be a problem with LTG and, indeed, patients often report an intriguing improvement in well-being, an effect that demands further investigation [46]. Although effective in partial seizures, LTG is also a promising treatment for the primary generalized epilepsies [18].

CONCLUSIONS
Complete abolition of seizures using anticonvulsant monotherapy can be expected in up to 80% of patients with newly diagnosed epilepsy. There is little evidence that more than 10% of those not responding to monotherapy will benefit substantially from treatment with more than one drug and much more evidence that polypharmacy produces cognitive impairment and complex drug interactions. Once all reasonable monotherapy options have been explored in patients with refractory epilepsy, VGB or CLB can be added if the main problem is complex partial seizures. For generalized seizures, adjuvant LTG should be tried first. In some patients, the law of diminishing returns will require doctor and patient to accept the persistence of a few fits each month. In this situation, the aim is to balance maximum seizure control with optimal quality of life. Combinations of high doses of sedative anticonvulsants will produce intolerable sedation and simplification of drug dosages and regimens may reduce seizure frequency.

A few simple rules should be followed in treating patients with anticonvulsant drugs:

1. Choose the correct drug for the seizure type using the accepted international classification.
2. Start at low dosage with all drugs in all patients.
3. Titrate slowly using 2–4 weekly increments to avoid concentration-dependent side-effects and allow tolerance to central nervous symptoms.
4. Keep the regimen simple with once or twice daily dosing in all patients.
5. Measure the drug concentration if seizure control is not readily attained.
6. Counsel the patient early regarding the implications of the diagnosis and prophylactic nature of the treatment.
7. As monotherapy is the preferred approach, a second or even a third anticonvulsant should be substituted before adding in a second drug.
8. If monotherapy fails, combine the best tolerated first-line drug with VGB or CLOB for partial seizures and with LTG for generalized tonic–clonic seizures.
9. Simplify dosage schedules and drug regimens as much as possible in patients receiving polypharmacy who are truly refractory to pharmacotherapy.

ACKNOWLEDGEMENT

My grateful thanks go to Anne Somers for expert secretarial assistance.

REFERENCES

1. Shorvon SD. Epidemiology, classification, natural history and genetics of epilepsy. *Lancet* 1990; 336: 93–96
2. Chadwick DW. Diagnosis of epilepsy. *Lancet* 1990; 336: 291–295
3. Brodie MJ. Established anticonvulsants and the treatment of refractory epilepsy. *Lancet* 1990; 336: 350–354
4. Editorial. Anticonvulsant drug withdrawal – hawks or doves? *Lancet* 1991; 337: 1193–1194
5. Schmidt D. Prognosis of chronic epilepsy with partial seizures. *J Neurol Neurosurg Psychiatry* 1984; 47: 1274–1279
6. Reynolds EH. Changing view of prognosis of epilepsy. *Br Med J* 1990; 301: 1112–1114
7. Commission on Classification and Terminology of the International League against Epilepsy. Proposal for revised classification of epilepsy and epileptic syndromes. *Epilepsia* 1989; 30: 389–399
8. Wallace SJ. Childhood epileptic syndromes. *Lancet* 1990; 336: 486–488
9. Rylance GW. Treatment of epilepsy and febrile convulsions in children. *Lancet* 1990; 336: 488–491
10. Editorial. Carbamazepine update. *Lancet* 1989; ii: 595–597
11. McKee RJW, McGinn G, Larkin JG, Brodie MJ. Myoclonic epilepsy – pitfalls in diagnosis and management. *Scot Med J* 1991; 36: 18–19
12. Mattson RH, Cramer JA, Collins JF et al. Comparison of carbamazepine, phenobarbital, phenytoin and primidone in partial and secondary tonic–clonic seizures. *N Engl J Med* 1985; 313: 145–151
13. Watts AE. A model of managing epilepsy in a rural community in Africa. *Br Med J* 1989; 298: 805–807
14. Specht V, Boenigk HE, Wolf P. Discontinuation of clonazepam after long-term treatment. *Epilepsia* 1989; 30: 458–463
15. Heller AJ, Ring HA, Reynolds EH. Factors relating to dramatic response to clobazam therapy in refractory epilepsy. *Epilepsy Res* 1988; 2: 276–280
16. Feely M, Gibson J. Intermittent clobazam for catamenial epilepsy: tolerance avoided. *J Neurol Neurosurg Psychiatry* 1984; 27: 1279–1282
17. Grant SM, Heel RC. Vigabatrin. *Drugs* 1991; 41: 889–926
18. Brodie MJ. Lamotrigine. *Lancet* 1992; 339: 1397–1400

19 Larkin JG, McKee PJW, Brodie MJ. Tolerance to psychomotor side-effects with carbamazepine. *Br J Clin Pharmacol 1992; 33*: 111–114
20 Brodie MJ, Feely J. Practical clinical pharmacology. Therapeutic drug monitoring and clinical trials. *Br Med J 1988; 296*: 1110–1114
21 Larkin JG, Herrick AL, McGuire GM et al. Antiepileptic drug monitoring at the epilepsy clinic: a prospective evaluation. *Epilepsia 1991; 32*: 89–95
22 Macphee GJA, Brodie MJ. Carbamazepine substitution in severe partial epilepsy: implication of autoinduction of metabolism. *Postgrad Med J 1985; 61*: 779–783
23 Larkin JG, McLellan A, Munday A et al. A double-blind comparison of conventional and controlled-release carbamazepine in healthy subjects. *Br J Clin Pharmacol 1989; 27*: 313–322
24 McKee PJW, Blacklaw J, Butler E et al. Monotherapy with conventional and controlled-disease carbamazepine: a double-blind, double-dummy comparison in epileptic patients. *Br J Clin Pharamacol 1991; 32*: 99–104
25 Gillham RA, Williams N, Wiedmann KD et al. Cognitive function in adult epileptic patients established on anticonvulsant monotherapy. *Epilepsy Res 1990; 7*: 217–225
26 Editorial. Sodium valproate. *Lancet 1988; ii*: 1229–1231
27 Dreifuss FE, Santilli N, Langer DH et al. Valproic acid hepatic fatalities: a retrospective review. *Neurology 1987; 37*: 379–385
28 Rowan AJ, Binnie CD, Warfield CA et al. The delayed effect of sodium valproate on the photoconvulsive effect in man. *Epilepsia 1979; 20*: 61–68
29 Woo E, Chan YM, Yu YL, Huang GM. If a well stabilised patient has a subtherapeutic antiepileptic drug level should the dose be increased? A randomised prospective study. *Epilepsia 1988; 29*: 129–139
30 Gannaway DJ, Mawer GE. Serum phenytoin concentration and clinical response in patients with epilepsy. *Br J Clin Pharmacol 1981; 2*: 833–839
31 Beghi E, Di Marcio R, Tognoni G. Drug treatment of epilepsy: outlines, criticism and perspectives. *Drugs 1986; 31*: 249–265
32 Schmidt D. Two anti-epileptic drugs for intractable epilepsy with complex partial seizures. *J Neurol Neurosurg Psychiatry 1982; 45*: 1119–1124
33 Brodie MJ, McPhail E, Macphee GJA et al. Psychomotor impairment and anticonvulsant therapy in adult epileptic patients. *Eur J Clin Pharmacol 1986; 31*: 655–660
34 Brodie MJ. Drug interactions and epilepsy. *Epilepsia 1992;* in press
35 Rogawski MA, Porter RJ. Antiepileptic drugs: pharmacological mechanisms and clinical efficacy with consideration of promising developmental stage compounds. *Pharmacol Revs 1990; 42*: 223–286
36 Rowan AJ, Meijer JWA, De Beer-Pawlikowski N et al. Valproate-ethosuximide combination therapy for refractory absence seizures. *Arch Neurol 1983; 40*: 797–802
37 Theodore WH, Porter RJ. Removal of sedative, hypnotic antiepileptic drugs from the regimes of patients with intractable epilepsy. *Ann Neurol 1983; 13*: 320–324
38 Spitz MC, Deasy DN. Conversion to valproate monotherapy in nonretarded adults with primary generalised tonic-clonic seizures. *J Epilepsy 1991; 4*: 33–38
39 Polkey CE. Surgical treatment of epilepsy. *Lancet 1990; 336*: 553–555
40 Editorial. Vigabatrin. *Lancet 1989; i*: 532–533
41 Sander JWAS, Hart YM, Trimble MR, Shorvon SD. Vigabatrin and psychosis. *J Neurol Neurosurg Psychiatry 1991; 54*: 435–439
42 Robertson MM. Current status of the 1,4 and 1,5-benzodiazepines in the treatment of epilepsy: the place of clobazam. *Epilepsia 1986; 27* (Suppl 1): S27–S41
43 Leach MJ, Marden CM, Miller AA. Pharmacological studies on lamotrigine, a novel potential antiepileptic drug: 2 Neurochemical studies on the mechanism of action. *Epilepsia 1986; 27*: 490–497
44 Binnie CD, Van Emde Boas W, Kasteleijn-Nolste-Trenite DGA et al. Acute effects of lamotrigine (BW 430C) in persons with epilepsy. *Epilepsia 1986; 27*: 248–254
45 Betts T, Goodwin G, Withers RM, Yuen AWC. Human safety of lamotrigine. *Epilepsia 1991; 32* (Suppl 2): S17–S21
46 Smith D, Baker GA, Dewey M, Chadwick DW. Lamotrigine-induced well-being in epilepsy: antiepileptic or psychotropic effect. *Epilepsia 1991; 32* (Suppl 1): 59 (abstract)

THE USE OF MRI IN DIAGNOSTIC NEUROLOGY

DH Miller
National Hospital for Neurology and Neurosurgery, London

INTRODUCTION
Within the last few years magnetic resonance imaging (MRI) has become an invaluable diagnostic tool for the practising neurologist. It is uniquely senstitive in detecting many central nervous system (CNS) pathologies and is non-invasive. It often replaces computed tomography (CT), myelography and even conventional angiography, as the preferred investigation in neurological practice. This paper will review the role of MRI in neurological practice. The background principles of MR will be mentioned briefly. There will also be a short discussion of MR angiography and future developments.

Background principles
Conventional MR images are constituted from the nuclear magnetic resonance (NMR) signals derived from mobile protons which are abundant in water and fat. Different tissues, normal or pathological, are discriminated by differences in the density and macromelecular environment of their mobile protons – in the brain these are almost all water protons since the lipid protons in myelin are immobile and thus do not produce an NMR signal.

Most MRI scanners have a field strength between 0.5 and 1.5T. Although 1.5T will better visualize small regions of interest (e.g. auditory canal, intervertebral foramina, pituitary fossa) the great majority of CNS disorders requiring MRI can be dealt with adequately at 0.5T.

The MR image intensity of any given tissue is mainly influenced by three parameters: its mobile proton density, T_1- and T_2- relaxation times. Sequences are employed to highlight one or other of these parameters. The intravenous MRI contrast agent, gadolinium-DTPA (Gd), produces enhancement on T_1-weighted images by reducing proton mobility in areas in which it accumulates (e.g. regions with an abnormal blood-brain barrier).

CURRENT INDICATIONS FOR MRI
It is appropriate to compare MRI with alternative investigations, and in doing so to consider both the site and pathological nature of the problem.

Cerebral hemisphere mass lesions
Most supratentorial gliomas, metastases and abscesses are visualized adequately on CT [1]. However, occasional tumours, especially low grade gliomas, are poorly defined on CT and display little mass effect. In such circumstances MRI may clearly identify the tumour and distinguish it from surrounding oedema [2]. In AIDS, MRI sometimes shows multiple lesions where only a single mass is visible on CT, which favours a diagnosis of toxoplasmosis over cerebral lymphoma. Gd-enhanced MRI is the most sensitive method for detecting meningiomas [3] but some small meningiomas are missed completely on non-enhanced MRI.

Vascular disease
Large cerebral infarcts are readily seen with either CT or MRI, and the former is generally adequate for diagnosis, although CT abnormalities may not appear for a day or two whereas MRI becomes abnormal within a few hours of the event. Haematomas, be they parenchymal, subdural or extradural, are detected better with MRI than CT. Because of the magnetic properties of deoxyhaemoglobin, methaemoglobin and haemosiderin, characteristic serial MRI changes are seen which identify the age of the haematoma [4]. MRI provides evidence of old haemorrhages at a time when CT has returned to normal. However, CT more readily detects subarachnoid haemorrhage [1].

Cavernous angiomas, which are small vascular malformations, are a frequent incidental finding on MRI. They occasionally produce symptoms due to bleeding. The MRI appearances are highly characteristic with a reticulated centre of mixed signal intensity, surrounded by an area of decreased signal on T_2-weighted sequences due to haemosiderin. With recent bleeding there may also be slight mass effect and high signal on T_1-weighted images due to methaemoglobin (Figure 1). Cavernous angiomas are often not visible or produce only non-specific changes on CT and angiography. Their diagnosis using MRI avoids invasive investigations such as angiography or even brain biopsy.

White matter disease
MRI is vastly superior to CT in detection of white matter abnormalities.

Multiple sclerosis, cerebrovascular disease and normal ageing
There are many causes of MRI white matter lesions (Table I) but the most common cause under the age of 50 is multiple sclerosis (MS), while cerebrovascular disease is most frequently responsible over 50 years. MRI also demonstrates asymptomatic white matter lesions in 30% of the general population aged over 50 years, due to asymptomatic vascular disease [5].

Although none of the differences is absolute, certain features favour vascular disease while others are more suggestive of MS [6]. In vascular disease continuous, smooth periventricular abnormalities are seen along with lesions in the centrum semiovale discrete from both the ventricles and cortex. In MS, periventricular lesions usually predominate and are asymmetrical, multifocal and irregular, but peripheral white matter lesions extending to the cortex are

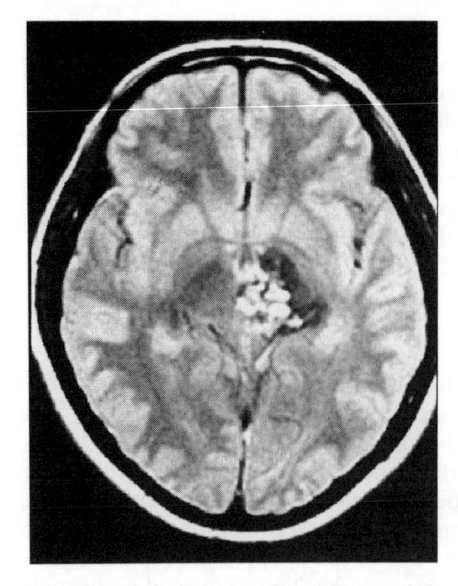

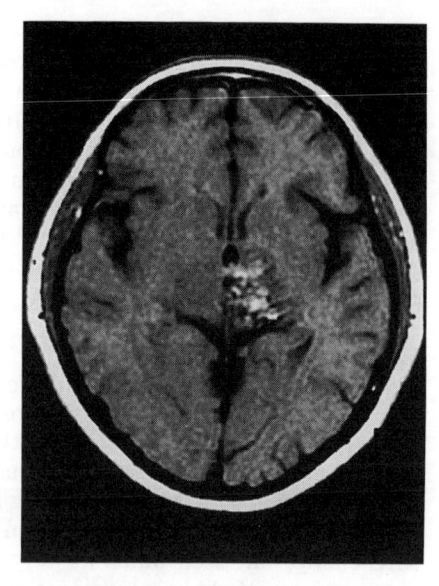

Figure 1. Unenhanced MRI (left) T_2-weighted and (right) T_1-weighted of a cavernous angioma.

also common (Figure 2). In the posterior fossa, a particularly characteristic site for MS plaques is the floor of the fourth ventricle.

The interpretation of MRI white matter lesions therefore requires consideration of the patient's age, the clinical context and the pattern of MR abnormalities. In those aged less than 50 years MRI is a reliable and sensitive method for confirming the diagnosis of MS. Ninety-five per cent of patients with clinically definite MS have multifocal white matter lesions; 60% have similar lesions at presentation with their first clinical episode of demyelination, the occurrence of which is associated with a substantial risk of progression to clinically definite MS within 5 years.

TABLE I. Causes of MRI white matter abnormalities

1 Age (particularly > 50 years)	12 Phenylketonuria
2 Cerebrovascular disease	13 Leucodystrophy
3 Multiple sclerosis	14 Subacute sclerosing panencephalitis
4 Cerebral trauma	15 Migraine
5 Cerebral irradiation	16 Motor neurone disease
6 Systemic lupus erythematosus	17 Progressive multifocal leucoencephalopathy
7 Behçet's disease	18 Cerebral fat embolism
8 Neurosarcoidosis	19 Decompression sickness
9 ADEM	20 Mitochondrial encephalopathy
10 HTLV-1 myelopathy	21 Hydrocephalus
11 AIDS	

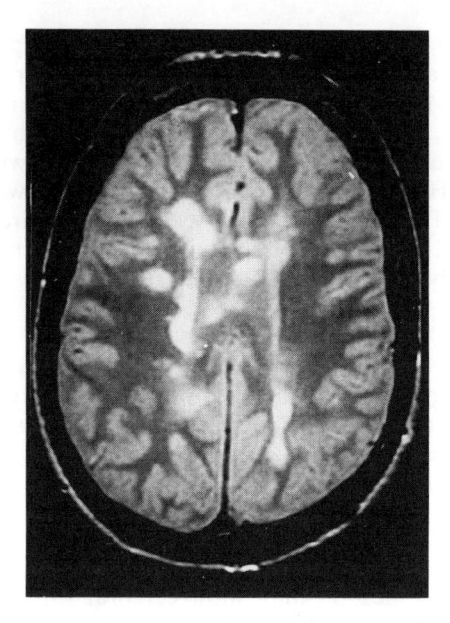

Figure 2. T_2-weighted MRI showing typical white matter lesions of MS.

For many of the other conditions listed in Table I, a consideration of both the clinical features and the pattern of MR lesions will clarify the diagnosis. Several disorders which may be difficult to distinguish clinically from MS are now discussed.

Acute disseminated encephalomyelitis (ADEM)
A single clinical episode of CNS demyelination (e.g. optic neuritis) may be due to either ADEM, which is monophasic, or MS. MRI may display multifocal asymmetrical white matter lesions in both disorders and, since it is not possible to age lesions on a single scan, their presence does not allow a distinction between the two disorders. Extensive symmetrical white or grey matter lesions are, however, more suggestive of ADEM but the major difference emerges with serial scanning: in ADEM the initial lesions partially resolve and no new lesions appear, while in MS new lesions appear in most patients [7].

Systemic lupus erythematosus (SLE)
Features such as optic neuropathy, internuclear ophthalmoplegia and subacute myelopathy, not infrequently seen in SLE, may lead to confusion with MS. MRI shows multifocal white matter lesions in SLE which are usually subcortical, whereas most MS lesions are periventricular [8]. Cortical lesions are more common in SLE and occasionally large infarcts are seen.

Sarcoidosis
Optic neuropathy, acute or chronic myelopathies and brain stem syndromes are seen in both MS and neurosarcoidosis. MRI in sarcoidosis may show large mass lesions, hydrocephalus and diffuse or patchy (and often basal) meningeal enhancement with Gd [9, 10], abnormalities which are clearly not expected in MS. However, multifocal periventricular white matter lesions indistinguishable from MS are also seen in one-third of patients with neurosarcoidosis [10] and may be the only abnormal finding. These lesions could be due to subependymal granulomas or secondary to a granulomatous angiitis.

Behçet's disease
Acute, relapsing/remitting and chronic brain stem syndromes are commonly seen in neuro-Behçet's disease. MRI often reveals brain stem lesions [8] which at times are extensive, sometimes associated with swelling or atrophy. Supratentorial white matter lesions, indistinguishable from MS, are also seen.

HTLV-1 associated myelopathy (HAM)
Brain MRI in this condition may show cerebral white matter lesions but these are few in number. Infratentorial lesions are rare in HAM but frequent in MS.

Motor neurone disease (MND)
When the initial presentation of MND is with a pure upper motor neurone syndrome confusion with MS may arise. Some MND patients display symmetrical lesions involving both corticospinal tracts extending from the centrum semiovale to the brain stem [11]. Such changes probably indicate degeneration of the pyramidal tracts and are not seen in MS.

Adrenomyeloneuropathy
This X-linked disorder presents as a slowly progressive spastic paraparesis in young adults (the female heterozygote may be symptomatic). Characteristic MR abnormalities have been found in symptomatic males, consisting of symmetrical lesions involving the optic radiations, posterior internal capsule and pyramidal tracts in the brain stem [12]. Elevation of very long chain fatty acids in the serum confirms the diagnosis.

Temporal lobes
MRI has considerable advantages over CT in this region with superior discrimination of normal and pathological anatomy, the absence of bone hardening artefact, and multiplanar imaging.

In patients with intractable seizures of temporal lobe origin, MRI occasionally detects tumours and hamartomas not seen on CT. The more common pathology in such patients is focal neuronal loss and gliosis in the hippocampus (medial temporal sclerosis). CT is usually normal, but MRI reveals abnormalities in over 80% of hippocampi which are suspected of being the epileptic focus from clinical and EEG findings. MRI reveals atrophy, altered signal and disordered internal architecture of the hippocampus [13], and is emerging as a very important tool in the work-up of patients being considered for surgical treatment of intractable epilepsy.

Posterior fossa/foramen magnum

The posterior fossa is also a difficult region to study with CT because of bone hardening artefacts. Brain stem tumours, arteriovenous malformations, haematomas, infarcts and plaques are readily identified with MRI but may be poorly visualized or missed altogether on CT [14]. Gd-enhanced MRI is the most sensitive method for detecting acoustic neuromas, and is now the investigation of choice in patients with unexplained unilateral sensorineural deafness. A variety of spinocerebellar degenerations show characteristic patterns of atrophy and signal change in the cerebellum and/or brain stem.

Congenital craniocervical junction anomalies can present with a mixture of spinal cord, cerebellar and brain stem signs simulating MS. The foramen magnum region is difficult to visualize with either CT or myelography. MRI clearly and unequivocally demonstrates such anomalies.

Spinal cord/cauda equina

Spinal cord compression due to extradural tumours, cysts, haematomas, abscesses and intervertebral disc prolapses is readily identified by MRI with a sensitivity equal to that of combined CT/myelography (Figure 3) and with

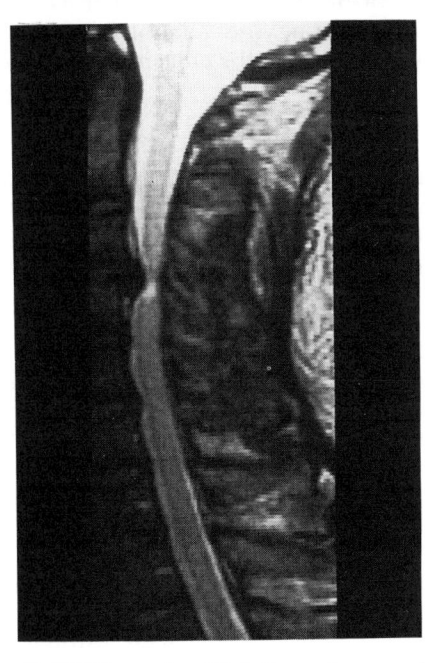

Figure 3. T_2-weighted sagittal MRI reveals a C3–4 disc prolapse producing cord compression, with signal change in the cord probably due to myelomalacia.

greater specificity. Gd-enhanced MRI demonstrates leptomeningeal metastases in up to two-thirds of patients with a proven malignant meningitis, which is considerably more sensitive than myelography [15].

MRI demonstrates other intradural extramedullary tumours such as neurofibroma or meningioma very clearly. Unenhanced and Gd-enhanced MRI is vastly better than CT and/or myelography in displaying intramedullary spinal cord lesions, including syringomyelia, gliomas, lipomas, haemangioblastomas, granulomas, abscesses, radiation necrosis and MS lesions. However, some spinal angiomas may be missed on MRI, and supine myelography followed by spinal angiography are required if an angioma is strongly suspected.

Lumbosacral intervertebral disc disease, or cauda equina tumours, are usually detectable with MRI. The overall sensitivity in this region is similar to combined CT/myelography and better than myelography alone.

In summary, given the frequent side-effects, possible complications and the need for admission associated with myelography, MRI should largely replace it before long.

Orbits and optic chiasm
MRI is hampered by the dominant signal and chemical shift effects of orbital fat, and high resolution CT remains the preferred investigation of the orbits. Conversely, Gd-enhanced MRI is the optimum method for detecting the intracranial extension of orbital pathology, such as optic nerve glioma or meningioma, and in depicting the relationship of pituitary and other tumours in the chiasmal region to the chiasm itself, such information being valuable to the neurosurgeon.

CNS infections
MRI is helpful in patients with undiagnosed meningoencephalitis. The characteristic inferior frontal and temporal lesions of herpes simplex encephalitis are more readily seen on MRI than CT. Meningeal inflammation and granuloma formation in tuberculous meningitis are better visualized with Gd-enhanced MRI than with iodine-enhanced CT.

MR ANGIOGRAPHY (MRA)
A number of strategies are available to collect NMR signals from flowing protons in a relatively specific manner, allowing the generation of MR 'angiograms'. Limitations of MRA include: (i) signal loss in areas of turbulent, complex or slow flow, e.g. vessel bifurcations, carotid siphon, beyond stenoses, and within some aneurysms; (ii) low resolution compared with conventional angiography; (iii) the need for the patient to be immobile for up to 30 minutes.

The full range of clinical applications of MRA remain to be determined. MRA reliably detects major stenoses at the carotid bifurcation [16] with a sensitivity similar to Doppler ultrasound [17]. It may therefore prove a useful non-invasive screening test in patients with carotid transient ischaemic attacks.

Intracranial MRA demonstrates about 70% of aneurysms seen with conventional angiography in patients with subarachnoid haemorrhage [18]. This suggests a possible role in the work-up of patients at high risk of berry aneurysm but invasive angiography is clearly still required in the evaluation of subarachnoid haemorrhage. MRA is excellent at demonstrating cortical venous sinus thrombosis and is perhaps the investigation of choice when this disorder is suspected.

FUTURE DEVELOPMENTS

Fast scanning

At present the amount of time required to perform conventional spin echo and inversion recovery imaging of the head is about 20 minutes and the spine takes a further 20–40 minutes. The benefits of reducing scan time include improved patient tolerance, reduced movement artefact, and increased patient throughput.

Faster scanning techniques already available or in development include gradient echo, fast spin echo, and echoplanar imaging, the latter obtaining images in a matter of milliseconds.

Specificity

Pathological specificity of conventional MRI is limited. Several approaches, e.g. diffusion/perfusion imaging, new contrast agents, image texture analysis, chemical shift imaging, and MR spectroscopy (MRS), may have a useful role in the future.

MRS allows the study of individual compounds which contain a specified atomic nucleus capable of producing an NMR signal, e.g. ^1H, ^{31}p, ^{13}C. A standard clinical high field imager (1.5T) can be used for spectroscopy.

In ^1H spectroscopy the major peaks are due to N-acetyl aspartate (NAA), choline containing compounds (Cho) and creatine/phosphocreatine. NAA is predominately contained within neurones and therefore may provide an indication of neuronal loss or dysfunction. Smaller peaks from glutamate and glutamine are also seen when short echo times are employed. Other peaks, not ordinarily visible in healthy brain, are produced by lactate and mobile lipids. It can be inferred that ^1H MRS may prove useful both in diagnosis and understanding the pathophysiology of CNS diseases. A variety of spectral abnormalities have already been described in preliminary studies of tumours [19], infarcts [20], MS [21], hepatic encephalopathy [22], and leucodystrophies [23]. The specificity and pathological basis of the changes is still uncertain and the role of MRS in clinical practice is yet to be defined. A clearer picture will emerge in the next few years.

Spinal cord imaging

Current limitations are the time required to study the whole cord, and the poor resolution of small intrinsic cord lesions, e.g. in MS. Potential solutions include the implementation of fast imaging methods and of phased array coils. The latter allow simultaneous imaging of the whole cord with improved signal to noise compared with conventional coils.

CONCLUSION

MRI is a powerful tool for the diagnosis of many neurological disorders. As it becomes more widely available it will increasingly replace other neuroradiological modalities leading to fewer invasive procedures and greater emphasis on outpatient management, which also implies economic benefits. The continuing rapid developments of MR technology promise further advances in clinical diagnosis.

REFERENCES

1. Brandt-Zawadski M. MR imaging of the brain. *Radiology 1988; 166*: 1–10
2. Robinson DA, Steiner RE, Young IR. The MR contribution after CT demonstration of supratentorial mass effect without additional localising features. *J Comput Assist Tomog 1988; 12*: 275–279
3. Schorner W, Schubeus P, Henkes H et al. Intracranial meningiomas. Comparison of plane and contrast-enhanced examinations in CT and MRI. *Neuroradiology 1990; 32*: 12–18
4. Gomori JM, Grossman RI, Goldberg HI et al. Intracranial haematomas: imaging by high field MR. *Radiology 1985; 157*: 87–93
5. Awad IA, Johnson PC, Spetzler RF et al. Incidental subcortical lesions identified on magnetic resonance imaging in the elderly. II. Postmortem pathological correlations. *Stroke 1986; 17*: 1090–1097
6. Ormerod IEC, Miller DH, McDonald WI et al. The role of NMR imaging in the assessment of multiple sclerosis and isolated neurological lesions: a quantitative study. *Brain 1987; 110*: 1579–1616
7. Kesselring J, Miller DH, Robb SA, McDonald WI. Acute disseminated encephalomyelitis: MRI findings and the distinction from multiple sclerosis. *Brain 1990; 113*: 291–302
8. Miller DH, Ormerod IEC, Gibson A et al. MR brain scanning in patients with vasculitis: differentiation from multiple sclerosis. *Neuroradiology 1987; 29*: 226–231
9. Seltzer S, Mark AS, Atlas SW. Sarcoidosis: evaluation with contrast-enhanced MR imaging. *Am J Neuroradiol 1991; 12*: 1227–1233
10. Miller DH, Kendall BE, Barter S et al. Magnetic resonance imaging in central nervous system sarcoidosis. *Neurology 1988; 38*: 378–383
11. Sales Luis ML, Hormigo A, Mauricio C et al. Magnetic resonance imaging in motor neurone disease. *J Neurol 1990; 237*: 471–474
12. van der Knaap MS, Valk J. The MR spectrum of paroxysmal disorders. *Neuroradiology 1991; 33*: 30–37
13. Jackson GD, Berkovic SF, Tress BM et al. Hippocampal sclerosis can be reliably detected by magnetic resonance imaging. *Neurology 1990; 40*: 1869–1875
14. Bradley WG, Waluch V, Yadley RA, Wycoff R. Comparison of CT and MR in 400 patients with suspected disease of the brain and spinal cord. *Radiology 1984; 152*: 695–702
15. Bronen R, Sze G. Magnetic resonance imaging contrast agents: theory and application to the central nervous system. *J Neurosurg 1990; 73*: 820–839
16. Masaryk AM, Ross JS, Di Cello MC et al. 3 DFT MR angiography of the carotid bifurcation: potential and limitations as a screening examination. *Radiology 1991; 179*: 797–804
17. Polak JF, Bajaklan RL, O'Leary DH et al. Detection of internal carotid artery stenosis: comparison of MR angiography, color doppler sonography, and arteriography. *Radiology 1992; 182*: 35–40
18. Ross JS, Masaryk TJ, Modic MT. Intracranial aneurysms: evaluation by MR angiography. *Am J Neuroradiol 1990; 11*: 449–456
19. Segebarth CM, Baleriaux DF, Luyten PR et al. Detection of metabolic heterogeneity of human intracranial tumours in vivo by ^{1}-H NMR spectroscopic imaging. *Magn Reson Med 1990; 13*: 61–76
20. Bruhn H, Frahm J, Gyngell ML et al. Cerebral metabolism in man after acute stroke: new observations using localized proton NMR spectroscopy. *Magn Reson Med 1989; 9*: 126–131

21 Arnold DL, Matthews PM, Francis G et al. Proton magnetic resonance spectroscopy of human brain in vivo in the evaluation of multiple sclerosis: assessment of the load of the disease. *Magn Reson Med 1990; 14*: 154-159
22 Kreis R, Ross BD, Farrow NA, Ackerman Z. Metabolic disorders of the brain in chronic hepatic encephalopathy detected with H-I MR spectroscopy. *Radiology 1992; 182*: 19-27
23 Austin SJ, Connelly A, Gadian DG et al. Localized 1H NMR spectroscopy in Canavan's disease: a report of two cases. *Magn Reson Med 1991; 19*: 439-445

RECENT ADVANCES IN DEMENTIA

GK Wilcock
Frenchay Hospital, Bristol

INTRODUCTION

Advances in our knowledge about the clinical manifestations and the pathological background to many dementias are progressing at such a rate that it is extremely difficult to keep up with the literature, let alone incorporate new findings into our clinical practice, where this is relevant. During 1991 there were on average between 150 and 180 relevant new publications each month. Some of these report findings that are of clinical relevance, whilst many others add to our knowledge of the pathogenetic mechanisms which may eventually help in developing new treatments or perhaps even one day the prevention of some of these diseases. It will be apparent to the reader that a modest chapter such as this limits the scope of the material that can be reviewed. I will therefore restrict myself to dementia that is caused by Lewy bodies, as this is becoming of increasing importance, and to some of the newer findings in Alzheimer's disease.

CORTICAL LEWY BODY DISEASE

Background

The association between Lewy bodies and Parkinson's disease was established in 1912 when Lewy first described them in the substantia nigra. In more recent years, particularly with the advent of more sophisticated staining techniques using immunocytochemistry with antibodies to ubiquitin, it has become increasingly apparent that in a proportion of people with dementia this may be also caused by Lewy bodies, especially in the cerebral cortex. There is still some controversy as to whether or not it is entirely appropriate to try and distinguish discrete disease entities within the overall umbrella of Lewy body dementia.

The alternative is that it is really a spectrum. At one end sits typical Parkinson's disease with predominantly brain stem Lewy bodies, and no dementia. At the other, numerous and diffuse Lewy bodies are present, involving the cortex as well as other sites, and also exhibiting a variable degree of plaque and tangle formation, in a patient with dementia. There is a transitional group with some spread of Lewy bodies into the cortex, who clinically can be divided into Parkinson's disease with and without dementia.

Clinical features

Descriptions of the clinical features of Lewy body dementia are hampered by the absence of large-scale prospective studies such as have been undertaken for conditions like Alzheimer's disease and multiple infarct dementia. Nevertheless some common ground is emerging from the literature which is beginning to produce a coherent clinical picture. There is much overlap with both the features of Alzheimer's disease and multiple infarct dementia.

The initial symptom is often memory impairment leading on to more global intellectual deficits, often associated with a motor disorder of extrapyramidal type, although other features have been reported, e.g. motor neurone disease, spastic tetraparesis and axial rigidity [1, 2]. The mental state fluctuates, sometimes widely from almost complete lucidity at one moment to gross disturbance an hour or two later. Hallucinations are more marked than in many other dementias and there is often an alteration of consciousness, suggesting the presence of delirium rather than dementia. The onset is often short in duration compared to, say, Alzheimer's disease and extrapyramidal symptoms may develop relatively early in the disease, but after the cognitive deficits appear.

It can be seen from the foregoing that there is no clear distinguishing feature, but an apparent case of Alzheimer's disease or multiple infarct dementia associated with these features should raise the clinical suspicion of cortical Lewy body disease.

The relatively sudden onset of the condition, its fluctuation and the rigidity often lead to misdiagnosis as multiple infarct dementia, but most reported series include subjects who have been misdiagnosed as Alzheimer's disease as well. This condition differs from the dementia associated with Parkinson's disease as the latter is usually subcortical, and appears some time after the movement disorder becomes apparent.

In summary, therefore, it should be suspected in those developing a cortical dementia with extrapyramidal signs at a later stage, especially when it is associated with a short course, fluctuating severity and hallucinations. Nevertheless, the diagnosis can only be confirmed at autopsy.

There is no specific treatment and although anti-Parkinsonian strategies for treating the associated extrapyramidal disorder may lead to some remission, there is no evidence as yet that this has any beneficial effect upon the dementia.

Senile dementia of Lewy body type (SDLT)

Some authors, e.g. Perry and colleagues [3, 4], believe that within this spectrum of disorders there is a discrete clinical entity that they have called senile dementia of Lewy body type, SDLT. Patients with this disorder present similarly to those described above, with a subacute/acute confusional state progressing to a fluctuating dementia associated with visual hallucinations and behavioural disturbances. Mild extrapyramidal features are present in many.

Neuropathological examination revealed Lewy body formation and selective neuronal loss in the brain stem and other subcortical nuclei with Lewy body formation in neo- and limbic cortex, but at densities well below those previously reported for diffuse Lewy body disease. In addition there was a variable degree of senile plaque and neurofibrillary tangle formation in most cases. Perry and colleagues reported that in a sequential series of autopsies such cases may comprise up to 20% of the hospitalized population of demented elderly subjects over the age of 70 years, thus rivalling multi-infarct dementia as the second commonest cause of dementia in the elderly. In general, Lewy body formation was much commoner in subjects with psychiatric symptoms. Whether these subjects really constitute a discrete clinical entity remains to be seen, and at present it is probably best to regard dementias associated with Lewy body formation as part of a continuous spectrum. Such cases are increasingly being discovered to have their own specific biochemical and neuropathological features which distinguish them from other dementias [5-7].

THERAPEUTIC ADVANCES IN ALZHEIMER'S DISEASE

Cholinergic enhancement therapies

The debate about the place of strategies designed to enhance cholinergic neurotransmitter function in Alzheimer's disease (AD) continues. It was established nearly twenty years ago that there was a significant depletion of acetylcholine from the Alzheimer brain, and that this appeared quantitatively to be the most significant neurotransmitter deficit. There were many early attempts to rectify this, using treatment pathways similar to those that are helpful in the treatment of people with Parkinson's disease. These included precursor loading in the hope that neurotransmitter production would be increased, anticholinesterase therapy with the object of reducing the rate of breakdown of the intrinsically produced acetylcholine, and receptor agonist strategies designed to increase sensitivity to the reduced quantities of acetylcholine produced. The results obtained from such approaches were disappointing and cholinergic approaches to treatment began to be viewed with some disillusionment until revitalized by the much debated study published by Summers et al [8] in 1986. The somewhat extravagant claims made for tetrahydroaminoacridine (THA) at that time have now been tempered by the more modest results reported in subsequent studies on the one hand, and the apparently negative studies on the other [9-12]. These studies have all been criticized on methodological grounds but in general the negative studies are in my opinion more flawed in design than some of the more positive ones, such as that reported from Professor Levy's group in London [11]. A modest benefit was shown in a small number of the variables assessed, producing an improvement in some outcome measures roughly equivalent to the deterioration which might have occurred over a 6 to 12 month period if the disease had progressed. This was only observed in a proportion of patients.

In all the reported studies there is a significant toxicity profile, particularly of peripheral cholinergic symptoms and a, usually, mild degree of hepatotoxicity that is reversible in those in whom it occurred.

In the author's opinion, the recent hearing by the FDA has further muddied the waters [13], rather than shedding light and objectivity on an issue that is of crucial importance to millions of sufferers and their families throughout the world.

Although it is difficult to be objective in the present climate, a consensus is beginning to emerge that THA and chemically related compounds may eventually find a useful niche in a sub-group of AD sufferers in whom modest benefits may accrue to the patient and their family. More work is needed to indicate which sub-groups are most likely to respond, and whether it is possible to predict those most likely to benefit, as has been claimed in at least one study where it was found that EEG changes from baseline recorded 90 minutes after a single oral dose of THA were of some discriminatory value.

The other major contender for consideration as of potential therapeutic value in this context is physostigmine, in one of its longer acting and orally available forms. Despite the disappointing results from earlier studies, more recent reports of long-term therapy appear to suggest, as is the case for THA, that appropriate forms of physostigmine may be of some benefit to at least a proportion of subjects with AD [14-18]. This would appear to be most marked after chronic rather than short-term administration and stabilization of symptoms as well as improvement have both been claimed.

Neurotrophic factors and the treatment of Alzheimer's disease
Attempts to improve symptomatology in sufferers with AD by rectifying neurotransmitter imbalances within the brain tacitly assume acceptance of the underlying cell death that occurs, since it is neuronal death that probably plays a significant part in causing the neurochemical changes that occur in this condition. Such an approach also makes the assumption that the neuronal death itself is of secondary importance when compared to the loss of the neurotransmitter. This is probably not the case, and in the longer term we have to seek methods of preventing or retarding neuronal degeneration. One approach that has been explored is that of the neuroprotective effect of a variety of trophic factors, especially nerve growth factor (NGF), but increasingly now others such as brain derived neurotrophic factor (BDNF) and neurotrophin-3 (NT-3). BDNF may be particularly important to our understanding of AD.

NGF was first described in the 1950s by Levi-Montalcini as a substance produced by mouse sarcomas which induced sensory and sympathetic fibre innervation of tumour material when the sarcoma was transplanted into chick embryos. It has subsequently been extensively investigated in many species, and its role in the peripheral and autonomic nervous system is now well described.

Many studies have now demonstrated that NGF has a neuroprotective effect on the important cells in the basal nucleus of Meynert and the diagonal band of Broca in some of the so-called animal models of AD. Furthermore, it has been demonstrated that administration of NGF to these neurones in vitro or in vivo leads to an increase in cholinergic output [19-24]. The thesis that NGF might be an important potential therapy in AD is also supported by studies on human post mortem brain, including the distribution of NGF receptors [25, 26], the changes in the basal forebrain in AD [27, 28], and the binding characteristics of NGF to membrane preparations from the basal forebrain in both AD and control subjects [29]. Using a sensitive and specific two-site enzyme-linked immunosorbent assay (ELISA) we have been able to show that there is no significant loss of NGF in four regions of cortex and hippocampus obtained at post mortem from patients with Alzheimer's disease and suitable control subjects [30]. As NGF passes retrogradely from target site back to neuronal perikaryon we now need to establish whether or not basal nucleus levels of NGF are normal in AD. If not, this would imply that an important part of the pathophysiology of AD lies in the failure of intraneuronal transport systems, possibly related to the appearance of neurofibrillary tangles in these cells, since the latter may well result from inappropriately assembled or synthesized cytoskeletal components of the cellular transport mechanism, i.e. the cytoskeleton. If on the other hand levels of NGF in the subcortical sites are normal, this does not exclude a potentially neuroprotective role for NGF since it may still have the same beneficial effects as those demonstrated in animal models and in tissue culture, and may enhance acetylcholine synthesis.

More recently it has become apparent that NGF is only one of a number of structurally related neurotrophic proteins which include BDNF and NT-3. These are also therefore now under investigation for a potential role in neurodegenerative diseases, including AD, and attention is also being turned to their receptors. All appear to bind equally to a low affinity receptor [31, 32]. A high affinity receptor for NGF has recently been shown to be a tyrosine receptor kinase (trk) [33, 34], and it is now known that there are two related receptor proteins, trkB and trkC, which have been identified as the receptors for BDNF and NT-3 respectively, although NT-3 also has some action at trk and trkB receptors. These receptors are important in the signal transduction processes initiated by the trophic factors and work via rapid and specific phosphorylation of trk tyrosine residues.

In summary, the family of neurotrophic factors and their receptors is under extensive investigation in the hope that this may lead to a neuroprotective therapy that would be particularly valuable in subjects with AD if diagnosed early in the course of their illness. There is also increasing evidence from animal studies that NGF may be particularly relevant to age-related memory impairment. This could indicate that such neurotrophic activity may be more relevant to elderly subjects with AD than those who are younger.

Amyloid and therapeutic strategies in Alzheimer's disease
Increasing evidence has accumulated over the 5 years, albeit mainly circumstantial, for the central involvement of the amyloid beta/A4 protein in the development of the pathological changes of AD. This consists of approximately 40 amino acid residues cleaved out of a much larger precursor protein, beta-APP, the latter existing in several different forms.

Several mutations at codon 717 of the gene encoding the beta-APP protein have been reported in affected members of a small number of families with autosomal dominant, predominantly presenile, AD. This firmly establishes beta amyloid as an important if not the main factor in the development of the condition in this small number of families.

Other studies of transgenic mice, developed from fertilized mouse eggs into which genes encoding different parts of the human beta-amyloid protein have been injected, have also emphasized the importance of the amyloid process. One of these models has proved particularly intriguing [35] as the mice have developed very similar changes to those described in the human brain in AD, i.e. beta/A4 deposition, plaque formation, neurofibrillary tangle formation and neuronal loss. Despite the fact that this model has its limitations, and is not entirely analogous with the Alzheimer pathology, it has created much excitement as it may lead to a model allowing the development of strategies to modify amyloid production, and which could also be used for screening promising compounds. This model may also have some importance for normal ageing as the elderly brain contains a similar but lesser deposition of amyloid, extracellular beta/A4 protein deposition and neurofibrillary tangle formation.

Finally, in relation to beta/A4 amyloid deposition, mention must be made of the work of Yankner and colleagues [36, 37]. They have shown that the beta/A4 amyloid is both neurotrophic and neurotoxic to neurones depending upon their stage of development and the concentration of the amyloid protein, and furthermore that neurones can be protected from this toxicity by tachykinin neuropeptides, and in particular substance P.

In summary, it would seem that amyloid in the form of the beta/A4 protein may play an important role in the development of AD and that we now have a potential animal model in which to investigate possible therapeutic strategies, although this model has important limitations. Interestingly, it may also be relevant to the normal cognitive changes of ageing as similar pathological changes, albeit to a lesser extent, are present in the normal elderly brain notwithstanding the fact that AD differs from normal ageing qualitatively as well as quantitatively.

CONCLUSION

Our understanding of the clinical presentation and underlying pathogenetic mechanisms of the important conditions that cause dementia is advancing rapidly. In particular, there would appear to be real potential on the horizon for the development of effective therapies worthy of evaluation in AD which would appear more promising than the present neurotransmitter based strategies. These should, however, not be discarded lightly as there are many sufferers with existing disease who are unlikely to be improved by strategies aimed at preventing the disease development or progression, and it is also probable that some degree of cognitive impairment will be the presenting feature of the disorder. The latter implies the need for treatment of those symptoms even if further progress of the condition can be ameliorated. Although I have concentrated on cholinergic strategies as these are most advanced, it should not be forgotten that there are equally important hypotheses revolving around the role of excitatory amino acids, particularly glutamate, and also the role of serotonin, especially 1A-receptor antagonists.

REFERENCES

1. Byrne EJ, Lennox G, Lowe J, Godwin-Austin RB. Diffuse Lewy body disease: Clinical features in fifteen cases. *J Neurol Neurosurg Psychiatry 1989; 52*: 709-717
2. Gibb WRG, Luthert PJ, Janota I, Lantos PL. Cortical Lewy body dementia: Clinical features and classification. *J Neurol Neurosurg Psychiatry 1989; 52*: 185-192
3. Perry RH, Irving D, Blessed G et al. Senile dementia of Lewy body type. A clinically and neuropathologically distinct form of Lewy body dementia in the elderly. *J Neurol Sci 1990; 95*: 119-139
4. Perry RH, Irving D, Tomlinson BE. Lewy body prevalence in the aging brain: relationship to neuropsychiatric disorders, Alzheimer-type pathology and catecholaminergic nuclei. *J Neurol Sci 1990; 100*: 223-233
5. Dickson DW, Ruan D, Crystal H et al. Hippocampal degeneration differentiates diffuse Lewy body disease (DLBD) from Alzheimer's disease: light and electron microscopic immunocytochemistry of CA2-3 neurites specific to DLBD. *Neurology 1991; 41*: 1402-1409
6. Leake A, Perry EK, Perry RH et al. Neocortical concentrations of neuropeptides in senile dementia of the Alzheimer and Lewy body type: comparison with Parkinson's disease and severity correlations. *Biol Psychiatry 1991; 29*: 357-364
7. Perry EK, Smith CJ, Court JA, Perry RH. Cholinergic nicotinic and muscarinic receptors in dementia of Alzheimer, Parkinson and Lewy body types. *J Neural Transm Park Dis Dement Sect 1990; 2*: 149-158
8. Summers WK, Majovski LV, Marsh GM et al. Oral tetrahydroaminoacridine in long-term treatment of senile dementia, Alzheimer type. *N Engl J Med 1986; 315*: 1241-1245
9. Gauthier S, Bouchard R, Lamontagne A et al. Tetrahydroaminoacridine-lecithin combination treatment in patients with intermediate-stage Alzheimer's disease. Results of a Canadian double-blind, crossover, multicenter study. *N Engl J Med 1990; 322*: 1272-1276
10. Chatellier G, Lacomblez L. Tacrine (tetrahydroaminoacridine; THA) and lecithin in senile dementia of the Alzheimer type: a multicentre trial. Groupe Francais d'Etude de la Tetrahydroaminoacridine. *Br Med J 1990; 300*: 495-499
11. Eagger SA, Levy R, Sahakian BJ. Tacrine in Alzheimer's disease. *Lancet 1991; 337*: 989-992
12. Weinstein HC, Teuninse S, van-Gool WA. Tetrahydroaminoacridine and lecithin in the treatment of Alzheimer's disease. Effect on cognition, functioning in daily life, behavioural disturbances and burden experienced by the carers. *J Neurol 1991; 238*: 34-38
13. Relman AS. Tacrine as a treatment for Alzheimer's dementia. *N Engl J Med 1991; 324*: 349
14. Alhainen K, Partanen J, Reinikainen K et al. Discrimination of tetrahydroaminoacridine responders by a single dose pharmaco-EEG in patients with Alzheimer's disease. *Neurosci Lett 1991; 127*: 113-116
15. Jenike MA, Albert M, Baer L, Gunther J. Oral physostigmine as treatment for primary degenerative dementia: a double-blind placebo-controlled inpatient trial. *J Geriatr Psychiatry Neurol 1990; 3*: 13-16
16. Harrell LE, Callaway R, Morere D, Falgout J. The effect of long-term physostigmine administration in Alzheimer's disease. *Neurology 1990; 40*: 1350-1354
17. Jenike MA, Albert MS, Baer L. Oral physostigmine as treatment for dementia of the Alzheimer type: a long-term outpatient trial. *Alzheimer Dis Assoc Disord 1990; 4*: 226-231
18. Tune L, Brandt J, Frost JJ et al. Physostigmine in Alzheimer's disease: effects on cognitive functioning, cerebral glucose metabolism analyzed by positron emission tomography and cerebral blood flow analyzed by single photon emission tomography. *Acta Psychiatr Scand Suppl 1991; 366*: 61-65
19. Gnahn H, Hefti F, Heumann R et al. NGF mediated increase on choline acetyltransferase (ChAT) in the neonatal rat forebrain: evidence for a phsyiological role of NGF in the brain? *Dev Brain Res 1983; 9*: 45-52
20. Mobley WC, Rutkowski JL, Tennekoon GI et al. Nerve growth factor increases choline acetyltransferase activity in developing basal forebrain neurones. *Mol Brain Res 1986; 1*: 53-62

21 Mobley WC, Rutkowski JL, Tennekoon GI et al. Choline acetyltransferase activity in striatum of neonatal rats increased by nerve growth factor. *Science 1986; 229*: 284-287
22 Honnegar P, Lenoir D. Nerve growth factor (NGF) stimulation of cholinergic telencephalic neurons in aggregating cell cultures. *Dev Brain Res 1982; 3*: 229-238
23 Hefti H, Hartikka J, Eckenstein F et al. Nerve growth factor (NGF) increases choline acetyltransferase but not survival or fiber growth of cultured septal cholinergic neurones. *Neuroscience 1985; 14*: 55-68
24 Martinez HJ, Dreyfus CF, Jonakeit M, Black IB. Nerve growth factor promotes cholinergic development in brain striatal cultures. *Proc Natl Acad Sci USA 1985; 82*: 7777-7781
25 Allen SJ, Dawbarn D, Wilcock GK et al. The distribution of Beta-nerve growth factor receptors in the human basal forebrain. *J Comp Neurol 1989; 289*: 626-640
26 Mufson EJ, Bothwell M, Hersh LB, Kordower JH. Nerve growth factor receptor immunoreactive profiles in the normal, aged human basal forebrain: colocalization with cholinergic neurones. *J Comp Neurol 1989; 285*: 196-217
27 Allen SJ, Dawbarn D, MacGowan SH et al. A quantitative morphometric analysis of basal forebrain neurones expressing Beta-NGF receptors in normal and Alzheimer's disease brains. *Dementia 1990; 1*: 125-137
28 Allen SJ, Dawbarn D, Wilcock GK. Morphometric immunochemical analysis of neurons in the nucleus basalis of Meynert in Alzheimer's disease. *Brain Res 1988; 454*: 275-281
29 Treanor JJS, Dawbarn D, Allen SJ et al. Nerve growth factor receptor binding in normal and Alzheimer's disease basal forebrain. *Neurosci Lett 1991; 121*: 73-76
30 Allen SJ, MacGowan SH, Treanor JJS et al. Normal NGF content in Alzheimer's disease cerebral cortex and hippocampus. *Neurosci Lett 1991; 131*: 135-139
31 Squinto SP, Stitt TN, Aldrich TH et al. TrkB encodes a functional receptor for brain-derived neurotrophic factor and neurotrophin-3 but not nerve growth factor. *Cell 1991; 65*: 885-893
32 Rodriguez-Tebar A, Dechant G, Barde Y-A. Binding of the brain-derived neurotrophic factor to the nerve growth factor receptor. *Neuron 1990; 4*: 487-492
33 Kaplan DR, Masrtin-Zanca D, Parada LF. Tyrosine phophorylation of tyrosine kinase activity of the trk proto-oncogene product induced by NGF. *Nature 1990; 350*: 158-160
34 Klein R, Jing S, Nanduri V et al. The trk proto-oncogene encodes a receptor for nerve growth factor. *Cell 1991; 65*: 189-197
35 Kawabata S, Higgins GA, Gordon JW. Amyloid plaques, neurofibrillary tangles and neuronal loss in brains of transgenic mice overexpressing a C-terminal fragment of human amyloid precursor protein. *Nature 1991; 354*: 476-478
36 Yankner BA, Duffy LK, Kinchner DA. Neurotrophic and neurotoxic effects of amyloid beta protein: reversal by tachykinin neuropeptides. *Science 1990; 250*: 279-282
37 Kowall NW, Beal MF, Busciglio J et al. An in vivo model for the neurodegenerative effects of beta amyloid and protection by substance P. *Proc Natl Acad Sci USA 1991; 88*: 7247-7251

IgA NEPHROPATHY

SJ Harper, MJR Feehally
Leicester General Hospital, Leicester

It is 25 years since the disease now called IgA nephropathy (IgAN) was first described [1]. It was a pathologist, Jean Berger, who made that report, and for some years the disease carried his name, although the term IgA nephropathy is now widely accepted.

It was the application of immunofluorescence techniques to renal biopsy material that allowed the identification of a group of patients with glomeruler disease in whom IgA was the dominant immune reactant present. Since the precise immune mechanisms underlying this and most other forms of glomerulonephritis remain elusive, classification of these diseases continues, as in IgAN, to be based on description of the biopsy findings.

DEFINITION
Nevertheless IgAN has proved a durable term describing patients with predominant deposition of IgA in the glomerular mesangium. The definition excludes other groups of patients with glomerular IgA deposition including those with lupus nephritis (who have IgA deposited along with multiple other immune reactants in a characteristic clinical and pathological setting) and patients with alcoholic liver disease (the mechanism for mesangial IgA deposition in this context will be discussed below).

The IgA deposition occurs with a wide range of glomerular damage defined by light microscopy and the intensity of IgA deposits does not correlate with the degree of structural damage. IgA may be found alone or coincidental with deposits of IgG, IgM or C3. The presence of these additional deposits likewise does not predict the degree of structural damage.

CLINICAL PRESENTATION
IgAN is three times as common in males as in females. Characteristic clinical presentations of IgAN vary with age (Figure 1).

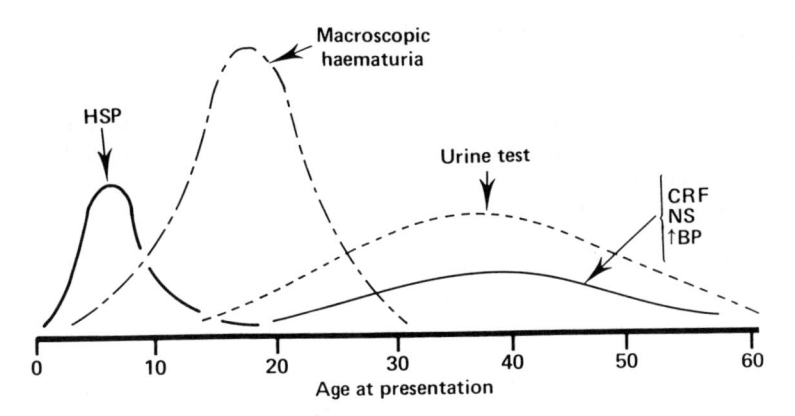

Figure 1. Age distribution of clinical manifestations of IgA nephropathy. Henoch-Schönlein purpura (HSP) typically occurs in the first decade. IgAN with macroscopic haematuria is the commonest presentation and is typically in the second and third decades. Those with clinically more advanced renal disease at presentation (chronic renal failure (CRF), nephrotic syndrome (NS), hypertension (↑BP)), along with those presenting with asymptomatic immune abnormalities, will be older.

Relationship of IgAN and Henoch-Schönlein purpura (HSP)

Use of the term IgAN implies that clinical manifestations are restricted to the kidney. When the same renal lesion occurs in the clinical context of systemic vasculitis with IgA deposition in the skin and other organs as well as the kidney, the term Henoch-Schönlein purpura (HSP) is used. HSP was of course described long before immunohistology allowed identification of tissue deposits of immunoglobulin and complement. It remains frequently a clinical diagnosis but it is preferable for the term to be reserved for those with proven tissue IgA deposition. Although HSP is characteristically a disease of the first decade it may occur at any age.

IgAN and HSP share many immune abnormalities and IgAN is often regarded as a forme fruste of HSP. An explanation for the development of systemic vasculitis in some patients while others have disease limited to the kidney may lie in the recent observation that antineutrophil cytoplasmic antibodies if IgA isotype (IgA-ANCA) occur in acute HSP but not IgAN [2].

Haematuria

Haematuria is the characteristic, although not universal, presenting clinical symptom of IgAN. Haematuria in IgAN may be persistent microscopic haematuria, identified by routine urine testing, or recurrent macroscopic haematuria, the latter characteristically induced by exercise or more commonly coinciding with intercurrent respiratory or other mucosal infection. Haematuria will often be the only manifestation of renal disease, occurring in the absence of proteinuria, raised blood pressure or raised serum creatinine. In contrast to the haematuria in post-streptococcal glomerulonephritis, which typically follows the infection by 2 to 3 weeks, frank haematuria in IgAN will occur within 24 hours of the onset of symptoms of the precipitating infection. The haematuria is painless and usually brown (like tea) rather than red. Haematuria is self-limiting, usually lasting only 2 or 3 days. Very occasionally an episode of haematuria will result in acute renal failure either because of tubular blockage by red cells [3] or because the frank haematuria marks transformation into acute severe glomerulonephritis [4]. Perhaps surprisingly there is no clear evidence that the frequency of macroscopic haematuria alters prognosis.

Proteinuria and renal impairment

Other patients will have proteinuria as well as haematuria detected on urine testing and occasionally (in no more than 5% of all IgAN) be frankly nephrotic. Still others will already have renal impairment with hypertension when first seen. They will tend to be older with more advanced damage on renal biopsy at presentation and a less good prognosis. These older patients presenting with chronic renal failure may well have longstanding IgAN not previously diagnosed because episodes of macroscopic haematuria did not occur or went unreported when younger, but this supposition will only be confirmed by very prolonged natural history studies.

PREVALENCE AND PROGNOSIS

IgAN is an important condition since it is now known to be the commonest form of glomerulonephritis found in countries where renal biopsy is widely practised [5]. Furthermore, despite its often innocent initial presentation, it is not a benign disease. After 20 years' follow-up some 20% of patients will require renal replacement therapy, while only 50% will still have a normal serum creatinine [6, 7]; findings of major importance in a disease with a peak incidence in the second and third decades of life.

These long-term implications are easily obscured by the initial straightforward clinical presentation. Until recently the term 'benign recurrent haematuria' was used in paediatric practice to describe patients presenting with isolated haematuria who were thought not to need renal biopsy and had a good prognosis. Many such patients would have IgAN and the fact that episodic macroscopic haematuria will stop within months or years is not necessarily evidence of resolution of the glomerular disease.

Therefore haematuria should not be taken lightly in otherwise fit young people. Such patients should remain under observation and many nephrologists now argue for an early renal biopsy to establish a diagnosis. Urological causes of haematuria are extremely uncommon in those under 40 if renal tract imaging is normal and therefore nephrological rather than urological assessment is preferable.

INCIDENCE OF IgAN

The worldwide distribution of IgAN is accompanied by great variations in apparent incidence: for example, high in Japan and Mediterranean countries, lower in the UK and USA. These may be true differences in incidence with a genetic or environmental basis, but there are other confounding factors. A country with widespread routine urine testing which will identify patients with microscopic haematuria or proteinuria is likely to have a higher perceived incidence of IgAN, particularly if it coincides with an aggressive attitude to the use of renal biopsy in patients with asymptomatic urine abnormalities. A conservative approach to renal biopsy may particularly be a factor in the low apparent incidence of IgAN in the USA. A survey of UK nephrologists revealed widely disparate attitudes to renal biopsy in this context and described an association between these attitudes and apparent incidence of IgAN in individual units [8]. In one centre changing attitudes to renal biopsy over time appeared to explain a rising incidence of IgAN [9].

PATHOGENESIS OF IgAN
Disease mechanisms in IgAN remain unclear. Since glomerular IgA is the hallmark of the disease, investigation has concentrated on abnormalities of IgA and the IgA immune system which might predispose to IgA deposition, whilst recognizing that a range of other mechanisms may be involved subsequent to IgA deposition in the progressive renal damage.

A number of concepts have emerged.

IgAN is a systemic disease
Numerous abnormalities of the IgA immune system have been described in IgAN which taken together suggest that IgAN is a systemic disease rather than one confined to the kidney [10]. This is supported by evidence that IgAN frequently recurs after renal transplantation [11]; and by unwitting experiments in which cadaver kidneys, thought to be normal and used for transplantation, turn out to have had IgA deposits at the time of grafting which subsequently disappear [12].

Characterization of glomerular IgA
The mesangial IgA is polymeric and mostly of the IgA1 subclass. The mucosal immune system is the chief source of polymeric IgA (p-IgA), whereas the great majority of circulating IgA is monomeric and bone marrow derived. The mucosal immune system would seem a likely source of deposited IgA in view of the coincidence of haematuria with mucosal infection. However, IgA1 is more likely to be of marrow origin.

Circulating IgA
Raised serum IgA levels may occur in IgAN, but more than 90% of circulating IgA is monomeric and more important are reports of increased p-IgA in the circulation in IgAN, which may be more marked during episodes of frank haematuria [13, 14]. An increased propensity for IgA production has also been shown in a range of in vitro culture systems using circulating immune cells from patients with IgAN [9].

However, a raised circulating IgA level is not sufficient of itself to produce glomerular IgA since patients with IgA myeloma do not develop IgAN.

Possible sites of abnormality in the IgA immune system
Whilst these observations indicate a disordered overactive IgA system in

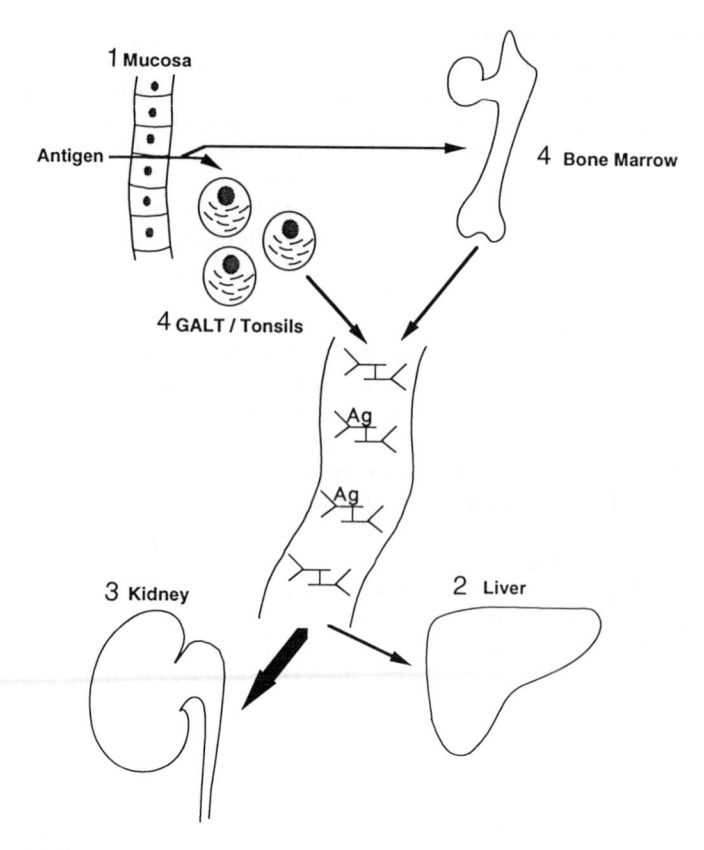

Figure 2. IgA immune system in IgA nephropathy. Possible sites of dysfunction which might predispose to increased circulating p-IgA or antigen (Ag)-antibody complexes and hence to glomerular p-IgA deposition. 1, Mucosal antigen penetration; 2, hepatic clearance of p-IgA; 3, glomerular abnormalities promoting IgA deposits; 4, increased p-IgA production in the mucosal immune system (e.g. gut-associated lymphoid tissue (GALT) and tonsil) or bone marrow.

IgAN, they do not indicate whether the source of the p-IgA is mucosa or bone marrow nor do they reveal where the primary abnormality lies in IgAN. Figure 2 indicates possible points in the sequence of immune events where abnormalities may lie.

(1) Mucosal antigen penetration
Whilst enhanced antigen penetration might overstimulate the IgA system, there is no evidence for this in IgAN [15]. Furthermore IgAN, although occasionally associated with coeliac disease, is not a frequent feature of other diseases where chronic inflammation might enhance antigen penetration (e.g. inflammatory bowel disease).

(2) Hepatic clearance
p-IgA is cleared from the circulation in health through the liver. Failure of hepatic clearance of IgA is the mechanism thought to explain the glomerular IgA deposits which accompany alcoholic liver disease (and which typically occur without clinical evidence of renal disease) but there is no evidence for defective clearance in IgAN.

(3) Role of the kidney
Mesangial immune deposits, such as are seen in IgAN, are usually thought typical of the deposition of circulating antigen–antibody complexes. In this model the glomerulus is often regarded as an 'innocent bystander' passively trapping circulating complexes.

Alternatively circulating p-IgA may accrete to antigen already present in the glomerulus: either extrinsic antigen such as food or viral antigen, or intrinsic neoantigen. Thirdly, the p-IgA may bind to the glomerulus by non-immune mechanisms, for example physicochemical linkage due to abnormalities in glomerular or antibody structure. There is at present no good evidence to distinguish between these possibilities. In particular there are only isolated reports of food antigens in association with deposits even though circulating antigliadin antibodies may be raised [16]. A report of cytomegalovirus in the glomeruli in IgAN has not been confirmed by molecular study [17, 18].

(4) Source of p-IgA
The favoured hypothesis that circulating polymeric IgA and circulating IgA immune cells are mucosally derived may prove wrong in the light of recent evidence that polymeric IgA production is downregulated in the duodenal mucosa and upregulated in the bone marrow in IgAN [19, 20]. If the marrow proves to be the source of p-IgA, a further explanation would then be required for the close link between mucosal infection and frank haematuria. Animal studies do suggest there is a mucosa–marrow immune axis perhaps mediated by cytokines, but as yet no evidence exists for this in man.

Role of IgG
By definition IgA deposits are the hallmark of IgAN, but IgA is poorly phlogistic compared to IgG and activates complement only weakly. Animal studies suggest that IgG and C3 deposition are required along with IgA to generate haematuria, although this is less clear cut from human biopsy data. However, a relationship has been shown between circulating IgG with antimesangial specificity and disease activity in IgAn [21] suggesting that involvement of other Ig isotypes may be needed for clinically detectable disease episodes to occur.

PROGRESSION OF IgAN
Although there is little doubt that mesangial deposition of IgA and other immune reactants is the primary event in IgAN, it is a very slowly progressive disease in which it would seem probable that, as in any form of chronic renal

disease, common non-immunological factors may determine progression of glomerular and interstitial scarring and eventual renal failure.

TREATMENT OF IgAN

As in other types of indolent immune renal disease, treatment with immune modifying regimens has proved very disappointing. There is evidence that steroids give benefit in the small minority (less than 5%) who are frankly nephrotic, but no evidence they influence the majority [22]. Cyclosporin has been used and will lower proteinuria, but only at the expense of falling glomerular filtration rate (GFR), suggesting a nephrotoxic effect due to cyclosporin rather than specific immune modulation [23]. Phenytoin (which lowers serum IgA levels) is ineffective [24].

Episodes of frank haematuria are self-limiting and, since the mucosal infections which stimulate them are various, there is no place for prophylactic penicillin. Tonsillectomy may sometimes be necessary but it is not widely thought to influence the natural history of IgAN. If haematuria is precipitated by exercise there is no evidence that inactivity is advantageous. Interest in the influence of dietary gluten has led to studies of dietary gluten exclusion which have not influenced the course of the disease [25].

On the rare occasions that severe glomerulonephritis with crescentic changes develops, it will usually respond to immunosuppression with steroids and cyclophosphamide with or without plasma exchange [26], in regimens used for crescentic glomerulonephritis without IgA.

For the great majority of patients with IgAN there is still no specific treatment to offer. Long-term follow-up and careful observation, treatment of blood pressure and measures applicable to any progressive renal disease are necessary. Renal replacement therapy will be needed in some patients. The frequent recurrence of IgA deposits should not militate against transplantation, since the deposits will rarely contribute to graft dysfunction.

THE FUTURE

Specific treatment of IgAN must await better understanding of the immune mechanisms which underlie it, and these mechanisms remain the major focus of current investigation. If progress toward specific treatment in the early immune phase of the disease is made, early recognition and diagnosis of this very common glomerular disease will become increasingly important, since intervention may prevent later progressive renal failure.

REFERENCES

1. Berger J, Nevell T, Morel-Maroger L et al. Applications de l'immunofluorescence en néphrologie localisation des immunoglobulines et fibrinogene dans les lésions glomérulaires. In Hammarion M, ed. *Act Nephrol Hop Necker.* Vol 1, Paris 1968: 141–154
2. Ronda N, Esnault VLM, Layward L et al. Association between Henoch-Schonlein purpura and anti-neutrophil cytoplasmic antibodies of IgA class. *J Am Soc Nephrol 1991; 2*: 603 (abstract)
3. Kincaid-Smith P, Bennett WM, Dowling SP, Ryan GB. Acute renal failure and tubular necrosis associated with haematuria due to glomerulonephritis. *Clin Nephrol 1983; 19*: 206–210
4. Kincaid-Smith P, Nicholls K. Mesangial IgA nephropathy. *Am J Kidney Dis 1983; 3*: 90–102

5   D'Amico G. The commonest glomerulonephritis in the western world: IgA nephropathy. *Q J Med 1987; 64*: 709-727
6   Rodicio JL. Idiopathic IgA nephropathy. *Kidney Int 1984; 25*: 717-729
7   D'Amico G, Imbasciati E, Barbiano de Belgioso G et al. Idiopathic IgA mesangial nephropathy. Clinical and histological study of 374 patients. *Medicine (Baltimore) 1985; 64*: 49-60
8   Feehally J, O'Donoghue DJ, Ballardie FW. Current nephrological practice in the investigation of haematuria: relationship to incidence of IgA nephropathy. *J Roy Coll Phys (London) 1989; 23*: 228-231
9   Ballardie FW, O'Donoghue DJ, Feehally J. Increasing frequency of adult IgA nephropathy in the UK? *Lancet 1987; ii*: 1205
10   Feehally J. Immune mechanisms in glomerular IgA deposition. *Nephrol Dialysis Transplant 1988; 3*: 361-378
11   Berger J, Noel LH, Nabarra B. Recurrence of mesangial IgA nephropathy after renal transplantation. *Contrib Nephrol 1984; 40*: 195-197
12   Sanfilippo F, Croker BP, Bollinger RR. Fate of four cadaveric donor allografts with mesangial IgA deposits. *Transplantation 1982; 33*: 214-216
13   Valentijn RM, Kauffmann RH, De La Riviere GB et al. Presence of circulating macromolecular IgA in patients with haematuria due to primary IgA nephropathy. *Am J Med 1983; 74*: 375-381
14   Feehally J, Beattie TJ, Brenchley PEC et al. Sequential study of the IgA immune system in relapsing IgA nephropathy. *Kidney Int 1986; 30*: 924-931
15   Layward L, Hattersley JM, Patel HR et al. Gut permeability in IgA nephropathy. *Nephrol Dial Transplant 1990; 5*: 569-571
16   Rostoker G, Chaumette MT, Wirquin E et al. IgA mesangial nephritis, IgA antigliadin antibodies and coeliac disease. *Lancet 1990; 336*: 824-825
17   Gregory MC, Hammond ME, Breward ED. Renal deposition of cytomegalovirus antigen in immunoglobulin A nephropathy. *Lancet 1988; i*: 11-14
18   Okamura M, Kanayama Y, Negoro N et al. Failure to detect cytomegalovirus-DNA in IgA nephropathy by in-situ hybridisation. *Lancet 1989; i*: 1265
19   Harper SJ, Pringle JH, Wicks ACB et al. Simultaneous in situ hybridisation of immunoglobulin J chain mRNA and conventional immunofluorescence in cells of the lamina propria in IgA nephropathy. *J Am Soc Nephrol 1991; 2*: 543 (abstract)
20   van den Wall Bake W, Daha MR, Radl J et al. The bone marrow as production site of the IgA deposited in the kidneys of patients with IgA nephropathy. *Clin Exp Immunol 1988; 72*: 321-325
21   Ballardie FW, Williams S, Brenchley PEC, O'Donoghue DJ. Autoimmunity in IgA nephropathy. *Lancet 1988; ii*: 588-591
22   Schena FP, Montenegro M, Scivittaro V. Meta-analysis of randomised controlled trials in patients with primary IgA nephropathy (Berger's Disease). *Nephrol Dial Transplant 1990; Suppl 1*: 47-52
23   Lai KN, MacMoune Lai F, Li PKT, Vallence Owen J. Cyclosporin treatment of IgA nephropathy. *Br Med J 1987; 295*: 1165-1168
24   Clarkson AR, Seymour AE, Woodroffe AJ et al. Controlled trial of phenythoin therapy in IgA nephropathy. *Clin Nephrol 1980; 13*: 215-218
25   Coppo R, Roccatello D, Amore A et al. Effects of gluten free diet in primary IgA nephropathy. *Clin Nephrol 1990; 33*: 72-86
26   Boobes Y, Baz M, Durrant C et al. Early start of intensive therapy in malignant form of IgA nephropathy. *Nephron 1990; 54*: 351-353

THE MANAGEMENT OF BONE DISEASE IN RENAL FAILURE

John Cunningham
Royal London Hospital and Medical College, London

INTRODUCTION
Patients with renal insufficiency invariably have demonstrable abnormalities of bone structure and function, accompanied by disturbances of vitamin D metabolism and usually by evidence of parathyroid gland over-activity also. If a sufficiently diligent assessment is carried out, even patients with mild renal impairment will be found to manifest at least some of the above abnormalities, and at the other extreme patients with end-stage renal disease being treated by haemodialysis or continuous ambulatory peritoneal dialysis (CAPD) show striking disturbances of bone and mineral metabolism.

At the level of bone itself, a number of changes may develop, either singly or in combination.

(1) Hyperparathyroid bone disease, in which excess parathyroid hormone (PTH) effect leads to high bone turnover with coupled increases in bone formation (osteoblast mediated) and bone resorption (osteoclast mediated), abnormally large amounts of osteoid (hyperosteoidosis), and peritrabecular fibrosis.

(2) Osteomalacia, with a marked reduction of both bone mineralization and usually bone resorption also. The rate of osteoid formation by osteoblasts exceeds the rate at which the new osteoid is mineralized (although both are reduced), leading to hyperosteoidosis, in this instance with osteomalacia and a very low bone formation rate (cf. hyperparathyroidism).

(3) Mixed osteodystrophy, in which features of hyperparathyroid bone disease and osteomalacic bone disease coexist.

(4) Adynamic bone disease, in which a profound reduction of the synthesis of osteoid, mineralization of osteoid, and bone resorption together result in a low bone turnover rate without excess osteoid, paucity of bone cells and reduced bone cell activity.

(5) *Aluminium bone disease*, in which aluminium derived from dialysate (in haemodialysis patients), or from aluminium containing phosphate binders (haemodialysis and CAPD patients) is deposited at the mineralization front where it interferes with the function of osteoblasts and prevents the mineralization of osteoid. Its frequency and severity are greatest in patients with low turnover bone lesions.

PATHOGENESIS OF RENAL OSTEODYSTROPHY

Hyperparathyroidism

This results from a real or threatened reduction of extracellular (ECF) fluid calcium concentration. The downward pressure on calcium triggers secondary hyperparathyroidism, and is driven by (a) decreased phosphaturia as the glomerulofiltration rate (GFR) falls and (b) a relative reduction of the renal synthesis of calcitriol (1,25-dihydroxyvitamin D), the active hormonal form of vitamin D.

Phosphate retention
The importance of phosphate retention as a drive to hyperparathyroidism in renal failure was demonstrated by Bricker and Slatopolsky [1]. Their 'trade off' hypothesis postulated that decrements of GFR would inevitably be associated with decrements of phosphaturia also, and a consequent tendency for renal phosphate retention. Phosphate retention would in turn exert downward pressure on ECF calcium concentration, triggering an increment of PTH secretion, leading to accelerated skeletal resorption, and compensatory phosphaturia. Thus with each decrement of GFR, both phosphate and calcium would be maintained at normal or near normal levels, but only at the expense of increased PTH secretion with its associated deleterious consequences for the skeleton.

Reduced renal synthesis of calcitriol
This results from a reduced mass of proximal tubular cells (which contain 25-hydroxyvitamin D 1α-hydroxylase), thereby reducing the capacity of the kidney to make calcitriol. The resulting intestinal calcium malabsorption exerts further downward pressure on ECF calcium concentration and consequently exacerbates hyperparathyroidism. Calcitriol synthesis is further compromised by phosphate retention (phosphate inhibits the 1α-hydroxylase enzyme) and possibly by other elements of the uraemic state as well. Because calcitriol directly inhibits PTH synthesis (see below), its lack adds further impetus to the development of hyperparathyroidism. This in turn stimulates the remaining 1α-hydroxylase, such that if measured the plasma concentrations of calcitriol are often maintained within the normal range in early renal impairment, only falling to subnormal levels when renal damage advances. The price paid for the maintenance of normal or near normal concentrations of calcitriol is further PTH excess.

Both experimentally and clinically the above sequences can be partially or completely reversed by prevention of phosphate retention by dietary restriction or use of oral phosphate binders [1, 2] and the provision of supplemental calcitriol to replace the deficient hormone [3]. Unfortunately the clinical reality of the treatment of patients with renal hyperparathyroidism is less straighforward, and although the majority of patients show excellent early responses to treatment with phosphate binders and calcitriol, the long-term results are often disappointing: inexorable hyperparathyroidism, accompanied by hypercalcaemia, often recurs, ultimately requiring parathyroidectomy [4]. The observed behaviour of the parathyroid glands in this clinical setting and also the results of many experimental studies indicate that in chronic uraemia there is a progressive change in the parathyroid response to ECF calcium concentration, and suggest also that a major factor determining this change is likely to be lack of calcitriol. The parathyroid glands are one of the major target organs for calcitriol, possessing abundant specific calcitriol receptors which mediate reduced prepro PTH mRNA and PTH secretion following exposure to calcitriol [5, 6] via binding of the receptor-calcitriol complex to the 5'-flanking region of the PTH gene [7]. This phenomenon was demonstrated for the first time in the clinical setting by Madsen et al who found that elevated PTH concentrations in patients with acute renal failure decreased strikingly following parenteral calcitriol administration, even while their blood ionized calcium concentrations were held constant and low by continuous peritoneal dialysis [8]. Subsequent studies have demonstrated convincingly that in chronic renal failure also, the administration of calcitriol can reduce the activity of the parathyroid glands independent of changes in ECF calcium concentration [9].

From in vitro experiments using human parathyroid tissue taken from patients with uraemia, it is clear that there is an increase in the parathyroid 'set point' (that extracellular calcium concentration at which 50% maximal PTH release occurs), an abnormality that was also found in parathyroid adenomas taken from patients with primary hyperparathyroidism [10]. The abnormal parathyroid tissue (whether from uraemic patients or adenomas) was responsive to changes in ambient calcium concentration, but over a range of concentrations slightly higher than for normal human parathyroid tissue. More recently the addition of calcitriol to a similar in vitro model was found to reduce the parathyroid response to ambient calcium concentration in a manner consistent with return of the set point for calcium towards physiological levels [6]. Careful dynamic testing of parathyroid function in uraemic patients subjected to acute perturbation of ECF calcium concentration has shown that calcitriol given parenterally [9] also modifies the parathyroid-calcium relationship in a manner consistent with normalization of the set point, and we have found similar changes (Figure 1) following weekly 'pulsed' oral dosing [11].

The above observations, however, while supporting the crucial role of calcitriol deficiency in the genesis of hyperparathyroidism, do not fully explain the parathyroid refractoriness to calcitriol that is frequently encountered in clinical practice. Such refractoriness develops partly as a result of progressive parathyroid hyperplasia leading in many cases to striking increases in parathyroid cell mass [12]. This also is likely to be the result of calcitriol

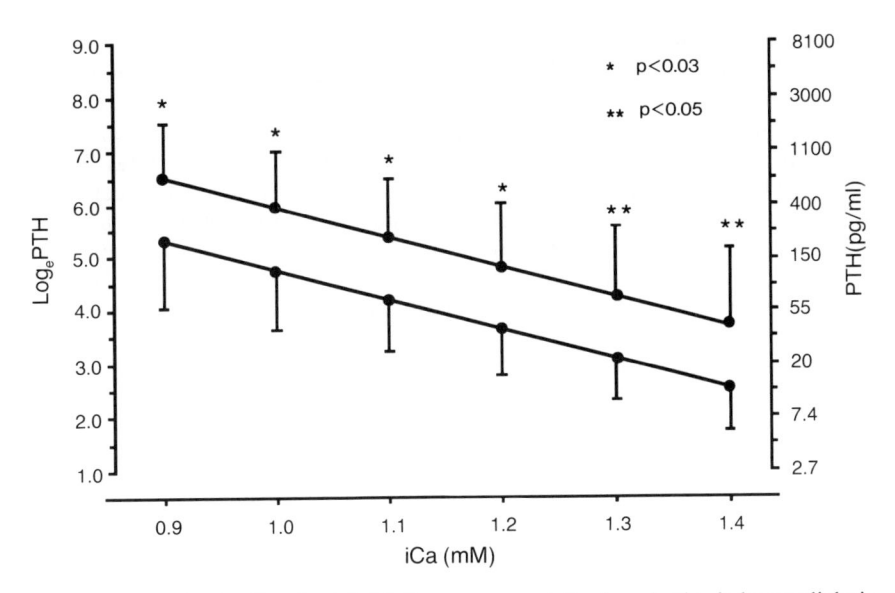

Figure 1. Effect of 'pulsed' oral calcitriol (6µg once a week for 4 weeks) in six haemodialysis patients. PTH was followed during acute perturbation of ionized calcium (iCa) before calcitriol therapy (upper line) and repeated after calcitriol (lower line). Normal range for PTH is 10–55 pg/ml. The curve shift represents a 70% decrease of PTH across the range of ionized calcium studied. From Kwan et al [11] with permission of *Nephrology Dialysis Transplantation*.

deficiency – parathyroid tissue taken from uraemic animals shows accelerated ^{3}H-thymidine incorporation which is attenuated by provision of exogenous calcitriol [13].

Osteomalacia and adynamic bone disease

The pathogenesis of these skeletal lesions is much less well understood than is that of hyperparathyroidism. Both are associated with low rates of bone turnover, often though not always accompanied by a surprising absence of PTH excess. In these conditions, skeletal metabolism is relatively quiescent, possibly reflecting a lack of hormonal drive to osteoblast function by PTH, and abnormal synthesis and/or action of bone cytokines. Furthermore, much evidence points to important adverse effects of aluminium deposition on the pathogenesis of low bone turnover renal bone disease. Approximately 90% of such patients have demonstrable aluminium at the mineralization front, whereas in patients with predominant hyperparathyroid bone disease (high skeletal turnover), only about 10% are found to have significant aluminium deposition [14]. The precise mechanism of these likely adverse effects of aluminium is poorly understood, but both experimental and clinical studies have demonstrated a strong association between the rate of bone turnover, and the amount of linear aluminium deposition at the mineralization front [14].

Metabolic acidosis

Metabolic acidosis resulting from renal tubular disorders is usually associated with osteomalacic bone disease, which may in some cases be severe. It is likely that the impact of acidosis is largely direct, and at the level of bone itself: bone mineral contributes significantly to buffering in acidotic states. This is achieved by mobilization of alkaline bone mineral, mediated by direct effects of pH on bone, and also by increased osteoclastic resorption. In addition acidosis almost certainly interferes with the mineralization of osteoid and with osteoblast cellular metabolism. Calcium regulating hormones show subtle changes in acidotic states – PTH is usually normal, but acidosis undoubtedly impairs the bioactivation of vitamin D by reducing 1α-hydroxylase activity [15], an effect that is particularly important in situations of deficient calcium supply when high rates of calcitriol synthesis are required.

Uraemic acidosis in patients with chronic renal failure or on dialysis is usually less severe and its consequences less striking, although recent evidence indicates that the rigorous correction of acidosis in these patients is associated with improvements in bone and mineral metabolism [16].

TREATMENT OF RENAL OSTEODYSTROPHY

Control of hyperphosphataemia

This is achieved by a combination of dietary phosphate restriction, removal of phosphate during dialysis procedures and the liberal use of oral phosphate binders which reduce the amount of dietary phosphate available for absorption in the intestine. Aluminium salts (aluminium hydroxide or aluminium carbonate) have been used to good effect for many years and when taken in sufficient dose at meal times, can reduce elevated serum phosphate concentrations to normal in virtually all patients. Elevated PTH concentrations are also reduced, though rarely completely normalized, by such therapy. However, in recent years concern with aluminium toxicity, both at the level of bone (see above), and also in brain (in severe cases leading to 'dialysis dementia') has led to a move away from aluminium salts and the evaluation of alternative phosphate binders. Of these, calcium carbonate and calcium acetate are widely used, and as well as achieving phosphate control without adding to aluminium burden, have the potential advantage of increasing calcium supply in these patients in whom intestinal calcium malabsorption is the rule [17]. The calcium salts are, however, associated with troublesome hypercalcaemia in some patients, in whom vitamin D independent intestinal calcium absorption becomes significant [18]. This can usually be dealt with satisfactorily by a reduction of calcium concentration in the dialysis fluid from about 1.65mM to 1.00–1.25mM [18]. Calcium acetate is superior to calcium carbonate in this respect [19], but although used widely in North America, does not at the time of writing have a product licence in the UK.

Calcitriol and alfacalcidol

Although effective phosphate control reduces PTH in virtually all patients, in only a few is hyperparathyroidism eliminated completely. The addition of calcitriol (or its 1α-hydroxylated analogue alfacalcidol), further reduces hyperparathyroidism, and in the short and medium term the combination of effective phosphate control and calcitriol therapy usually deals satisfactorily with the problem of hyperparathyroidism. However as mentioned above, many patients subsequently 'escape', and attention has therefore been focused on refinements to calcitriol regimens, and also to the development of new analogues of calcitriol that are less prone to cause dose limiting hypercalcaemia. To do this, the regimen needs to target the parathyroid glands selectively, with relatively less effect on the two major calcaemic target organs of calcitriol, namely the intestine and bone, thereby allowing larger doses of the vitamin D analogue to be given.

A number of reports suggest that when calcitriol is given as intravenous pulses thrice weekly (a highly unphysiological form of hormone replacement therapy), the tendency to hypercalcaemia may be reduced, with maintenance of effective PTH suppression [9]. Further, it appears that 'pulsed' oral calcitriol, with large doses being given once per week (Figure 1), may also achieve this result [11], although in both cases formal comparisons with conventional daily oral therapy are lacking.

However, although intravenous or 'pulsed' oral administration of calcitriol may achieve a degree of target organ specificity, a much better prospect lies in the development of new analogues of calcitriol with intrinsically different potencies on the respective target organs, such that selective parathyroid suppression can be achieved. Several such analogues are being evaluated, the initial thrust for their development being in the field of oncology where calcitriol and its analogues can act as promoters of mononuclear cell differentiation. Amongst these, 22-oxacalcitriol shows great promise, suppressing the parathyroids with a potency similar to that of calcitriol itself, while demonstrating only 1–2% of the potency of calcitriol when used to raise blood calcium in vivo or to mobilize calcium from bone in vitro [20]. Early studies in uraemic animals have also confirmed striking suppression of PTH, again without changing blood calcium [21].

Although the mechanisms underlying the specificity for the parathyroids of 22-oxacalcitriol are not fully understood at present, there is increasing evidence that differences between the pharmacokinetics of calcitriol and 22-oxacalcitriol may be important. Physiological vitamin D metabolites, including calcitriol, circulate in plasma attached to a globulin carrier protein (vitamin D binding protein – DBP). Virtually all the circulating calcitriol is present in bound form and only a very small amount exists as free hormone. In contrast, 22-oxacalcitriol exhibits binding affinity to DBP several orders of magnitude lower than that of calcitriol, and one consequence of this is that exogenous 22-oxacalcitriol has an extremely short half-life in plasma (a few minutes only) compared with that of calcitriol. It is conceivable, although not established with certainty, that the abrupt and abbreviated presentation of 22-oxacalcitriol to its potential target tissues results in apparent selectivity reflecting differences in the uptake of ligand during its brief period of availability, or the limited duration of biological effect in rapidly turning over cell populations (intestinal mucosa) compared with those turning over slowly (parathyroids). Alternative possibilities are that 22-oxacalcitriol may be catabolized rapidly in some, although not all, target tissues, or finally that there are organ specific differences of the intracellular stability of the ligand or the receptor-ligand complex.

When should treatment start?
Although the disturbances to bone and mineral metabolism parallel the reduction in GFR, becoming striking only in moderate and advanced renal failure, careful analysis has indicated quite clearly that the behaviour of parathyroid-vitamin D axis is disturbed even when GFR is reduced by as little as 20% [22] and that bone metabolism reflects these changes early in the progression of chronic renal disease. Given these observations, and the knowledge that relative lack of calcitriol sets the stage for parathyroid overactivity and hyperplasia, it is logical to propose therapy very early in the natural history of progressive renal failure. A number of studies have shown that early use of phosphate binders can partially reverse the above hormonal abnormalities [2], and because phosphate retention is also implicated in the progression of chronic renal disease, it makes sense to start therapy with calcium carbonate or calcium acetate even when the GFR has only fallen to 70-80% of normal. However, even rigorous phosphate control at this stage cannot completely restore vitamin D metabolism to normal and there is accumulating evidence that the state of subtle calcitriol deficiency can even at this early stage be corrected with benefit by administration of small doses of calcitriol [22].

Differences between haemodialysis and CAPD
Bone disease seen in association with these therapies differs quantitatively rather than qualitatively. Thus, haemodialysis patients, in whom phosphate removal by dialysis is less than that achieved by CAPD, are more likely to manifest significant hyperparathyroid bone disease and because of their greater requirement for phosphate binders are more likely to develop significant aluminium deposition in bone if aluminium containing binders have been used. Despite these differences, however, the overall approach to therapy, centred upon the use of calcium containing phosphate binders (with reduction of dialysate calcium concentration) and calcitriol, remains common to both.

Who should have a parathyroidectomy?
Indications for parathyroidectomy in chronic renal disease are restricted to patients with intractable hypercalcaemia that is demonstrably the result of PTH excess and is refractory to non-surgical therapies. Under no circumstances should parathyroidectomy be performed in patients manifesting:

1 PTH excess without hypercalcaemia – these individuals require calcitriol or similar vitamin D metabolites to raise blood calcium to the upper normal range and reduce PTH secretion.
2 Hypercalcaemia that is definitely or possibly the result of calcaemic vitamin D analogues and/or calcium containing phosphate binders – these patients require in the first instance withdrawal or reduction of the calcaemic therapy.

3 Low turnover bone disease in whom there is a high probability of significant aluminium deposition – these patients nearly always have relatively low parathyroid activity and there is good evidence that in this setting parathyroidectomy leads to yet more reduction in bone cell activity and to intractable osteomalacia or adynamic bone disease [23]. The degree of aluminium deposition and its likely impact on bone metabolism should be assessed by a bone biopsy, followed in severely affected cases by therapeutic removal of aluminium using desferrioxamine. Such therapy can undoubtedly improve bone metabolism in parallel with aluminium removal [24], but should not be undertaken lightly given the rare but serious side-effects attributable to desferrioxamine.

FUTURE PROSPECTS

More careful correction of uraemic acidosis, by use of oral alkali in predialysis patients and dialysate with higher concentrations of bicarbonate (in haemodialysis) or lactate (in CAPD), is likely to evolve.

The first clinical studies of 22-oxacalcitriol are expected in 1992 and there is every reason to believe that its striking efficacy in controlling hyperparathyroidism in animals will be reproduced in man also. As a result the treatment of uraemic hyperparathyroidism should become a great deal easier in the future.

There remains, however, a need for an effective, palatable and safe phosphate binder and as yet no single agent satisfies these criteria. Aluminium is likely to be used less and less and at present calcium salts offer the best compromise, with calcium carbonate as the current imperfect standard and calcium acetate likely to enter the clinical arena in the UK in the future.

REFERENCES

1 Slatopolsky E, Calglar S, Pennell JP et al. On the prevention of secondary hyperparathyroidism in experimental chronic renal disease using proportional reductions of dietary phosphorus intake. *Kidney Int 1972; 2*: 147–151
2 Portale AA, Booth BE, Halloran BP, Morris RC. Effect of dietary phosphorus on circulating concentrations of 1,25-dihydroxyvitamin D and immunoreactive parathyroid hormone in children with moderate renal insufficiency. *Kidney Int 1984; 73*: 1580–1589
3 Wilson L, Felsenfeld A, Drezner MK, Llach F. Altered divalent ion metabolism in early renal failure: role of $1,25(OH)_2D$. *Kidney Int 1985; 27*: 565–573
4 Sharman VL, Brownjohn AM, Goodwin FJ et al. Longterm experience of alfacalcidol in renal osteodystrophy. *Q J Med 1982; 203*: 271–278
5 Silver J, Russell J, Sherwood LM. Regulation by vitamin D metabolites of messenger ribonucleic acid pre-pro parathyroid hormone in isolated bovine parathyroid cells. *Proc Natl Acad Sci USA 1985; 82*: 4270–4273
6 Chan YL, McKay C, Dye E, Slatopolsky E. The effect of 1,25-dihydroxycholecalciferol on parathyroid hormone secretion by monolayer cultures of bovine parathyroid cells. *Calcif Tiss Int 1986; 38*: 27–32
7 Okazaki T, Igarashi T, Kronenberg HM. 5'-flanking region of the parathyroid hormone gene mediates negative regulation by $1,25\text{-}(OH)_2$ vitamin D_3. *J Biol Chem 1988; 263*: 2203–2208
8 Madsen S, Olgaard K, Ladefoged J. Suppressive effect of $1,25(OH)_2D_3$ on circulating parathyroid hormone in acute renal failure. *J Clin Endocrinol Metab 1981; 53*: 823–827
9 Dunlay R, Rodriguez M, Feldsenfeld AJ, Llach F. Direct inhibitory effect of calcitriol on parathyroid function (sigmoidal curve) in dialysis. *Kidney Int 1989; 36*: 1093–1098

10 Brown EM. Four-parameter model of the sigmoidal relationship between parathyroid hormone release and extracellular calcium concentration in normal and abnormal parathyroid tissue. *J Clin Endocrinol Metab* 1983; 56: 572–581
11 Kwan JTC, Almond MK, Beer J et al. Pulsed oral calcitriol in uraemic patients: rapid modification of parathyroid response to calcium. *Nephrol Dial Transplant* 1992; in press
12 McCarron DA, Muther RS, Lenfesty B, Bennett WF. Parathyroid function in persistent hyperparathyroidism: relationship to gland size. *Kidney Int* 1982; 22: 662–670
13 Szabo A, Merke J, Beier E et al. 1,25-$(OH)_2$ vitamin D_3 inhibits parathyroid cell proliferation in experimental uremia. *Kidney Int* 1989; 35: 1049–1056
14 Malluche HH, Faugere M. Renal bone disease 1990: an unmet challenge for the nephrologist. *Kidney Int* 1990; 38: 193–211
15 Cunningham J, Bikle DD, Avioli LV. Acute, but not chronic, metabolic acidosis disturbs 25-hydroxyvitamin D_3 metabolism. *Kidney Int* 1984; 25: 47–52
16 Lefebvre A, de Vernejoul MC, Gueris J et al. Optimal correction of acidosis changes progression of dialysis osteodystrophy. *Kidney Int* 1989; 36: 1112–1118
17 Fournier A, Moriniere P, Sebert JL et al. Calcium carbonate an aluminium-free agent for control for hyperphosphatemia, hypocalcemia, and hyperparathyroidism in uremia. *Kidney Int* 1986; 29: S114–S119
18 Cunningham J, Beer J, Coldwell RD et al. Dialysate calcium reduction in CAPD patients treated with calcium carbonate and alfacalcidol. *Nephrol Dial Transplant* 1990; 7: 63–68
19 Sheik MS, Maguire JA, Emmett M et al. Reduction of dietary phosphate absorption by phosphorous binders. A theoretical in vitro and in vivo study. *J Clin Invest* 1989; 83: 66–73
20 Brown AJ, Ritter CR, Finch JL et al. The non-calcemic analog of vitamin D, 22-oxacalcitriol, suppresses parathyroid hormone synthesis and secretion. *J Clin Invest* 1989; 84: 728–732
21 Brown AJ, Finch JL, Lopez-Hilker et al. New active analogues of vitamin D with low calcaemic activity. *Kidney Int* 1990; 38: S22–S27
22 Ritz Ceidel A, Ramisch H et al. Attenuated rise of 1,25-$(OH)_2$ vitamin D_3 in response to parathyroid hormone in patients with incipient renal failure. *Nephron* 1991; 57: 314–318
23 Felsenfeld AJ, Harrelson JM, Gutman RA et al. Osteomalacia after parathyroidectomy in patients with uremia. *Ann Intern Med* 1982; 96: 34–39
24 Malluche HH, Smith AJ, Abreo K, Faugere MC. The use of desferrioxamine in the management of aluminium accumulation in bone in patients with renal failure. *N Engl J Med* 1984; 311: 140–144

THE HAEMOLYTIC URAEMIC SYNDROMES

CM Taylor
The Children's Hospital, Birmingham

INTRODUCTION
A review of Gasser's report [1], from which the term haemolytic uraemic syndrome (HUS) was born, serves to illustrate the heterogeneity of the conditions covered by this title. It is worth noting that the precise translation of the German title is haemolytic uraemic *syndromes*. Of the five cases, all fatal, one infant had a post-enteropathic form closely resembling that which is prevalent today in North America and Europe [2]. By contrast an older girl developed HUS without any apparent prodrome. A child of 1 year had red cell polyagglutination following pneumonia and one suspects that she had exposure of the Thomsen–Friedenreich antigen following removal of sialic acid from cell membranes, perhaps by bacterial neuraminidase; an uncommon but well described form of HUS [3]. The boundary with previously described thrombotic thrombocytopenic purpura (TTP) is indistinct [4]. For example, fluctuating neurological involvement is a cardinal feature of TTP in adults, and yet 20% of children with HUS will have some neurological involvement, usually seizures related to hyponatraemia and hypertension. Moreover, patients with TTP may develop acute oliguric renal failure resembling HUS. The distinctive histological finding of arteriolo-capillary thrombosis, 'thrombotic microangiopathy', which had been reviewed by Symmers [5] some 3 years before Gasser's paper, is typical of both.

The scientific aim is to understand each of the component forms of HUS as specific disease entity with clearly defined aetiology and pathogenesis. Until the early 1980s there had been little progress with this approach. However, an important step forward was to recognize two broadly different clinical groups of patients; those with an antecedent, presumably infective illness and those without [6]. The former typically have diarrhoea, often bloody, in the 2 weeks before anaemia or renal impairment is noted. Like other diarrhoeal diseases, these cases present more often in the summer months and there are small outbreaks of the syndrome which suggest an infective cause. With improved management of fluid and electrolyte disturbance, this 'extrinsic' group has a high recovery rate. This contrasts with the other group, itself heterogeneous, in which microangiopathy and renal impairment occur without diarrhoea. These patients tend to have recurrences of the syndrome. Some cases are familial and there is a tendency for siblings to develop the syndrome at similar ages. This 'intrinsic' sub-group has a poor prognosis with more than 80% progressing to end-stage renal failure. Much of the confusion regarding claims of treatment has been caused by the failure to specify which forms of HUS are being considered. A simple mnemonic is to separate patients on clinical grounds into diarrhoea-associated (D+) and non-prodromal (D−) groups. In a recent national survey of childhood HUS in the UK [7] in which nearly 300 patients were reported, 95% of cases were D+ and 5% were D−. Very rarely patients present with other forms of HUS, for example induced by drugs (e.g. Mitomycin C, metronidazole, cyclosporin A), following radiation, other primary renal diseases or red cell polyagglutination.

It is widely held that endothelial cell injury is common to all forms of HUS. Endothelial swelling, detachment and microvascular thrombosis suggests that target organ damage is to a large extent explained by ischaemia. The erythrocyte fragmentation has been previously explained by mechanical damage as red cells pass through fibrin-containing vessels. However, red cell membrane lipid abnormalities suggest that oxidative damage may also participate in the haemolytic process [8–10]. Platelet survival is reduced. Plasma levels of beta thromboglobulin and platelet factor 4 are elevated, whereas platelets themselves show reduced aggregation in vitro and lower intracellular serotonin content. This is strong evidence of platelet activation and release in vivo, effete platelets being removed from the circulation by the liver and spleen [4, 11].

D+ HUS: RECENT ADVANCES
As most of the recent progress has been made in this sub-group the remainder of this paper will concentrate on diarrhoea-associated HUS, which in the last decade has become the commonest medical cause of acute renal failure in children of the developed world.

Epidemiology
During the 1980s, two epidemiological leads converged. The first recognized the association between *Shigella dysenteriae* type 1 infection and HUS in the Asian subcontinent [12]. The second followed the discovery by Konowalchuk et al [13] that certain strains of *Escherichia coli* produce an exotoxin to which Vero cells (a primate kidney cell line) were especially vulnerable: verocytotoxin (VT). The initial association between VT-producing *E. coli* (VTEC) infection and childhood HUS was made by Karmali et al [14] in Canadian children in 1983, and subsequently reported by others in both North and South America and Europe [2]. By combining serological and bacteriological techniques it appears that 80% of British children with D+ HUS have evidence of VTEC infection, usually with VT2-producing organisms of serotype 0157:H7 [15]. There are clinical and bacteriological parallels between VTEC and *Shigella dysenteriae* induced HUS.

The exotoxins

At least two VTs are known, VT1, VT2 and a VT2 variant. All closely resemble Shiga exotoxin produced by *Shigella dysenteriae* type 1. VT1 and Shiga toxin are homologous and some authors use the term Shiga-like toxin interchangeably with VT [16]. The intact toxins consist of a single A-subunit, surrounded by five B-subunits. In VT1 and Shiga toxin the A-subunit molecular weight is 32kDa, and each B-subunit is 7.7kDa. The latter have high affinity receptors for the terminal moiety galactose (alpha 1–4 beta) galactose of the human cell membrane glycoprotein Gb_3 [17]. Glycoprotein Gb_3 is the blood group antigen Pk which is expressed on many cells including the kidney cortex [18]. The same terminal disaccharide motif occurs in the red cell antigen P1 which is variably expressed in man. Interestingly, there are correlations between P1 blood group expression and susceptibility to HUS [19]. Following binding, the toxin gains entry to the cell by endocytosis. Lysosomes cleave the toxin to release the A-subunit fragment which, through its *N*-glycosidase activity, interrupts RNA transcription in the 60S ribosomes [20]. Cell death results from the failure of protein synthesis (Figure 1). It is noteworthy that whereas in *Shigella dysenteriae* type 1, Shiga toxin production is encoded in the bacterial chromosome, in *E. coli* a bacteriophage is responsible. It is therefore not surprising that a number of *E. coli* serotypes are known to be capable of producing VT1 and VT2. In North America and Europe the strain 0157:H7 is the one most closely linked with haemorrhagic colitis and childhood HUS.

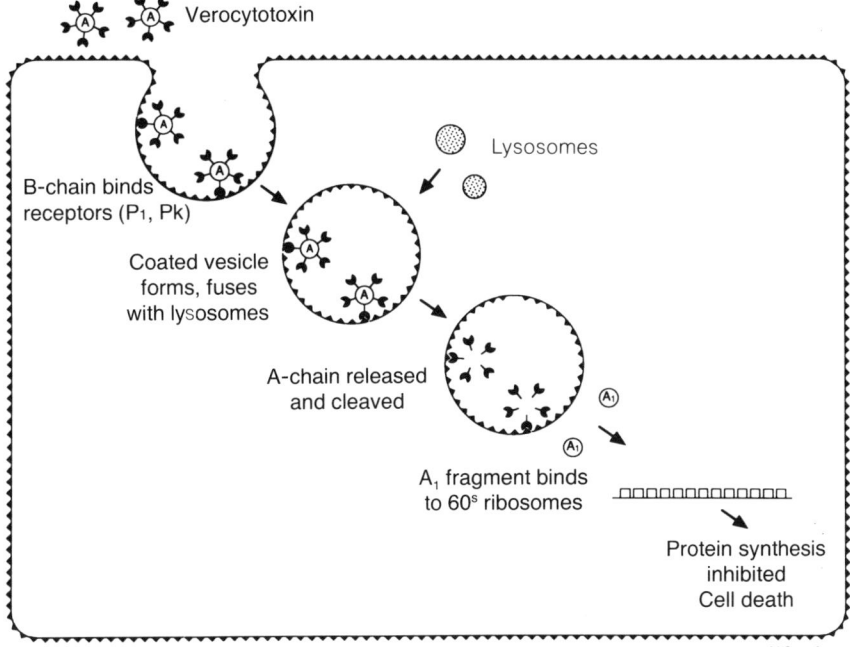

Figure 1. The action of verocytotoxin. Reproduced with permission from Milford and Taylor [2].

There is little evidence that Shiga toxin or VT plays a direct role in the epithelial lesion of the colitis. However, human endothelial cells in vitro are susceptible and it is likely that the haemorrhagic aspects of the colitis are attributable to the local effects of exotoxin in blood vessels. It is not known whether systemic toxicity occurs; specifically it is not known whether glomerular endothelial damage is *directly* caused by VT or Shiga toxin. Injection of purified VT into rodent laboratory animals does not cause HUS, the probable explanation being that they do not express Gb_3 on cells. VT has not been administered to primates.

Pathogenesis
In *Shigella dysenteriae* type 1 infection, the complication of HUS is associated with endotoxaemia, circulating immune complexes and a leukaemoid response [21, 22]. As yet no reports of plasma lipopolysaccharide (LPS) concentration have been reported from VTEC HUS cases, but an elevated neutrophil leucocyte count at onset correlates strongly with poor outcome as with *Shigella* induced HUS [7, 23, 24]. Moreover, plasma concentrations of elastase are elevated in the acute phase of the illness and also correlate with poor renal outcome [25, 26]. Neutrophils from patients with HUS show increased adhesion in endothelium in vitro [27], and appear degranulated on ultrastructure [25]. Together these observations suggest that neutrophils are actively involved in the pathogenesis.

Present knowledge of the actions of the exotoxins, VT and Shiga, do not explain the clinically important neutrophil response. However, there are well recognized pathways by which lipopolysaccharide may induce renovascular lesions and in these models, all variations on the generalized Schwartzman reaction, neutrophils play an essential role [28, 29]. Neutropenia induced by busulphan, for example, can block the reaction, and in one model neutrophils transferred from animals injected with LPS were capable of inducing the generalized Schwartzman reaction in recipients [30]. LPS primes neutrophils to release more elastase [31] and oxygen metabolites [32] when stimulated by chemoattractants. LPS injection into man stimulates the release of the cytokine tumour necrosis factor (TNF) [33], which in turn renders endothelium adhesive for neutrophils by the expression of surface receptors such as endothelial leucocyte adhesion molecule (ELAM) and intercellular adhesion molecule (ICAM) [34, 35]. In an elegant isolated rat kidney model, both LPS and the chemoattractant formyl-methionyl-leucyl-phenylalanine (FMLP) were required for neutrophils to cause renal injury, and the observed abrupt fall in glomerular filtration rate (GFR) was shown to be mediated by both elastase and oxygen metabolites together [36].

Lipopolysaccharide may also be responsible for the microvascular thrombosis. Without being directly toxic to endothelial cells in vitro, LPS stimulates them to produce tissue factor (thromboplastin) [37] and plasminogen activator inhibitor [38], and suppresses thrombomodulin expression [39]. Furthermore, monocytes exposed to LPS release TNF which also signals for pro-coagulant changes in endothelium [40].

These observations are beginning to join up to make a convincing pathogenic hypothesis involving LPS and neutrophils. However, significant gaps remain. To be robust, an hypothesis involving LPS dependent pathways must also encompass the epidemiological correlation with the exotoxins VT and Shiga. A simplistic explanation may be that VT, a virulence factor causing the vascular component of the haemorrhagic colitis, so damages the colonic mucosa that LPS is absorbed into the circulation. However, to look for other interactions between LPS and VT would seem a profitable line of enquiry. Recently, Tesh et al [41] have shown that LPS itself has no demonstrable effect on the cytotoxicity of VT on human endothelium in vitro. However, stimulation of endothelial cells by TNF augments their susceptibility to VT a hundred fold. In that TNF release via LPS is a likely, although as yet unconfirmed, accompaniment of VTEC induced HUS, this observation may go some way to explain the synergism between toxins.

Clinical aspects

Valuable clinical insights were gained from the survey of childhood HUS conducted jointly by the Division of Enteric Pathogens, Central Public Health Laboratory, the Communicable Disease Surveillance Centre and the British Association for Paediatric Nephrology [7]. D+ HUS was reported in 273 children over a 3 year period. Those shown to have VTEC infection had similar clinical features to the others, allowing all D+ cases to be analysed together. A typical course is shown in Figure 2. Cases occurred predominantly in the summer months. There was an excess of girls in the age group >10 years; otherwise both sexes were equally affected. The highest incidence was in children aged 1-2 years. The mean duration of diarrhoea was 7 days and the mean time from onset of prodrome to the diagnosis of HUS 8 days.

The diarrhoea was described as bloody in 73% of cases. Typically the onset of oliguria was first noted on the day the diagnosis was made, and seldom more than 3 days either side of this point. Seizures affected 19% of children and correlated with hyponatraemia. The latter was a common finding, 74% of children having a plasma sodium <130 mmol/l during their acute illness. Dialysis was required in more than half of the group.

Therapeutic strategies

Space does not allow a detailed review of treatment. The improvement of survival during the 1970s and 1980s was largely due to better management of fluid and electrolyte disturbances and the control of hypertension, although there is also the suggestion that the nature of D+ HUS changed to a more common but less aggressive disorder with the arrival of VTEC [24]. From the foregoing it seems certain that by the time the diagnosis is made, intoxication has already occurred and the microangiopathic process is well established. Anticoagulant and thrombolytic treatments have not shown benefit [42]. Treatment with plasma, which has anecdotal success in some adult cases of TTP, at best provides marginal benefit [43, 44] and lacks a credible rationale. It deserves comment that there is no evidence of a deficiency of endothelial prostacyclin production restorable by plasma in D+ HUS. Moreover, pooled plasma and IgG contain negligible amounts of antibody against

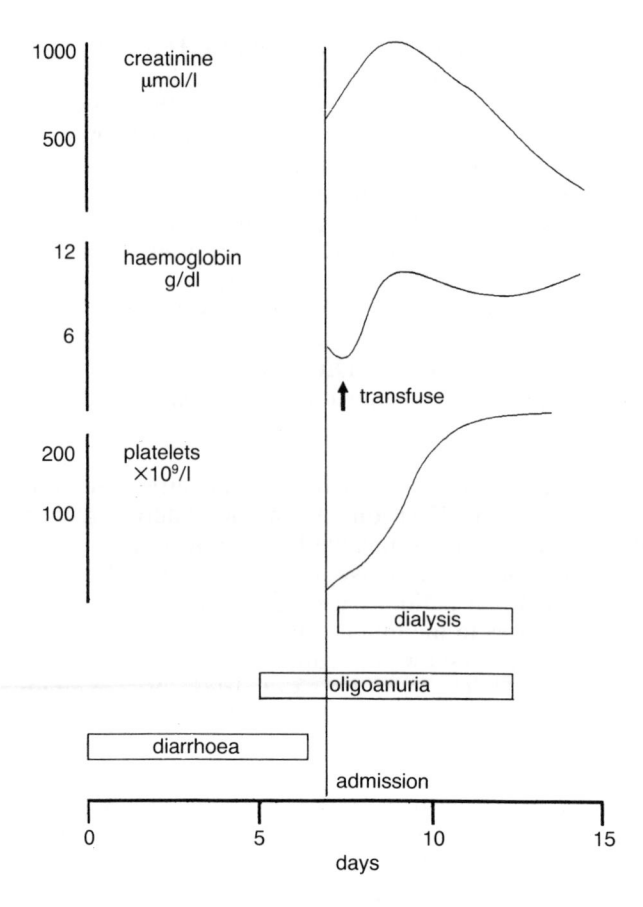

Figure 2. Typical clinical course of childhood diarrhoea-associated HUS.

VT2. Because 80% of children with D+ HUS are destined to recover with appropriate supportive management only, treatment trials are at risk of type 2 error unless huge numbers of patients are recruited. One way forward may be to design studies enrolling cases predicted to have a poor outcome, for example those with a high neutrophil count. If at diagnosis it is too late to block the action of toxins or prevent thrombosis, there is a case for exploring alternative treatments aimed at improving blood flow and preserving cell survival during ischaemia and reperfusion. Nevertheless, prevention of VTEC and *Shigella* induced HUS through immunization may be a more attractive strategy for the future.

Outcome

The outcome for children with D+ HUS is becoming clearer. There is an early mortality of 5%, and neurological complications are the usual cause of death. A further 5–10% of children are left with chronic renal failure or isolated hypertension. The early morning urine protein/creatinine ratio is a useful screening test with which to monitor survivors. In patients with good renal function there is a steady reduction of proteinuria so that normal protein excretion rates are achieved by 1 year of follow-up. By contrast all patients with reduced GFR continue to have significant proteinuria at this time [45]. Follow-up studies of patients more than 5 years from presentation give grounds for concern. Some cases with no significant proteinuria and near normal GFR in the years immediately after HUS develop proteinuria and declining function. Cross-sectional long-term follow-up studies show that within a decade a third of survivors have proteinuria, a fifth renal impairment, and hypertension is correlated with both these parameters [46]. Diarrhoea-associated HUS is relatively common (3.3 × 10^5 children per year in the 1–2 year age group) and an important cause of end-stage renal failure in childhood. However, these data suggest that after an interval there will be a further increase in end-stage renal failure attributable to this disorder with resource implications for adult renal services.

REFERENCES

1. Gasser C, Gauthier E, Steck A et al. Hamolytisch-uramische Syndrome: bilaterale Nierenrindennekrosen bei akuten erworbenen hamolytischen Anamien. *Schweiz Med Wochenschr* 1955; *38*: 905–909
2. Milford DV, Taylor CM. New insights into the haemolytic uraemic syndrome. *Arch Dis Childh* 1990; *65*: 713–715
3. McGraw ME, Lendon M, Stevens RF et al. Haemolytic uraemic syndrome and the Thomsen Friedenreich antigen. *Pediatr Nephrol* 1989; *3*: 135–139
4. Fong JSC, de Chadarevian JP, Kaplan BS. Hemolytic-uremic syndrome. Current concepts and management. *Pediatr Clin North Am* 1982; *29*: 835–856
5. Symmers W St C. Thrombotic microangiopathic haemolytic anaemia (thrombotic microangiopathy). *Br Med J* 1952; 897–903
6. Dolislager D, Tune B. The hemolytic-uremic syndrome. Spectrum of severity and significance of prodrome. *J Dis Child* 1978; *132*: 55–58
7. Milford DV, Taylor CM, Guttridge B et al. Haemolytic uraemic syndromes in the British Isles 1985–88, association with verocytotoxin producing *Escherichia coli*. Part 1: clinical and epidemiological aspects. *Arch Dis Childh* 1990; *65*: 716–721
8. O'Regan S, Chesney RW, Kaplan BS, Drummond KN. Red cell membrane phospholipid abnormalities in the hemolytic uremic syndrome. *Clin Nephrol* 1982; *15*: 14–17
9. Powell HR, Groves V, McCredie DA et al. Low red cell arachidonic acid in hemolytic uremic syndrome. *Clin Nephrol* 1987; *27*: 8–10
10. Taylor CM, Powell HR. Oxygen-derived free radicals in the pathogenesis of the hemolytic uremic syndrome. In Kaplan B, Trompeter R, Moake J, eds. *Hemolytic Uremic Syndrome: Thrombotic Thrombocytopenic Purpura*. New York: Marcel Dekker. 1992: 355–372
11. Walters MDS, Levin M, Smith C et al. Intravascular platelet activation in the hemolytic uremic syndrome. *Kidney Int* 1988; *33*: 107–115
12. Raghupathy P, Date A, Shastry JC et al. Haemolytic-uraemic syndrome complicating shigella dysentery in south Indian children. *Br Med J* 1978; *i*: 1518–1521
13. Konowalchuk J, Speirs JI, Stavric S. Vero response to a cytotoxin of *Escherichia coli. Infect Immun* 1977, *18*: 775–779
14. Karmali MA, Steele BT, Petric M, Lim C. Sporadic cases of haemolytic uraemic syndrome associated with faecal cytotoxin and cytotoxin–producing *Escherichia coli* in stools. *Lancet* 1983; *i*: 619–20.
15. Chart H, Smith HR, Scotland SM et al. Serological identification of *Escherichia coli* 0157:H7 infection in haemolytic uraemic syndrome. *Lancet* 1991; *i*: 138–140

16 O-Brien AD, Holmes RK. Shiga and Shiga-like toxins. *Microbiol Rev 1987; 51*: 206–220
17 Lingwood CA, Law H, Richardson S. Glycolipid binding of purified and recombinant *Escherichia coli* produced verotoxin in vitro. *J Biol Chem 1987; 262*: 34–39
18 Boyd B, Lingwood C. Verotoxin receptor glycolipid in human renal tissue. *Nephron 1989; 51*: 207–210
19 Taylor CM, Milford DV, Rose PE et al. The expression of blood group P1 in post-enteropathic haemolytic uraemic syndrome. *Pediatr Nephrol 1990; 4*: 59–61
20 Endo Y, Tsurgi K, Yatsudo T et al. Site of action of verotoxin (VT2) from *Escherichia coli* 0157:H7 and of Shiga toxin on eukaryotic ribosomes. *Eur J Biochem 1988; 171*: 45–50
21 Koster F, Levin J, Walker L et al. Hemolytic-uremic syndrome after shigellosis: relation to endotoxemia and circulating immune complexes. *N Engl J Med 1978; 298*: 927–933
22 Butler T, Islam MR, Azad MAK, Jones PK. Risk factors for the development of hemolytic uremic syndrome during shigellosis. *J Pediatr 1987; 110*: 894–897
23 Walters MDS, Matthei IU, Kay R et al. The polymorphonuclear leucocyte count in childhood haemolytic uraemic syndrome. *Pediatr Nephrol 1989; 3*: 130–134
24 Coad NAG, Marshall T, Rowe B, Taylor CM. Changes in the postenteropathic form of the hemolytic uremic syndrome in children. *Clin Nephrol 1991; 35*: 10–16
25 Milford DV, Taylor CM, Rafaat F et al. Neutrophil elastases and haemolytic uraemic syndrome. *Lancet 1989; ii*: 1153
26 Fitzpatrick MM, Shah V, Filler G et al. Neutrophil activation in the haemolytic uraemic syndrome: free and complexed elastase in plasma. *Pediatr Nephrol 1992; 6*: 50–53
27 Forsyth KD, Simpson AC, Fitzpatrick MM et al. Neutrophil-mediated endothelial injury in haemolytic uraemic syndrome. *Lancet 1989; ii*: 411–414
28 Butler T, Rahaman H, Al-Mahmud KA et al. An animal model of haemolytic-uraemic syndrome in Shigellosis: lipopolysaccharides of *Shigella dysenteriae 1* and *S. Flexneri* produce leucocyte-mediated renal cortical necrosis in rabbits. *Br J Exp Pathol 1985; 66*: 7–15
29 Vedanarayanan VV, Kaplan BS, Fong JSC. Neutrophil function in an experimental model of hemolytic uremic syndrome. *Pediatr Res 1987; 21*: 252–256
30 Niemetz J, Fani K. Thrombogenic activity of leukocytes. *Blood 1973; 42*: 47–59
31 Fittschen C, Sandhaus RA, Worthen GS, Henson PM. Bacterial lipopolysaccharide enhances chemoattractant-induced elastase secretion by human neutrophils. *J Leukocyte Biol 1988; 43*: 547–556
32 Guthrie LA, McPhail LC, Henson PM, Johnston RB. Priming of neutrophils for enhanced release of oxygen metabolites by bacterial lipopolysaccharide. Evidence for increased activity of the superoxide-producing enzyme. *J Exp Med 1984; 160*: 1656–1671
33 Michie HR, Manogue KR, Spriggs DR et al. Detection of circulating tumor necrosis factor after endotoxin administration. *N Engl J Med 1988; 318*: 1481–1486
34 Pober JS, Cotran RS. The role of endothelial cells in inflammation. *Transplantation 1990; 50*: 537–544
35 Pober JS, Gimbrone MA, Lapierre LA. Overlapping patterns of activation of human endothelial cells by interleukin 1, tumor necrosis factor, and immune interferon. *J Immunol 1986; 137*: 1893–1896
36 Linas SL, Whittenburg D, Repire JE. Role of neutrophil derived oxidants and elastase in lipopolysaccharide-mediated renal injury. *Kidney Int 1991; 39*: 618–623
37 Colucci M, Balconi G, Lorenzet R et al. Cultured human endothelial cells generate tissue factor in response to endotoxin. *J Clin Invest 1983; 71*: 1893–1896
38 Colucci M, Paramo JA, Collen D. Generation in plasma of a fast acting inhibitor of plasminogen activator in response to endotoxin stimulation. *J Clin Invest 1985; 75*: 818–824
39 Moore K, Andreoli SP, Esmon NL et al. Endotoxin enhances tissue factor and suppresses thrombomodulin expression of human vascular endothelium in vitro. *J. Clin Invest 1987; 79*: 124–130
40 Bevilacqua MP, Pober JS, Majeau GR, Fiers W et al. Recombinant tumor necrosis factor induces procoagulant activity in cultured human vascular endothelium: characterization and comparison with the actions of interleukin 1. *Proc Natl Acad Sci USA 1986; 83*: 4533–4537
41 Tesh VL, Samuel JE, Perera LP et al. Evacuation of the role of Shiga and Shiga-like toxins in mediating direct damage to human vascular endothelial cells. *J Infect Dis 1991; 164*: 344–352

42 Proesmans W, Eeckels R. The hemolytic uremic syndrome. *Ergebrisse der Inneren Medizin und Kinderheilkund 1989; 58*: 55–82
43 Loirat C, Sonsino E, Hinglais N et al. Treatment of the childhood haemolytic uraemic syndrome with plasma. *Pediatr Nephrol 1988; 21*: 279–285
44 Cole BR. Plasma infusion therapy in hemolytic uremic syndrome: is it warranted? *Pediatr Nephrol 1988; 2*: 286–287
45 Milford DV, White RHR, Taylor CM. Prognostic significance of proteinuria one year after onset of diarrhoea-associated hemolytic-uremic syndrome. *J Pediatr 1991; 118*: 191–194
46 Fitzpatrick MM, Shah V, Trompeter RS et al. Long term renal outcome of childhood haemolytic uraemic syndrome. *Br Med J 1991; 303*: 489–492

HYPERTENSION AND RENAL FAILURE

AEG Raine
Royal Hospital of St Bartholomew, London

Although it has been recognized for many years that hypertension, often severe, is common in patients with renal failure, the importance of the kidney in the pathogenesis of hypertension, and of hypertension in the progression of renal disease, has been recognized only recently. The associations between the kidney, hypertension and renal failure are particularly close, and may be expressed in several possible ways, as summarized in Figure 1. First, much evidence now suggests that an abnormality within the kidney, thought to be inherited, plays an important role in the pathogenesis of essential hypertension. This belief has grown from studies in the past two decades in several different animal models of hypertension, which have all shown that cross-transplantation of a kidney from a hypertensive donor to a normotensive recipient confers hypertension on the recipient, and vice versa [1].

Once essential hypertension is established, it may in some cases lead to appreciable renal dysfunction, although there are major ethnic differences in this respect (see below). The reverse situation arises when a specific renal disease such as chronic glomerulonephritis causes renal failure, which in turn causes secondary hypertension. Lastly, when hypertension and renal failure coexist, the presence of hypertension accelerates the rate of progression of renal disease, resulting in more severe renal failure; this in turn predisposes to greater severity of hypertension. The aim here is to review briefly these interrelationships, with particular reference to the impact of hypertension and its treatment on the progression of renal disease, and to the relationship between hypertension and cardiovascular morbidity in patients with renal failure.

ESSENTIAL HYPERTENSION AS A CAUSE OF RENAL FAILURE

Renal disease is a rare cause of hypertension in unselected hypertensive populations, being present in less than 5% of patients [2]. The reverse is also largely true; hypertension is a relatively rare cause of chronic renal failure in the UK and Europe, and was given as the aetiology of end-stage renal disease in only 6.1% of cases in the European Dialysis and Transplantation Registry

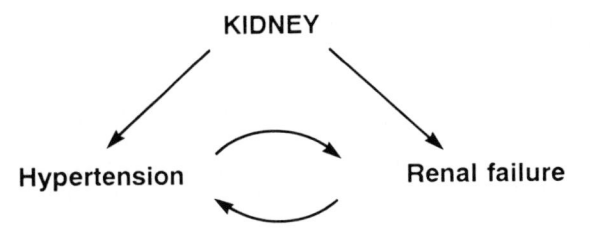

Figure 1. Associations between the kidney, hypertension and renal failure.

[3]. In contrast, hypertension is much more frequently a cause of progressive renal impairment in black and Afro-Caribbean patients. Surveys in Alabama, USA, suggest that end-stage renal failure due to hypertension is some 18-fold commoner in blacks than in whites [4]. This racial difference in morbidity persists even when equal and adequate blood pressure control is achieved [5], suggesting that more fundamental environmental or genetic factors may account for it.

Although benign essential hypertension rarely causes renal failure, this is not the case in accelerated and malignant hypertension. Kincaid-Smith et al [6] observed in a series of 89 patients that 73 had impaired renal function at presentation. Uraemia was, consequently, much the commonest cause of death in malignant hypertension before maintenance dialysis became available. Even now, impaired renal function at presentation and blood pressure achieved during treatment remain the most important adverse prognostic indicators in malignant hypertension [7], 5 year survival in patients free of renal involvement being little different to that of the general population [8]. The outlook for renal function in malignant hypertension depends very much on whether hypertension was initially caused by underlying renal disease. In one series, 1.5 year renal survival was 4% in patients with the malignant phase complicating glomerulonephritis, whereas 5 year survival of renal function was 60% in patients with malignant essential hypertension [9]. In the latter group, ultimate renal outcome may be roughly predicted by the serum creatinine at presentation. Prospects for recovery are good if it is 300µmol/l or less; above this level most patients progress to end-stage renal failure, although considerable overlap exists [10].

RENAL FAILURE AS A CAUSE OF HYPERTENSION

Nearly all patients with end-stage renal failure ultimately become hypertensive, though the pattern of development of hypertension depends in part on the primary cause of renal impairment. As a rule, hypertension is more severe and develops earlier in association with renal failure due to glomerular diseases than due to tubulo-interstitial disease. [11]. The relationship of hypertension to specific forms of glomerulonephritis is less predictable. Although earlier reports emphasized a high prevalence of hypertension in patients with focal glomerular sclerosis [12], IgA nephropathy, now recognized as one of the commonest forms of glomerulonephritis (see paper by Harper and Feehally in this volume), appears to be especially associated with hypertension, particularly accelerated hypertension [13]. Hypertension is more common in polycystic kidney disease than other diseases of tubulo-interstitial origin, and often appears early in its course [14].

It is commonly, though incorrectly, believed that hypertension in patients with renal impairment is due solely to hypervolaemia secondary to salt and water retention. In most cases of hypertension in end-stage disease, fluid removal by dialysis effectively controls blood pressure, in support of this belief. However, over 20 years ago it was recognized that in a substantial minority of patients blood pressure remained unaffected by fluid loss during dialysis, and in these cases inappropriate activation of the renin–angiotensin system was a major factor [15].

More extensive analyses of the contributions of volume expansion and renin system activation to hypertension in renal failure have yielded conflicting results, some studies showing a relationship between blood pressure and the product of blood volume and renin [16], whereas others do not [17]. In normovolaemic uraemic patients, blood pressure was unrelated to plasma renin activity [18]. The implication is that other factors may play a part in renal hypertension. These may include adrenergic mechanisms [19] and hyperparathyroidism, which in experimental studies contributed to the development of hypertension in chronic uraemia [20]. A further possibility of current interest is that abnormalities of the nitric oxide pathway may be involved. Inhibition of nitric oxide synthesis in normal rats by the L-arginine analogue L-NMMA causes a substantial and long-lasting increase in blood pressure [21], and thus the recent demonstration [22] that up to 10-fold increases in circulating levels of endogenous inhibitors of nitric oxide synthesis occur in uraemic patients may be of considerable importance. Accumulation of the vasoconstrictor peptide endothelin in uraemia is an alternative potential mechanism of hypertension, but so far less supported by experimental evidence. Although increased plasma levels of endothelin-1 have been observed in hypertensive end-stage renal failure patients [23], the absolute concentrations are low (1–3pg/ml), an order of magnitude below those which produce vasoconstriction experimentally [24]. However, enhanced local tissue accumulation of endothelin in uraemia, sufficient to cause vasoconstriction, remains a possibility.

HYPERTENSION AND PROGRESSION OF RENAL DISEASE
It is now universally accepted that coexistence of hypertension with renal impairment worsens the progression of renal failure, and it is remarkable how greatly perceptions have altered in just two decades. Guidance at one time in standard texts was that patients with chronic renal failure and hypertension who were asymptomatic – i.e. free of encephalopathy or symptomatic heart failure – should be given no treatment [25]. The basis for such a major change in thinking came largely from experimental studies. These showed that when secondary hypertension (e.g. DOCA salt or Goldblatt) was superimposed on experimental nephritis (immune complex or nephrotoxic), deterioration of renal function accelerated, sometimes dramatically [26]. Renal function was known to remain normal in the

spontaneously hypertensive rat, and micropuncture studies showed that afferent arteriolar resistance was increased, preventing transmission of elevated systemic arterial pressure to the renal circulation [27].

Observations such as these led Azar and colleagues to suggest that when the number of functioning nephrons is reduced, by whatever disease process, adaptive alterations in renal vascular resistance might result in increased blood flow and transmission of systemic hypertension to surviving nephrons [28] with an increase in glomerular capillary pressure and single-nephron glomerular filtration rate. Brenner and co-workers have argued, with experimental support from micropuncture studies in rats, that glomerular hypertension and hyperfiltration may then lead to increasing proteinuria and glomerular scarring [29, 30].

The weight of evidence thus suggests that, in rat models of renal failure at least, coexistence of hypertension exacerbates glomerular injury. Early studies by Purkerson et al [31] indicated the converse was also true; antihypertensive therapy with reserpine, hydralazine and hydrochlorothiazide was shown in a renal ablation model to reduce the degree of uraemia and of glomerular sclerosis. Similar reductions in renal injury produced by antihypertensive therapy in experimental renal failure have been reported in nephrotoxic nephritis [26], in immune complex nephritis induced in spontaneously hypertensive rats, and in streptozotocin-induced diabetes [32].

Interest was subsequently aroused by the demonstration by Anderson, Brenner and colleagues that, in a rat renal ablation model, both enalapril treatment and triple therapy (reserpine, hydralazine, hydrochlorothiazide) reduced blood pressure equally, whereas proteinuria and glomerular scarring were reduced only by enalapril [33]. Micropuncture studies showed that enalapril but not triple therapy reduced intraglomerular hypertension and glomerular transcapillary hydraulic pressure and hyperfiltration [33]. The conclusion was that reduction in renal mass leads to adaptive increases in perfusion, transmission of systemic hypertension to glomerular capillaries, and hence glomerular hypertension and hyperfiltration, postulated in turn to lead to glomerular injury. In accordance, the particular ability of converting enzyme inhibitors to protect against renal injury in experimental renal ablation [33] and diabetic nephropathy [32] was attributed to their reduction of intrarenal angiotensin-II mediated efferent arteriolar tone, thus reducing intraglomerular capillary pressure.

Although these theories have been widely accepted, more recent studies have cautioned that glomerular hyperfiltration and hypertension cannot provide a unifying explanation for the progression of all forms of chronic renal disease [34]. Increasing evidence now suggests that glomerular hypertrophy may be the consistent change which precedes progressive glomerular scarring [35]. Nevertheless, there is little doubt that the intensive study of glomerular haemodynamics and morphology in experimental renal failure in the past decade has greatly increased awareness of the importance of hypertension in progressive renal disease, and of the potential benefit of its treatment.

Despite this, well-controlled studies of treatment of hypertension in clinical progressive renal disease have to date been relatively few, and in the main confined to patients with insulin-dependent diabetes and nephropathy. Mogensen [36] first reported in an open study that adequate treatment of hypertension over 6 years with metoprolol, frusemide and hydralazine more than halved the rate of decline of renal function and reduced urinary albumin excretion in a small group of patients with diabetic nephropathy. Further studies, employing historical controls, showed that captopril therapy over 2 years was associated with a reduction in decline in glomerular filtration rate [37]. In a recent controlled study, evidence was obtained that converting enzyme inhibitors may delay progression to overt diabetic nephropathy in normotensive diabetic patients with microalbuminuria [38].

Several controlled treatment trials of blood pressure reduction in chronic renal impairment and in patients with proteinuria have now been carried out. In one, no differential effect of a converting enzyme inhibitor and a calcium entry blocker on reduction of microalbuminuria in patients with early diabetic nephropathy was observed [39]. However, Apperloo et al [40], in one of the few studies performed in non-diabetic renal failure, showed that in patients with moderate renal impairment (creatinine clearance 30–90ml/min) both enalapril and atenolol reduced blood pressure equally over 4 months, but reduction in proteinuria was restricted to patients receiving enalapril. Bjork and colleagues [41] have now shown in a prospective randomized study that enalapril therapy for 3 years in patients with established diabetic nephropathy resulted in a greater reduction in the rate of decline of renal function than equally effective antihypertensive therapy with metoprolol (Figure 2).

Although encouraging, these findings emphasize the need for large-scale well-conducted randomized studies to evaluate the benefit of treatment of hypertension in both incipient and established renal disease, and to determine whether some classes of antihypertensive therapy are superior to others. The answers to a number of important questions are still required. Does reduction in proteinuria equate to protection of renal function? How great is the long-term benefit of antihypertensive therapy in non-diabetic progressive renal failure? What is the optimum level of blood pressure control? Is the apparent superiority of converting enzyme inhibitors over other agents confirmed? Until these questions are answered, clear therapeutic guidelines for the treatment of hypertension in renal failure cannot be given, beyond the need for early and adequate blood pressure reduction.

HYPERTENSION AND CARDIOVASCULAR MORTALITY IN RENAL FAILURE

In addition to its impact on progression of renal disease, hypertension in patients with renal failure may be of major importance in determining their susceptibility to cardiovascular disease. Deaths from cardiovascular disease account for more than half of all mortality in patients with end-stage renal failure, whether treated by dialysis or transplantation [42]. Moreover, the rate of cardiovascular mortality in these patients is extremely high. Data from the Registry of the European Dialysis and Transplant Association show that in the UK, for example, the relative risk of death from myocardial infarction in patients aged 35–44 years is some ninety times that of the general population

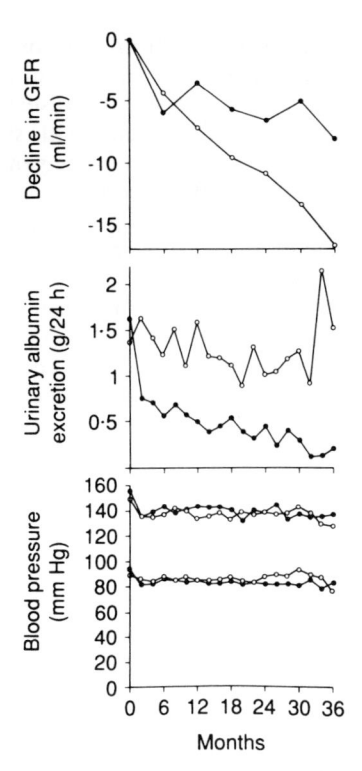

Figure 2. Change in glomerular filtration rate, urinary albumin excretion and blood pressure during treatment with enalapril (●) or metoprolol (○) in 40 patients with insulin-dependent diabetes and diabetic nephropathy. Reproduced with permission from Bjork et al [41].

[43]. Mortality from ischaemic heart disease is four- to five-fold higher in diabetic than non-diabetic patients with end-stage renal failure [43].

The mortality for myocardial infarction experienced by end-stage renal failure patients is equal to or exceeds that of other groups more commonly perceived as being at high risk of cardiovascular death, such as patients with hyperlipidaemia or those who have survived a myocardial infarction. In the ISIS-2 postmyocardial infarction trial, for example, myocardial infarction death rate over 4 years of follow-up in 1241 post-myocardial infarction patients receiving placebo averaged 26/1000 patients/year (A Keech, R Collins, personal communication). This compares with a death rate for myocardial infarction of 65/1000 patients/year in diabetic end-stage renal failure patients in the UK, and 20/1000 patients/year in non-diabetic renal failure patients (EDTA Registry data). Despite these high rates, mortality from myocardial infarction in dialysis patients does not increase with the duration of dialysis treatment, but remains stable once patients are established on renal replacement therapy [44]. The implication is that the risk factors which predispose to cardiovascular death arise during the development of progressive renal impairment, before dialysis commences.

The reasons for the high mortality from cardiovascular disease in renal failure have not been fully clarified. Prospective studies from the USA have indicated that the incidence of cardiovascular disease in dialysis patients is no higher than that of non-uraemic patients with similar risk profiles [45]. The risk factors which are well established in the general population include hypertension, especially with left ventricular hypertrophy, hypercholesterolaemia, diabetes and cigarette smoking [46]. Of these, the major role of hypertension as a risk factor for cardiovascular disease is undisputed. For any given set of risk factors, increasing blood pressure confers an exponential increase in risk of cardiovascular morbidity. This is illustrated by the interaction between hypertension and age. The Framingham study showed that with increasing age, itself a major risk factor for cardiovascular disease, the increase in risk associated with increasing systolic blood pressure rose dramatically (Figure 3) [47].

It is likely that similar interrelationships exist in uraemic patients, where hypertension would greatly augment any underlying risk of cardiovascular morbidity. In a single-centre study, a considerably reduced survival rate in hypertensive patients was observed, compared with those who were normotensive [48]. In addition, in a clinicopathological study, the presence of atherosclerosis assessed histologically in the iliac arteries of non-diabetic dialysis patients at the time of transplantation was related to age and degree of hypertension, but not to serum cholesterol level nor to duration of dialysis [49]. Although specific epidemiological data are lacking, it appears very likely that persistent hypertension and poor blood pressure control are major factors predisposing to the excess of cardiovascular death apparent in the renal failure population.

Thus there are cogent, though indirect, arguments in favour of effective blood pressure control in patients with renal failure. Extrapolation from the results of multicentre controlled trials of treatment in essential hypertension suggests that adequate blood pressure control in these patients may prove to be of major benefit. The findings of the trials are summarized in Table I, and show that when the underlying risk of cardiovascular mortality is low, as in the Medical Research Council trial of treatment of mild and moderate essential hypertension [50], little or no reduction in cardiovascular mortality is achieved by active therapy. In contrast, in the more recent trials of treatment of hypertension in the elderly, basal cardiovascular mortality was considerably higher (11-48 cardiovascular deaths per thousand patients per year), and here, active blood pressure reduction resulted in marked reductions in mortality of up to 58%. The cardiovascular death rate (myocardial infarction and stroke) of end-stage renal failure patients of all ages in the UK is similar to that of the elderly patients in the EWPHE [51], STOP-hypertension [52] and SHEP [53] studies. The implication is that effective blood pressure reduction in renal failure may achieve a similar beneficial reduction in absolute mortality. Clearly, this expectation requires testing through intervention trials in the renal failure population.

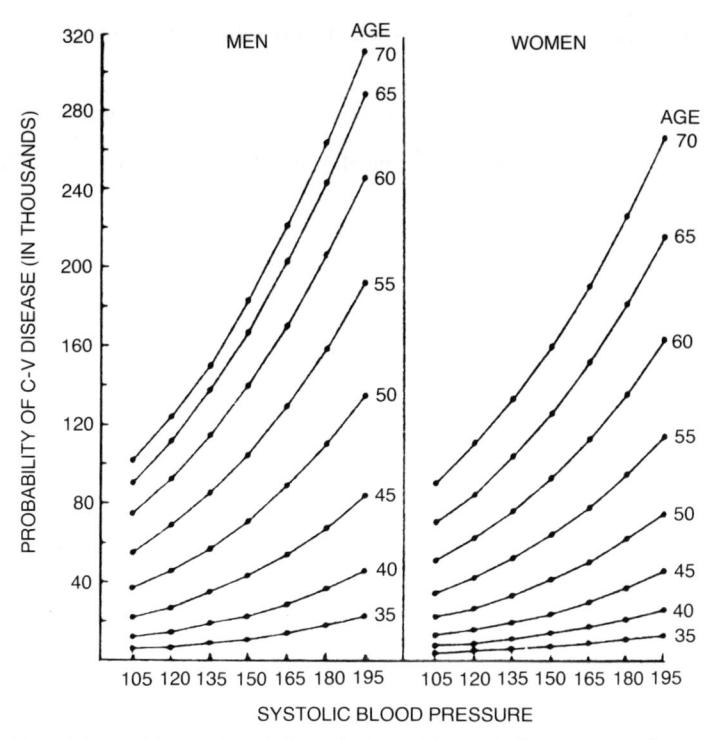

Figure 3. Probability of developing ischaemic heart disease in 8 years according to systolic blood pressure in low-risk persons aged 35 to 65 in the Framingham study. Reproduced with permission from Dawber and Kannel [47].

CONCLUSIONS

There is much evidence from animal models that coexistence of hypertension accelerates the progression of chronic renal disease, and that adequate treatment of hypertension may retard or even prevent this process. Adequately controlled long-term trials of blood pressure reduction in progressive renal failure are currently in progress, and the hope is that these will provide clinical evidence that effective antihypertensive therapy is of major benefit in retarding progression of renal disease. The possibility that therapy with converting enzyme inhibitors offers a specific additional benefit also awaits confirmation. It is apparent too that a more fundamental goal of effective blood pressure management in progressive renal disease is the reduction of cardiovascular mortality in these patients. The experience in treatment trials of high risk patients – the elderly – in essential hypertension suggests that the benefit may be substantial, though here too it awaits evaluation by formal controlled trials.

TABLE I. Cardiovascular mortality in essential hypertension and benefit of treatment: controlled trials

	No. of patients	Age range (yr)	Initial BP (mmHg)	Placebo CVS mortality (1000 pts/year)	BP reduction on treatment (mmHg)	CVS mortality reduction (%)
MRC [50]	17354	35–64	158/98	3	−11/6	Nil
EWPHE [51]	840	60–97	182/101	48	−23/9	38%
SHEP [53]	4736	60–80+	170/77	11	−11/3	19%
STOP-hypertension [52]	1627	70–84	195/102	23	−19/9	58%
ESRF, UK (EDTA data)	6742	15–74		26		?

CVS: cardiovascular; ESRF: end-stage renal failure.

REFERENCES

1. De Wardener HE. The primary role of the kidney and salt intake in the aetiology of essential hypertension. *Clin Sci 1990; 79*: 193–200
2. Berglund G, Andersson O, Wilhelmsen L. Prevalence of primary and secondary hypertension: studies in a random population sample. *Br Med J 1976; ii*: 554
3. European Dialysis and Transport Association Registry. Demography of dialysis and transplantation in Europe, 1984. *Nephrol Dial Transplant 1986; 1*: 1
4. Rostand SG, Kirk KA, Rutsky EA et al. Racial differences in the incidence of treatment for end-stage renal disease. *N Engl J Med 1982; 306*: 1276
5. Rostand SG, Brown G, Kirk KA et al. Renal insufficiency in treated essential hypertension. *N Engl J Med 1989; 320*: 684
6. Kincaid-Smith P, McMichael J, Murphy EA. Clinical course and pathology of hypertension with papilloedema. *Q J Med 1958; 37*: 117
7. Isles CG, Lim KG, Bouton-Jones M et al. Factors influencing mortality in malignant hypertension. *J Hypertension 1985; 3*: S405–S407
8. Bing RF, Heagerty AM, Russell GI et al. Prognosis in malignant hypertension. *J Hypertension. 1986; 4*: S42–S44
9. Kawazoe N, Eto T, Abe I et al. Long-term prognosis of malignant hypertension; difference between underlying diseases such as essential hypertension and chronic glomerulonephritis. *Clin Nephrol 1988; 29*: 53–57
10. Herlitz H, Gudbrandsson T, Hansson L. Renal function as an indicator of prognosis in malignant essential hypertension. *Scand J Urol Nephrol 1982; 16*: 51–55
11. Blythe WB. Natural history of hypertension in renal parenchymal disease. *Am J Kidney Dis 1985; 4*: A50
12. Vendemia F, Fornasieri A, Velis O et al. Different prevalence rates of hypertension in various reno-parenchymal diseases. In Blaufox MD, Bianchi C, eds. *Secondary Forms of Hypertension*. New York: Grune and Stratton. 1981: 89
13. Yu S-H, Whitworth JA, Kincaid-Smith PS. Malignant hypertension: aetiology and outcome in 83 patients. *Clinical and Experimental – Theory and Practice 1986; A8*: 1211–1230
14. Bell PE, Hossack KF, Gabow PA et al. Hypertension in autosomal dominant polycystic kidney disease. *Kidney Int 1988; 34*: 683
15. Vertes V, Cangiano JL, Berman LB, Gould A. Hypertension in end-stage renal disease. *N Engl J Med 1969; 180*: 978
16. Weidmann P, Berreta-Piccoli C, Steffeb P et al. Hypertension in terminal renal failure. *Kidney Int 1976; 9*: 294
17. McGrath BP, Ledingham JGG. Renin, blood volume and response to saralasin in

patients on chronic hemodialysis: evidence against volume- and renin-dependent hypertension. *Cli Sci Mol Med 1978; 54*: 305
18 Boer P, Koomans HA, Dorhout Mees EJ. *Nephron 1987; 45*: 7
19 Schohn D, Weidmann P, Jahn H, Beretta-Piccoli C. *Kidney Int 1985; 28*: 814
20 Iseki K, Massry SG, Campese VM. Effects of hypercalcemia and parathryoid hormone on blood pressure in normal and renal-failure rats. *Am J Physiol 1986; 250*: F924–F929
21 Rees DD, Palmer RMJ, Moncada S. Role of endothelium-derived nitric oxide in the regulation of blood pressure. *Proc Natl Acad Sci USA 1989; 86*: 3375–3378
22 Vallance P, Leone A, Calver A et al. Accumulation of an endogenous inhibitor of nitric oxide synthesis in chronic renal failure. *Lancet 1992; 339*: 572–575
23 Schichiri M, Hirata Y, Ando K et al. Plasma endothelin levels in hypertension and chronic renal failure. *Hypertension 1990; 15*: 493–496
24 Firth JD, Ratcliffe PJ, Raine AEG, Ledingham JGG. Endothelin: an important factor in acute renal failure? *Lancet 1988; ii*: 1179–1182
25 Wintrobe MM, Thorn GW, Adams RD et al (eds). *Harrison's Principles of Internal Medicine*, 6th edition. New York: McGraw-Hill. 1970: 1393–1394
26 Baldwin DS, Neugarten J. Treatment of hypertension in renal disease. *Am J Kidney Dis 1985; 5*: A57–A70
27 Azar S, Johnson MA, Scheinman J et al. Regulation of glomerular capillary pressure and filtration rate in young Kyoto hypertensive rats. *Clin Sci 1979; 56*: 203
28 Azar S, Johnson MA, Hertel B et al. Single-nephron pressures, flows and resistances in hypertensive kidneys with nephrosclerosis. *Kidney Int 1977; 12*: 28
29 Brenner BM. Nephron adaptation to renal injury or ablation. *Am J Physiol 1985; 249*: F324
30 Brenner BM, Meyer TW, Hostetter TH. Dietary protein intake and the progressive nature of kidney disease: the role of hemodynamically mediated glomerular injury in the pathogenesis of progressive glomerular sclerosis in ageing, renal ablation, and intrinsic renal disease. *N Engl J Med 1982; 307*: 652
31 Purkerson ML, Hoffsten PE, Klahr S. Pathogenesis of the glomerulopathy associated with renal infarction in rats. *Kidney Int 1976; 9*: 407
32 Zatz R, Dunn BR, Meyer TW et al. Prevention of diabetic glomerulopathy by pharmacological amelioration of glomerular capillary hypertension. *J Clin Invest 1986; 77*: 1925
33 Anderson S, Meyer TW, Rennke HG, Brenner BM. Control of glomerular hypertension limits glomerular injury in rats with reduced renal mass. *J Clin Invest 1985; 76*: 612
34 Klahr S, Schreiner G, Ichikawa I. Mechanisms of disease: the progression of renal disease. *N Engl J Med 1988; 318*: 1657
35 Yoshida Y, Fogo A, Ichikawa I. Effects of antihypertensive drugs on glomerular morphology. *Kidney Int 1989; 36*: 626–635
36 Mogensen CE. Long-term anti-hypertensive treatment inhibiting progression of diabetic nephropathy. *Br Med J 1982; 285*: 685
37 Parving H-H, Hommel E, Smidt UM. Protection of kidney function and decrease in albuminuria by captopril in insulin dependent diabetics with nephropathy. *Br Med J 1988; 297*: 1086
38 Mathieson ER, Hommel E, Giese J, Parving HH. Efficacy of captopril in postponing nephropathy in normotensive insulin dependent diabetic patients with microalbuminuria. *B Med J 1991; 303*: 81–87
39 Melbourne Diabetic Nephropathy Study Group. Comparison between perindopril and nifedipine in hypertensive and normotensive diabetic patients with microalbuminuria. *Br Med J 1991; 302*: 210–216
40 Apperloo AJ, de Zeeuw D, Sluiter HE, de Jong PE. Differential effects of enalapril and atenolol on proteinuria and renal haemodynamics in non-diabetic renal disease. *Br Med J 1991; 303*: 821–824
41 Bjork S, Mulec H, Johnsen S et al. Renal protective effect of enalapril in diabetic nephropathy. *Br Med J 1992; 304*: 339–343
42 Raine, AEG. Cardiovascular complications after renal transplantation. In Morris PJ, ed. *Kidney Transplantation, Principles and Practice*, 3rd Edition. WB Saunders 1988: 575–601

43 Raine AEG, MacMahon S, Selwood NH et al. Mortality from myocardial infarction in patients on renal replacement therapy in the UK. *Nephrol Dial Transplant 1991;* 6: 902
44 Brunner FP, Brynger H, Chantler C et al. Combined report on regular dialysis and transplantation in Europe. IX, 1978. *Proc EDTA 1979; 16*: 4-104
45 Rostand SG, Gretes JC, Kirk KA et al. Ischaemic heart disease in patients with uraemia undergoing maintenance dialysis. *Kidney Int 1979; 16*: 600-611
46 Kannel WB. Importance of hypertension as a major risk factor in cardiovascular disease. In Genest J, Koiw E, Kuchel O, eds. *Hypertension; Pathophysiology and Treatment*. New York: McGraw Hill. 1977: 888-909
47 Dawber TR, Kannel WB. Current status of coronary prevention. *Prev Med 1972; 1*: 499-512
48 Eliahou HE, Iaina A, Reisen E, Shapira J. *Israel J Med Sci 1977; 13*: 33-38
49 Vincenti F, Amend WJ, Abele J et al. The role of hypertension in hemodialysis-associated atherosclerosis. *Am J Med 1980; 68*: 363-369
50 Medical Research Council Working Party. MRC trial of treatment of mild hypertension: principal results. *Br Med J 1985; 291*: 97-104
51 Amery A, Birkenhager WH, Brixko P et al. Mortality and morbidity results from the European Working Party on High Blood Pressure in the Elderly trial. *Lancet 1985; i*: 1349-1354
52 Dahlof B, Lindholm IH, Hannson I et al. Morbidity and Mortality in the Swedish trial in old patients with hypertension (STOP-Hypertension). *Lancet 1991; 338*: 1281-1285
53 SHEP Cooperative Research Group. Prevention of stroke by antihypertensive drug treatment in older persons with isolated systolic hypertension: final results of the systolic hypertension in the elderly program. *JAMA 1991; 265*: 3255-3264

CLINICAL ASPECTS OF RENAL ARTERY STENOSIS

*LE Ramsay, *WW Yeo, *LA Brawn, *HA Cameron, †CF Close, ‡PC Waller, *PR Jackson

*Royal Hallamshire Hospital, Sheffield,
†General Hospital, Birmingham,
‡Medicine Controls Agency, London

INTRODUCTION
Surgical treatment of renovascular disease was reported to cure hypertension in one-half of cases, improve the blood pressure in about 15%, and have no effect in one-third [1]. Patients with fibromuscular disease had better responses than those with atherosclerotic renal artery stenosis [1]. The surgical mortality was 6% and 13% of patients had major complications [2]. Mortality was particularly high in those with atherosclerotic renovascular disease (9%), older patients, those with renal impairment and patients with generalized vascular disease [2]. About 50% of patients had nephrectomy performed as a primary or secondary procedure [1, 3–5]. Many physicians considered the mortality, morbidity and loss of functioning renal tissue with a surgical approach unacceptable in light of the improved acceptability of newer antihypertensive drugs, and gave up the search for renovascular disease except in young patients or those with severe and resistant hypertension.

Successful dilatation of renal artery stenosis by balloon catheter [6] rekindled interest in renovascular disease, and several large series of patients treated by percutaneous transluminal angioplasty have since been reported [7–16]. The blood pressure response to angioplasty appeared similar to that for surgery, but the procedure seemed simpler, safer and uncommonly led to loss of functioning renal tissue. It has become necessary to reconsider appropriate policies for the detection, investigation and management of renal artery stenosis, and these aspects are reviewed in this chapter.

CLINICAL FEATURES OF RENAL ARTERY STENOSIS
Renal artery stenosis is uncommon in unselected hypertensive patients, with a prevalence probably lower than 1% [17] and screening of all patients is not warranted [18]. It should be sought only in hypertensive patients who have clinical features or abnormalities in simple investigations which suggest its presence [19]. These features are shown in Table I. Among these the presence

TABLE I. Features of hypertension which should prompt investigation for underlying renovascular disease

Recent onset or recent worsening of hypertension
Accelerated (malignant) phase
Treatment resistance: uncontrolled by a three-drug regimen
Bruit in abdomen or loin
Proteinuria, haematuria or elevated serum creatinine
Hypokalaemia not otherwise explained e.g. by diuretics
Renal failure caused by angiotensin-converting enzyme (ACE) inhibitor
Severe peripheral vascular disease
Pulmonary oedema not otherwise explained

of a vascular bruit in the abdomen or loin is the most difficult to evaluate. Systolic bruits in patients over 50 are common and have low predictive value for renovascular disease. A continuous or systolic–diastolic bruit is virtually diagnostic of renal artery stenosis but extremely rare. In practice our policy is to investigate patients with a bruit further only if they are less than 50 years old. In a consecutive series of patients in the Sheffield Hypertension Clinic with these features (Table I), renal artery stenosis was confirmed in 29% of those with a bruit; 17% with accelerated hypertension; 15% with recent onset hypertension; 14% with resistant hypertension; 8% with renal impairment; and 4% with proteinuria or haematuria [20]. Young age (e.g. <35 years) is often considered an indication for seeking renal artery stenosis but in our series was not per se predictive of the condition [20]. The overall prevalence of renal artery stenosis in patients with the features listed in Table I is approximately 20% [20].

DIAGNOSING RENAL ARTERY STENOSIS

The rapid sequence intravenous urogram (IVU) was used as the screening test of choice for renal artery stenosis for many years, but recently some have favoured other screening methods such as digital subtraction angiography, captopril isotope renography, or Doppler ultrasound scanning [21, 22]. Others have suggested that screening tests should be abandoned altogether, and that renal arteriography [23], or intra-arterial digital subtraction angiography [24], should be the first and only test in all patients suspected of having renovascular disease. We disagree with these views and believe that the rapid sequence IVU remains the screening method of choice [20]. Its predictive value has been extensively investigated [25], and of the various screening tests proposed it alone is capable of detecting renal causes of hypertension other than renovascular disease, for example renal scarring, obstructive uropathy, renal tuberculosis or mass lesions [20]. In consecutive patients with features suggesting renal artery stenosis 5% had hydronephrosis and 5% renal scarring as the probable cause of hypertension [20]. Furthermore the rapid sequence IVU unlike many alternatives proposed is widely available. It is, however, an imperfect test for renovascular disease, with a sensitivity of 80% and specificity of 85% [25]. Of the non-invasive alternatives only intravenous digital subtraction angiography has been thoroughly validated. This has sensitivity and specificity similar to those for the rapid sequence IVU, but has no clear advantage [25]. In any event it is not universally available. The predictive value of other procedures such as captopril renography [26] and Doppler ultrasound scanning to record velocity profiles from the renal arteries [27] has not been examined in large series of consecutive patients.

Should all patients with features suggesting renal artery stenosis be investigated by more invasive procedures such as renal angiography [23], or intra-arterial digital subtraction angiography [24]? The sensitivity (80%) and specificity (85%) of the rapid sequence IVU are well established [25], and the prevalence of renovascular disease in patients selected appropriately (Table I) is about 20% [20]. Given these figures the rapid sequence IVU will diagnose correctly 80% of patients with renal artery stenosis, miss 20% of cases, and give a false positive result in 12% of those investigated. It will identify correctly the 10% of patients who have renal lesions other than renal artery stenosis such as hydronephrosis or scarring [20]; 28% of all patients screened would proceed to renal angiography. A policy of renal arteriography for all patients would entail the morbidity, inconvenience and expense of renal arteriography in the remaining 72% of patients. Arteriography without any initial screening procedure would result in the 10% of patients with other renal pathology [20] having an entirely inappropriate invasive procedure performed.

The price paid for relying entirely on screening by the rapid sequence IVU would be failure to diagnose renovascular disease in 20% of patients with the condition. Because of this it is important to proceed to renal arteriography *despite* a normal IVU when the clinical suspicion of renal artery stenosis is very high, or when it is *essential* to exclude the condition. This should be done in patients with severe and resistant hypertension, declining renal function of unknown cause, or pulmonary oedema which is not readily explained [28]. In summary, the rapid sequence IVU remains a suitable screening procedure for patients with suggestive features (Table I), but renal arteriography should be performed regardless of the result of the IVU in a small minority who have the specific indications described above.

BLOOD PRESSURE RESPONSE TO TRANSLUMINAL ANGIOPLASTY

The eventual blood pressure responses to angioplasty have been classed as cure, 'improvement', or no change, following the convention which was used to assess the outcome after surgery for renovascular disease. This classification is unsatisfactory in many ways, and the results cited for the outcome of angioplasty, and indeed surgery, have to be viewed with considerable caution. The definition of 'improvement' has differed between studies; the series reported have been uncontrolled; and no account has been taken of factors such as altered compliance, regression to the mean, placebo response, and observer bias, which all confound the assessment of response in hypertension [29]. Furthermore as many as 33% of patients with a similar degree of hypertension who had no intervention show 'improvement' in blood pressure control [30]. The figures for 'improvement' of hypertension cited in published series of angioplasty or surgery are therefore likely to be unreliable, and may even be entirely spurious [30]. These reservations do not, however, apply to the results of cure of hypertension, as the criteria for cure have been fairly uniform between studies [29], and without intervention 'cure' in hypertension of this severity is uncommon [30]. When assessing the results for angioplasty the figures for cure should therefore be given greater weight [30].

The blood pressure responses to angioplasty in 10 large published series have been reviewed [29]. The outcome has differed considerably for fibromuscular disease (Figure 1) and atherosclerotic renal artery stenosis (Figure 2). After technically successful angioplasty the cure rate for hypertension in fibromuscular disease is approximately 50% (Figure 1), whereas that in atherosclerotic disease is only 19%. A further 52% of patients with atherosclerotic renal artery stenosis were thought to have 'improved', but the reservations mentioned previously about the validity of 'improvement' must be borne in mind. In completely unselected patients with atherosclerotic disease the technical failure rate is about 60% [10, 30], and this means that the 'intention to treat' cure rate of hypertension is as low as 7% (Figure 2)[29]. This disappointing outcome is not really unexpected, because atheroma of the renal arteries is often a consequence of longstanding hypertension, and not its cause [22], and furthermore renal artery stenosis is common in normotensive patients who have extensive vascular disease [31].

In the clinical setting the initial blood pressure response to angioplasty can be quite misleading. Response to angioplasty may be delayed for as long as one month, while on the other hand hypertension can recur after an apparently good early response [8]. For this reason blood pressure must be monitored closely after discharge from hospital, particularly as these patients have often had severe hypertension, may be discharged on no treatment, and could have a rapid and dangerous rise in blood pressure. The long-term blood pressure response is intimately related to the technical success of angioplasty [10] and improvement should not be expected if the remaining stenosis after angioplasty is greater than 50% of the lumen.

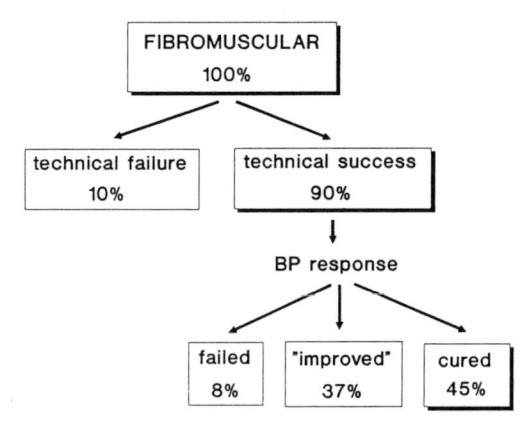

Figure 1. Response of blood pressure to percutaneous transluminal angioplasty of fibromuscular renal artery stenosis in 10 large series [29]. Note that 'improvement' of blood pressure is an unrealiable end-point [30].

```
                    ┌─────────────────┐
                    │ ATHEROSCLEROTIC │
                    │      100%       │
                    └─────────────────┘
                       ↙         ↘
        ┌──────────────────┐  ┌──────────────────┐
        │ technical failure│  │ technical success│
        │       60%        │  │       40%        │
        └──────────────────┘  └──────────────────┘
                                       ↓
                                  BP response
                              ↙       ↓       ↘
                      ┌──────┐ ┌──────────┐ ┌──────┐
                      │failed│ │"improved"│ │cured │
                      │ 12%  │ │   21%    │ │  7%  │
                      └──────┘ └──────────┘ └──────┘
```

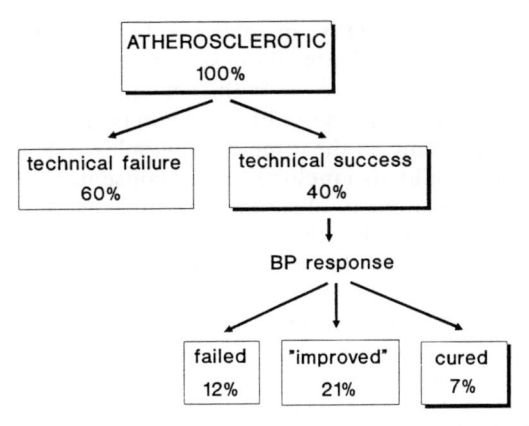

Figure 2. Response of blood pressure to percutaneous transluminal angioplasty of atherosclerotic renovascular disease in 10 large series [29]. Note that 'improvement' of blood pressure is an unreliable end-point [30].

PREDICTING CURE OF BLOOD PRESSURE

Over the years prediction of the blood pressure response to angioplasty or surgery in renovascular disease has been attempted by the use of numerous tests, for example measurement of renal vein renins, divided renal function tests, and the response to saralasin. Of these the renal vein renin ratio proved the most satisfactory [3], but its predictive power is too low to be of practical value [3-5, 9]. For this reason and also because of the low morbidity associated with angioplasty, use of the renal vein renin ratio and other predictive tests has been abandoned in most centres. The usual policy now is to dilate any significant renal artery stenosis (>50%) without further investigation [8, 9]. This policy seems justified as, in any case, the best predictors of the blood pressure response to angioplasty, or surgical intervention, are two simple variables – age and renal function [1, 30, 32]. The blood pressure of patients over the age of 60 years or those with elevated serum creatinine is less likely to respond well to angioplasty [30].

EFFECT OF ANGIOPLASTY ON RENAL FUNCTION

There are few data on the effects of angioplasty on renal function and those available are inconsistent. It can improve renal function substantially in patients with critical stenosis of the artery supplying a single functioning kidney [33], and some small series have suggested a more general improvement in renal function after angioplasty [16, 34]. However, this effect has not been observed in other series [30, 32, 35], and detailed study of the outcome of angioplasty on renal function is needed.

PERFORMING PERCUTANEOUS TRANSLUMINAL ANGIOPLASTY

Angioplasty should be performed at the same time as the diagnostic arteriogram whenever possible, otherwise the patient is subjected to two invasive procedures. Severe hypotension may occur immediately after dilatation of the stenosis [8, 36], especially in patients taking potent diuretic and antihypertensive therapy. Patients taking such treatment should be admitted 48 hours before the procedure to withdraw diuretics and reduce other antihypertensive drugs as far as possible. The aim is to control blood pressure with minimum treatment at the time of angioplasty. Routine procedures before angioplasty should also include written consent; a formal record of all peripheral pulses; measurement of serum creatinine, haemoglobin, urinalysis, and blood group; and ensuring that a vascular surgeon is available at short notice when the procedure is to be performed.

The technical aspects of angioplasty have been described elsewhere [37]. Briefly, the stenotic lesion is crossed by a balloon-tipped catheter and the balloon is then inflated to compress and abolish the stenosis. The procedure is performed most commonly through the femoral artery using local anaesthesia and under cover of infused heparin. It remains unclear whether bilateral lesions are best dealt with at a single or two separate sessions. Attempting to dilate both sides at once carries a small risk of causing bilateral renal artery thrombosis or dissection, which could leave the patient functionally anephric. It is probably safer to dilate the more severely affected artery and leave the contralateral artery to a later date. However, some groups perform bilateral angioplasties at a single session, apparently without serious complications [11, 38].

TECHNICAL FAILURE OF ANGIOPLASTY
In large series of renal angioplasties the procedure has been technically unsuccessful in 12% of patients, but the rate of failure has varied widely between series, from 3 to 24% [29]. This may well be a consequence of patient selection in tertiary referral centres. These figures are for all forms of renovascular disease, and there are important differences in technical success rate with angioplasty between fibromuscular and atherosclerotic forms of renovascular disease. Renal artery lesions can be dilated satisfactorily in 80–90% of patients with fibromuscular dysplasia. However, in unselected patients with atherosclerotic renovascular disease complete correction can be achieved in only 40% of cases [10, 30] (Figure 2). Short proximal atherosclerotic stenoses which do not involve the ostium are generally amenable to dilatation [10–12, 38, 39]. Technical failure in atherosclerotic renal artery stenosis is most commonly due to occlusion, long atherosclerotic lesions, or ostial stenosis, i.e. encroachment of an aortic plaque upon the origin of the renal artery.

RECURRENCE OF STENOSIS
Restenosis occurs in about 15% of patients [11, 38]. It is more common and occurs earlier in atherosclerotic disease [40]. Restenosis is also more likely if there is residual narrowing of 30% or more at the original angioplasty [11, 38]. Various measures have been employed to prevent thrombosis or restenosis after angioplasty [29]. We use aspirin because it is simple, economic and acceptably safe. Patients free of recurrence after 6 months are apparently likely to remain so in the long-term [11, 38]. Recurrent stenotic lesions can be

dilated readily and repeatedly if necessary [11, 38, 40]. Quite apart from restenosis, patients with hypertension which has been 'cured' by angioplasty need to be followed up long-term, as they may develop new stenosing lesions [41].

COMPLICATIONS OF ANGIOPLASTY
A complication rate of 9.1% and mortality of 0.43% were reported in an overview of 10 large series of renal artery angioplasty in 691 patients [29]. It was difficult to determine from the published reports what proportions of complications were major and minor. According to the classification of Mahler et al [42] 89% of complications were a direct consequence of the procedure, and 11% an indirect consequence. The most common direct complications of angioplasty are renal artery dissection, renal artery thrombosis, segmental renal infarction, haematoma or puncture trauma, retroperitoneal haemorrhage, profound hypotension, and acute tubular necrosis. The most feared direct complication is cholesterol embolism (athero-embolic disease). Serious indirect complications include stroke, myocardial infarction, spinal artery thrombosis, and bowel infarction. The services of a vascular surgeon should be available immediately if required. Following angioplasty patients should be monitored in hospital for about 5 days, paying particular attention to the urine output, urinalysis, serum creatinine, haemoglobin, puncture site and peripheral pulses.

ROLE OF ANGIOPLASTY IN THE MANAGEMENT OF RENAL ARTERY STENOSIS
Angioplasty is clearly the treatment of choice for fibromuscular renal artery stenosis. The chance of technically successful dilatation is high, complications in this group are relatively infrequent, and the cure rate of hypertension is approximately 50%. The role of transluminal angioplasty in the treatment of atherosclerotic renovascular disease is much less clear. For these patients the technical failure rate is high, the risk of complications is substantial, and the cure rate for hypertension is a disappointing 7–8% on an intention to treat principle. Benefit in this group hinges largely on 'improvement' of hypertension, and this is distinctly questionable. In any event those with 'improved' blood pressure have to continue on antihypertensive therapy (by definition). It is usually possible to control blood pressure adequately with modern antihypertensive therapy, without intervention, and it might be argued that those who have 'improved' are little better off. There is plainly a need for a prospective controlled trial comparing angioplasty to conservative medical management in atherosclerotic renovascular disease [29, 30]. However, in certain groups of patients with atherosclerotic renal artery stenosis there are clear indications for attempting angioplasty, for example in those with severe and uncontrollable hypertension, declining renal function despite adequate blood pressure control, and pulmonary oedema caused by advanced bilateral renovascular disease [28]. Although angioplasty should be attempted in these circumstances the outcome has been disappointing in our experience. A case can also be made for dilating discrete proximal non-ostial atherosclerotic lesions.

ROLE OF SURGERY

Surgical techniques used in renovascular disease have been reviewed by Novick [43]. Surgical intervention should be considered in the 10-20% of patients with fibromuscular disease which is not amenable to angioplasty, for example those with distal aneurysms or intrarenal lesions. In atherosclerotic renovascular disease surgery might be considered in the 60% or so of patients whose disease cannot be corrected by angioplasty, most often because of ostial stenosis, renal artery thrombosis, or long atherosclerotic lesions. However, such lesions are generally found in older subjects with renal impairment and generalized vascular disease, precisely the patients who have the highest mortality [2] and least satisfactory blood pressure responses [1] to surgery. When angioplasty cannot be performed in such patients we generally advise conservative medical management, and recommend surgery only when hypertension is severe and uncontrollable, when renal function declines, or in patients with pulmonary oedema.

CONCLUSIONS

Efforts to diagnose renovascular disease should be directed particularly at hypertensive patients aged 60 years or less who have the suggestive clinical features listed in Table I. The diagnosis should also be considered in older patients if there is severe and uncontrollable hypertension, declining renal function, or pulmonary oedema. The rapid sequence IVU remains the best screening test generally available, and also provides information on other renal causes of hypertension. However, it is an imperfect screening test, and renal arteriography should be performed when it is essential to exclude renovascular disease. In fibromuscular renal artery stenosis the lesion can usually be dilated by transluminal angioplasty, with few complications and a 50% cure rate of hypertension. In atherosclerotic renovascular disease technical failure is common, complications of angioplasty are frequent, the cure rate of hypertension is very low, and conservative management may be preferable. Patients unsuitable for angioplasty are generally those who are the least likely to do well with surgical management.

REFERENCES

1. Foster GH, Maxwell MH, Franklin SS et al. Renovascular occlusive disease. Results of operative treatment. *JAMA 1975; 231:* 1043-1048
2. Franklin SS, Young JD, Maxwell MH et al. Operative morbidity and mortality in renovascular disease. *JAMA 1975; 231:* 1148-1153
3. Mackay A, Boyle P, Brown JJ et al. The decision on surgery in renal artery stenosis. *Q J Med (New Series) 1983; 52*: 363-381
4. Sellars L, Siamopoulos K, Hacking PM et al. Renovascular hypertension: ten years experience in a regional centre. *Q J Med (New Series) 1985; 56*: 403-416
5. Sellars L, Shore AC, Wilkinson R. Renal vein renin studies in renovascular hypertension - do they really help? *J Hypertens 1985; 3*: 177-181
6. Gruntzig A, Kuhlmann U, Vetter W et al. Treatment of renovascular hypertension with percutaneous transluminal dilatation of a renal-artery stenosis. *Lancet 1978; i*: 801-802
7. Martin EC, Mattern RF, Baer L et al. Renal angioplasty for hypertension: predictive factors for long-term success. *Am J Roentgenol 1981; 137:* 921-924
8. Colapinto RF, Stronell RD, Harries-Jones EP et al. Percutaneous transluminal dilatation

of the renal artery. Follow-up studies on renovascular hypertension. *Am J Roentgenol 1982; 139:* 722-732
9   Geyskes GG, Puyleart CBA, Oei HY et al. Follow up study of 70 patients with renal artery stenosis treated by percutaneous transluminal dilatation. *Br Med J 1983; 287:* 333-336
10 Sos TA, Pickering TG, Sniderman K et al. Percutaneous transluminal renal angioplasty in renovascular hypertension due to atheroma or fibromuscular dysplasia. *N Engl J Med 1983; 309:* 274-279
11 Tegtmeyer CJ, Kellum CD, Ayers C. Percutaneous transluminal angioplasty of the renal artery. *Radiology 1984; 153:* 77-84
12 Miller GA, Ford KK, Braun SD et al. Percutaneous transluminal angioplasty vs surgery for renovascular hypertension. *Am J Roentgenol 1985; 144:* 447-450
13 Martin LG, Price RB, Casarella WJ et al. Percutaneous angioplasty in clinical management of renovascular hypertension: initial and long-term results. *Radiology 1985; 155:* 629-633
14 Kaplan-Pavlobcic S, Koselj M, Obrez I et al. Percutaneous transluminal renal angioplasty: follow up studies in renovascular hypertension. *Przegl Lek 1985; 42:* 342-344
15 Kuhlmann U, Greminger P, Gruntzig A et al. Long-term experience in percutaneous transluminal dilatation of renal artery stenosis. *Am J Med 1985; 79:* 692-698
16 Bell GM, Reid J, Buist TAS. Percutaneous transluminal angioplasty improves blood pressure and renal function in renovascular hypertension. *Q J Med (New Series) 1987; 63:* 393-403
17 Berglund G, Andersson O, Wilmhelmsen L. Prevalence of primary and secondary hypertension: studies in a random population sample. *Br Med J 1976; iii:* 554-556
18 Atkinson AB, Kellett RJ. Value of intravenous urography in investigating hypertension. *J Roy Coll Phys Lond 1974; 8:* 175-181
19 Simon N, Franklin SS, Bleifer KH, Maxwell MH. Clinical characteristics of renovascular hypertension. *JAMA 1972; 220:* 1209-1218
20 Cameron HA, Close CF, Yeo WW et al. Role of the rapid sequence intravenous urogram in investigating hypertension: diagnostic yield and effect on outcome. *Lancet,* in press
21 Thornbury JR, Stanley JC, Fryback DJ. Hypertensive urogram: nondiscriminatory test for renovascular hypertension. *Am J Roentgenol 1982; 138:* 43-49
22 Pickering TG. Renovascular hypertension. Medical evaluation and non-surgical treatment. In Laragh JH, Brenner BM, eds. *Hypertension: Pathophysiology, Diagnosis and Management.* New York: Raven Press. 1990: 1539-1559
23 Carmichael DJS, Mathias CJ, Snell ME, Peart S. Detection and investigation of renal artery stenosis. *Lancet 1986; i:* 667-670
24 Thornbury JR, Stanley JC, Fryback DG. Optimizing work-up of adult hypertensive patients for renal artery stenosis. Observations about hypertensive urography, digital subtraction arteriography, and patient selection. *Radiol Clin North Am 1984; 22:* 333-339
25 Havey RJ, Krumlovsky F, del Greco F, Martin HG. Screening for renovascular hypertension. Is renal digital-subtraction angiography the preferred noninvasive test? *JAMA 1985; 254:* 388-393
26 Fommei E, Ghione S, Palla L et al. Renal scintigraphic captopril test in the diagnosis of renovascular hypertension. *Hypertension 1987; 10:* 212-220
27 Kohler TR, Zierler E, Martin RL et al. Noninvasive diagnosis of renal artery stenosis by ultrasonic duplex scanning. *J Vasc Surg 1986; 4:* 450-456
28 Pickering TG, Herman L, Devereux RB et al. Recurrent pulmonary oedema in hypertension due to bilateral renal artery stenosis: treatment by angioplasty or surgical revascularisation. *Lancet 1988; ii:* 551-552
29 Ramsay LE, Waller PC. Blood pressure response to percutaneous transluminal angioplasty for renovascular hypertension: an overview of published series. *Br Med J 1990; 300:* 569-572
30 Brawn LA, Ramsay LE. Is 'improvement' real with percutaneous transluminal angioplasty in the management of renovascular hypertension? *Lancet 1987; ii:* 1313-1316

31 Choudhri AH, Cleland JGF, Rowlands PC et al. Unsuspected renal artery stenosis in peripheral vascular disease. *Br Med J 1990; 301:* 1197-1198
32 Marshall FI, Hagen S, Mahaffy RG et al. Percutaneous transluminal angioplasty for atheromatous renal artery stenosis - blood pressure response and discriminant analysis of outcome predictors. *Q J Med (New Series) 1990; 75:* 483-489
33 Sutters M, Al-Kutoubi MA, Mathias CJ, Peart S. Diuresis and syncope after renal angioplasty in a patient with one functioning kidney. *Br Med J 1987; 295:* 527-528
34 Pickering TG, Sos TA, Saddekni S et al. Renal angioplasty in patients with azotemia and renovascular hypertension. *J Hypertens 1986; 4 (Suppl 6):* S667-S669
35 Luft FR, Grim CE, Weinberger NJ. Intervention in patients with renovascular hypertension and renal insufficiency. *J Urol 1983; 130:* 645-656
36 Schwarten DE. Transluminal angioplasty of renal artery stenosis: 70 experiences. *Am J Roentgenol 1980; 135:* 969-974
37 Tegtmeyer CJ, Dyer R, Teates CD. Percutaneous transluminal dilatation of the renal arteries. Techniques and results. *Radiology 1980; 135:* 589-599
38 Tegtmeyer CJ, Kofler TJ, Ayers CA. Renal angioplasty: current status. *Am J Roentgenol 1984; 142:* 17-21
39 Cicuto KP, McLean GK, Oleaga JA et al. Renal artery stenosis: anatomic classification for percutaneous transluminal angioplasty. *Am J Roentgenol 1981; 137:* 599-601
40 Grim CE, Luft FC, Yune HY et al. Percutaneous transluminal dilatation in the treatment of renal vascular hypertension. *Ann Intern Med 1981; 95:* 439-442
41 Jones EOP, Wilkinson R, Taylor RMR. Contralateral renal artery fibromuscular dysplasia after nephrectomy for renal artery stenosis. *Br Med J 1978; ii:* 825-826
42 Mahler F, Triller J, Weidmann P, Nachbur B. Complications in percutaneous transluminal dilatation of renal arteries. *Nephron 1986; 44(suppl 1):* 60-63
43 Novick AC. Renovascular hypertension. Surgical treatment. In Laragh JH, Brenner BM, eds. *Hypertension: Pathophysiology, Diagnosis and Management.* New York: Raven Press. 1990: 1561-1571

INDEX

Acetyl-CoA 1
Achondroplasia 214
Acne, psychological impact 175–6
Acne Disability Index 178
Acromegaly, octreotide in 276–7
Acute disseminated encephalomyelitis (ADEM), MRI in 307
Acyl-CoA dehydrogenase deficiency 4, 6
Acyl-CoA esters 1–3
   intramitochondrial accumulation of 5
Acylglycines in urine 5
Adenosine 55
Adenosine deaminase (ADA) deficiency 75
Adenosine triphosphatase (ATPase) 180
Adrenomyeloneuropathy, MRI in 308
Adult polycystic kidney disease 214, 218
Adynamic bone disease 330, 333
Age-related diseases 25
Ageing
   normal physiological 194
   premature 194
   skin in. See Skin ageing
AIDs-related diarrhoea, octreotide in 279
Alcoholic cirrhosis 104
Alcoholic liver disease 95
   liver transplantation in 137
Alfacalcidol in hyperparathyroidism 334–5
Allergic contact hypersensitivity response 180
Alpha interferon 98–9
Aluminium bone disease 331
Alzheimer's disease 314, 315
   amyloid and therapeutic strategies 318
   cholinergic enhancement therapies 316–17
   neurotrophic factors 317–18
   therapeutic advances 316–19

Ambrosia artemisiifolia 236
Aminoglycosides in ulcerative colitis 150
5-Aminosalicylic acid (5-ASA) 144, 146, 148, 149
Aminotransferase (ALT) 91, 96, 98
Angelman syndrome 215, 220
Angioplasty. *See* Coronory angioplasty
Angiotensin converting enzyme (ACE) inhibitors 41
Antiarrhythmic drugs 55
Antiarrhythmic equipment 55
Antiarrhythmic facilities 55
Antibodies 80–8
   responses to immunotoxins 84
   specificity of 80
Antibody deficiency 70–3
Antibody dependent cellular cytotoxicity (ADCC) 81
Anticoagulation in TIAs and stroke 291
Antimitochondrial antibody (AMA) 154–6
Antineutrophil cytoplasmic antibodies (ANCAs) 60–2, 162
   clinical usefulness 61–2
   patterns of 61
Antineutrophil nuclear antibody (ANNA) 162
Antiphospholipid antibodies (APAs) 60
   clinical usefulness of 62–3
Antiplatelet agents (APT), randomized trials of 291
APC 243–7
Apert's syndrome 214
Aplastic anaemia 96
Asacol in ulcerative colitis 147
Asthma
   bronchial inflammation in 232
   characterization of 232

Asthma, *continued*
  diagnosis of 233
  genetics 232–9
Atherosclerosis 47
Atopic eczema 173
  psychological impact 175–6
Atopy 232
  and chromosome 11q 236–7
  familial clustering of 233
  IgE responsiveness 234–5
  sensitization 234
Atrial natriuretic factor (ANF) 257–62
  in heart failure 261
  in hypertension 260
Autoantibodies in the elderly 197–8
Autoantibody tests 60–3
Autoimmune hepatitis 95
Autoimmune liver disease 95
Azathioprine
  in primary biliary cirrhosis (PBC) 157
  in ulcerative colitis 148

Balloon angioplasty. *See* Coronary angioplasty
Behçet's disease, MRI in 308
BELD in malignant melanoma 171
Benzyl benzoate in scabies infection 209
Beta-blockers
  combinations of nitrovasodilators with 107–8
  complications of 113
  effect on kidney, liver and brain function in cirrhotic patients 113
  haemodynamic changes in systemic and portal circulations with 104–6
  in portal hypertension 103–18
  in prevention of re-bleeding from varices 111–13
  randomized clinical trials 109–13
β-cells 22–4, 26
Birth weight and diabetes 23
Blood
  intermediary metabolites in 4–5
  metabolic fuels in 4–5
Blood pressure
  predicting cure of 363
  response to percutaneous transluminal angioplasty 361–2
Blood transfusions 69
Body lice 205–6
  treatment 206
Bone density
  and fracture threshold 264
  measurements of 265, 267
Bone disease in renal failure 330–8
Bone formation, factors influencing 266
Bone loss, prevention of 265

Bone marrow transplantation 73–5
Bone mass
  and fracture 264–5
  calcium in 268
  genetic and mechanical factors in 263–4
  vitamin D in 269
Bone mass density (BMD) 264
Bone multicellular units (BMUs) 264
Bone resorption, prevention of 266
Brain derived neurotrophic factor (BDNF) 317–18
Brain natriuretic peptide (BNP) 261
Budesonide in ulcerative colitis 142
Bystander effect 82

Calcitriol
  in hyperparathyroidism 334–5
  reduced renal synthesis 331
Calcium in bone mass 268
Candoxatril in NEP inhibition 259
Candoxatrilat in NEP inhibition 258
CAPD 250, 251, 330, 336
Carbamazepine (CBZ) in epilepsy 294, 297
Carbaryl
  in crab louse infection 206
  in head louse infection 203–4
Carcinoid syndrome 278–9
Cardiac arrhythmias. *See* Life-threatening arrhythmias
Cardiac failure. *See* Heart failure
Cardiologists, number of 33
Cardiovascular disease 22, 47
  hypertension and renal failure in 352–4
Carnitine palmitoyltransferase I (CPT I) 1
Carnitine therapy 6
Carnitine transport, measurement of 5
Carniture palmitoyltransferase (CPT) deficiency 4
Carotid endarterectomy in TIAs and stroke 291
Cauda equina, MRI 309–10
CD antigen profile
  of neoplastic lymphoid proliferations 66
  of T- and B-cells 65
Cellular senescence, mechanisms of 194
Cerebral hemisphere mass lesions, MRI in 305
Cerebrovascular disease, MRI in 305–7
CGG triplets 216, 217, 221
Cholangiocarcinoma in primary sclerosing cholangitis (PSC) 159
Cholecystectomy, combination with laparoscopy 119
Cholelithiasis, treatment of 119–20
Cholesterol reduction
  clinical trials 48
  consequences of 50

Cholesterol reduction, *continued*
   strategies for 49–50
Cholestyramine 48
Chromosome 7 238
Chromosome 11q 236–7
Chromosome abnormalities 215
Chronic ambulatory peritoneal dialysis.
   See CAPD
Chronic granulomatous disease (CGD) 75–6
   general measures 76
   interferon therapy 76–7
Chronic progressive external
   ophthalmoplegia (CPEO) 10
Clobazam (CLB) in epilepsy 295, 300–1
Clonazepam (CLON) in epilepsy 295
Clothing lice 205–6
   treatment 206
CNS infections, MRI in 310
Colchicine 162
   in primary biliary cirrhosis (PBC) 157
Colestipol 49
Common variable immunodeficiency
   (CVI) 73
Complement mediated cell lysis 80–1
Complex I 6–7, 13
Complex II 6–7
Complex III 2, 6–7, 13
Complex IV 6–7, 11, 13
Complex V 6–7
Congenital heart disease 230
Congenital hypertrophy of the retinal pigment epithelium (CHRPE) 240–3, 244, 247
Connective tissue diseases 188–93
Continuous ambulatory peritoneal dialysis.
   See CAPD
Coronary angioplasty 30–7
   cost of 33–5
   current practice 30–3
   disposable materials 33–4
   future developments 36
   indications 31
   number of patients needing 35
   resources required for expansion of
      activity 35–6
   results 31
   total cost 34–5
Coronary artery disease in IDDM 250
Coronary heart disease (CHD) 47–8
   age-specific risk 50
   risk factors 48
Cortical Lewy body disease 314–16
Corticosteroids
   in primary biliary cirrhosis (PBC) 157
   in ulcerative colitis 142
   side effects 141
Cotrimoxazole in ulcerative colitis 150

CPT I 4
CPT II 2, 4
Crab louse infection 206
   eyelashes 206
Craniofacial osteomas 240
Crusted scabies 210–11
Cryoglobulinaemia 96
Cushing's syndrome 278
Cyclic AMP 273
Cyclic GMP 259–60
Cyclosporin
   adverse effects 149
   in ulcerative colitis 148–9
Cyclosporin A 162
   in liver transplantation 138
   in primary biliary cirrhosis (PBC) 157
Cylindrocapa lucidum 148
Cystic fibrosis (CF) 233, 238

Delayed dumping syndrome 280
Dementia 314–21
Deoxycorticosterone acetate (DOCA) 258
Dermatology Disease Disability Index 178
DeToni-Fanconi-Debré syndrome 12
Diabetes 249–56
   abnormalities in association with 21
   and birth weight 23
   and pregnancy 249, 252
   complications 249
   delivery of care 253–4
   foot problems 252
   genetic factors and inheritance 20
   glycaemic control 254
   incidence of 249
   inpatient costs 249
   insulin-dependent (IDDM) 19, 250, 254, 281
   macrovascular complications 250–1
   microvascular complications 251–3
   mortality 249–51
   non-insulin-dependent (NIDDM) 19–29, 251, 254, 281
   non-traumatic lower limb amputations 252
   octreotide in 281
   prevalence of 20, 249
   renal disease in 251
   risk of developing 24
   type II 252
Diabetes Centre, Manchester 253–4, 255
Diabetes Centres 253–4
Diabetic retinopathy 252
Dicarboxylic acids in urine 5
Diet in ß-oxidation disorders 6
DiGeorge's syndrome 230
Dilated cardiomyopathy (DCM) 229
Dinitrochlorobenzene (DNCB) 182, 184

Dipentum in ulcerative colitis 147
Discoid lupus erythematosus (DLE) 188–93
  features of patients 189
Disodium etidronate (EHDP) in osteoporosis 268
Disodium-cromoglycate, in ulcerative colitis 150
District general hospitals (DGHs) 54–9
  arrhythmia diagnosis and management 56–8
  management of life-threatening arrhythmias 58–9
Diuretics in portal hypertension 108–9
DNA analysis 230, 243, 247
DNA damage, UV-induced 196
DNA replication 213
DNA sequences 218, 225, 227
DNA synthesis in ageing cells 196
Down's syndrome 214, 230
DTIC in malignant melanoma 171
Duchenne muscular dystrophy (DMD) 218

Eczema 233
Effector mechanisms 80–5
Eicosapentaenoic acid in ulcerative colitis 150
Electron transfer flavoprotein (ETF) 2
Electrophysiological diagnosis 56, 57
Encephalopathies 10–11
Endoscopic retrograde cholangiopancreatography (ERCP) 122, 125, 159
Endothelial leucocyte adhesion molecule (ELAM) 342
Enzyme activity, measurement of 5
Enzyme and prodrug combinations 85
Enzyme replacement 75
Epidermoid cysts 240, 241
Epilepsy
  anticonvulsant monitoring 297
  choice of drug 294–5
  classification of seizure type 294
  diagnosis 293
  incidence 293
  monotherapy 295–9
  pharmacological management 293–303
  polypharmacy 299–300
  primary 293
  rules for anticonvulsant drug use 301–2
  secondary 293
Erythromycin in ulcerative colitis 150
Escherichia coli 156, 340, 341
Essential hypertension 260
ETF:ubiquinone oxidoreductase 2
Ethosuximide (ETH) in epilepsy 295

European Atrial Fibrillation Trial 291
Eysenck Personality Questionnaire 177
Familial adenomatous polyposis (FAP) 240–8
  clinical markers 240–3
  identification of mutations 245–7
  molecular genetic markers 243–7
  preclinical diagnosis 240, 243, 246
Familial hypertrophic cardiomyopathy (FHC) 227–9
FK506 138–9
Flavin adenine dinucleotide 1, 2
Flow cytometry 64
Fluticasone in ulcerative colitis 142
FMR-1 gene 221
Focal pigmentation of the retina 240
Foramen magnum, MRI 309
Fracture and bone mass 264–5
Fragile X expression 221
Fragile X mental retardation (FMR-1) 216–18
Fragile X mutation 216, 221
Fragile X phenotype 218
Fragile X syndrome 216, 221
Free hepatic venous pressure (FHVP) 108
Fulminant hepatic failure 135–6

Gallbladder
  dissection of 125–6
  surgical removal of 120
Gallstones, ideal therapy 121
Gamma-aminobutyric acid (GABA) 300
Gamma-benzene hexachloride in scabies infection 209
Gastrinoma, octreotide in 279
Gastroenteropancreatic endocrine tumours, octreotide in 278–9
Gastrointestinal bleeding
  octreotide in 280
  prevention of 109–10
Gene defects 229–30
Gene expression 225–7
Gene therapy 75
Genetic counselling 230
Genetic disease
  heart in 227–30
  molecular biology in 213–24
  parental origin of 214–15
Genetic heterogeneity 237
Genetic lesions, clinical relevance 230–1
Genetic linkage 236, 238
Genetic markers for polyposis coli 240–8
Genetics
  heart 225–31
  in asthma 232–9
Genomic imprinting 210–22

Genomic imprinting, *continued*
  and fragile X syndrome 221
  and oncogenesis 221-2
  and parental origin 220
Glomerular filtration rate (GFR) 328, 331, 336, 342, 345
Glucagenomas, octreotide in 279
Glucose tolerance test 26
Glycaemic control 254
Gonadotrophin releasing hormone (GnRH) analogues 277
Graft-versus-host disease (GVHD) 74
Growth hormone (GH) releasing factor 272
Growth hormone (GH) secretion physiology 274-6

Haematological disease 12
Haematuria in IgAN 323-4
Haemodialysis 330, 336
Haemolytic uraemic syndromes (HUS) 339-47
  diarrhoea-associated (D+) 340
    clinical aspects 343
    epidemiology 340
    exotoxins 341-2
    outcome 344-5
    pathogenesis 342-3
    recent advances 340-5
  non-prodromal (D-) 340
  therapeutic strategies 343-4
Harvey ras-1 (H-ras-1) gene locus 229-30
Head louse infection 202-5
  treatment 203-5
Heart
  genetic diseases 227-30
  genetics 225-31
Heart failure 38-46
  aetiology of 40
  ANF levels 261
  cost versus benefit analysis for treatment of 42-4
  definitions 38-9
  efficacy of treatment 41-2
  epidemiology 39-40
  immediate causes of 39
  implications for management 44-5
  investigations in 44
  multiple objectives of treatment of 43
  prevalence of 40
  prognosis in 40-1
Henoch-Schönlein purpura (HSP) and IgAN 323
Hepatic artery thrombosis 133
Hepatic venous pressure gradient (HVPG) 104-6, 109
Hepatitis B and HIV 95

Hepatitis B cirrhosis, liver transplantation in 136
Hepatitis B surface antigen (HBsAg) 136
Hepatitis C virus (HCV) 72, 89-102
  and HIV 95
  antibodies 90-1
  clinical features
    acute hepatitis C 96
    chronic hepatitis C 96-7
  community-acquired transmission 92-3
  diagnosis of 90-2
  epidemiology 92-6
  high risk populations 94
  intrafamilial transmission 93
  management
    acute hepatitis C 97
    chronic hepatitis C 97-8
  maternal-infant transmission 93
  population studies 93
  post-transfusion 94
  prevalence of anti-HCV in chronic liver disease 94
  RNA testing 91
  serological diagnosis
    acute hepatitis C 91-2
    chronic hepatitis C 92
  supplemental antibody tests 91
  transmission 92-3
  virology of 89-90
Hepatocellular carcinoma (HCC) 95
Herpes zoster 197
High density lipoprotein (HDL) 49
Histamine bronchial responsiveness 233
HIV 197
  and HCV 95
HLA Class II 236, 237
Hormone replacement therapy (HRT) 266-8
HTLV-1 associated myelopathy (HAM), MRI in 308
Huntington's chorea 215
Hybridoma technology 60
Hydrocortisone in ulcerative colitis 142
Hydroxychloroquine in ulcerative colitis 151
Hydroxylamine and osmium tetroxide (HOT) 246
3-Hydroxy-3-methylglutaryl coenzyme A (HMG CoA) reductase inhibition 49, 51
Hypercholesterolaemia 51
  risk factors 49
  treatment of 48
Hyperinsulinaemia 280
Hyperlipidaemia 51, 52
Hyperparathyroid bone disease 330
Hyperparathyroidism 331, 334-5

Hyperphosphataemia in renal
 osteodystrophy 334
Hypertension 22, 24, 348–58
 and progression of renal disease 350–2
 ANF levels 260
 as cause of renal failure 348–9
 atrial natriuretic factor (ANF) in 260
 in cardiovascular disease 352–4
 neutral endopeptidase (NEP) in 260
 renal failure as cause of 349–50
Hypogammaglobulinaemia 70
Hypoglycaemia 280
Hypoketotic hypoglycaemic episodes 3

ICAM-1 182, 184
Idiopathic dilated cardiomyopathy 229
Idiopathic lymphadenopathy/
 lymphocytosis 64–6
Idiotype network 81
IgA deficiency 70
IgA nephropathy (IgAN) 322–9
 circulating 325
 clinical presentation 322–4
 definition 322
 glomerular 325
 haematuria in 323–4
 immune system 325–7
 incidence 324–5
 pathogenesis 325–7
 polymeric 327
 prevalence and prognosis 324
 progression of 327–8
 relationship with Henoch–Schönlein
  purpura (HSP) 323
 treatment 328
IgE levels 232–3, 234
IgE responsiveness
 allergen specific 235
 in atopy 234–5
IgG
 and IgAN 327
 deposition 198
 subclass deficiency 72
IgG levels 71, 72
Immune function of the skin 180
Immune response
 antimicrobial, of the skin 180
 induction of 180
Immune sensitivity, expression of 182–6
Immunoconjugates, Phase I clinical
 responses 86
Immunodeficiency disorders, evaluation
 and monitoring of 66
Immunogenicity 86
Immunoglobulin replacement therapy 71–2
Immunology
 and the skin 180–7

Immunology, *continued*
 multidisciplinary nature of 60
 primary biliary cirrhosis (PBC) 155–7
 primary sclerosing cholangitis (PSC)
  160–2
 tests 60–8
Immunophenotyping of lymphocytes 63–7
Immunotoxins 83
 handling 87
 maximum tolerated dose (MTD) 84
 mode of action 87
 Phase I clinical responses 86
 potency 87
 principal forms of toxicity seen 85
 selection of 87
Impaired glucose tolerance (IGT) 23, 24
Infestations 202–12
Inflammatory bowel disease (IBD) 159
Insulin
 administration of 21
 assay methodology 22
 deficiency 21
 radio-immunoassays 21
 resistance 21
 secretion 21
Insulin-like growth factor-1 (IGF-1) 274–5
Insulinoma, octreotide in 279
Intercellular adhesion molecule (ICAM)
 342
Intercellular adhesion molecule-1 (ICAM-
 1) 181
Interferon-γ (IFN-γ) 76–7
Interleukin-2 (IL-2) 73
Intermediary metabolites in blood 4–5
Intramuscular immunoglobulin 71
Intravenous immunoglobulin (IVIG) 71–2
Intravenous urogram (IVU) 360–1, 366
Ischaemic heart disease 24
Isolated myopathy 10
Isoniazid in ulcerative colitis 150
Isosorbide 5 mononitrate (ISMN) 107–8
Isosorbide dinitrate 107
Isosorbide mononitrate 107

Kearns–Sayre/CPEO phenotype 12
Kearns–Sayre syndrome (KSS) 10
Ketoconazole in ulcerative colitis 150
Ketotifen in ulcerative colitis 151
Klinefelter's syndrome 215
Koch postulates 73

Lactic acidosis in infancy 13
Lamotrigine (LTG), in epilepsy 295, 301
Langerhans' cells (LCs) 180–2
Laparoscopic cholecystectomy 119–29
 collected experience with 122
 complications 127

Laporoscopic cholecystectomy, *continued*
  indications for 122
  introduction of 121-2
  patient details 127
  results 127
  technique 122-7
  working relationship with
    gastroenterological colleagues 125
Laparoscopy
  combination with cholecystectomy 119
  history of 119
Leber's optic atrophy 12
Leigh's syndrome 11
Leukaemia/lymphoma
    immunophenotyping 64-7
Leukotriene B4 (LTB4) in ulcerative colitis
  150
Lewy bodies 314
Life-threatening arrhythmias 54-9
  programmed electrical stimulation 55-7
  requirements for management in DGH
    58-9
Lignocaine 55
Lindane
  in crab louse infection 206
  in scabies infection 209
Linked DNA markers 243-5
Lipid clinic 47-53
  alternatives to 51-2
  goals of 51
  work of 50-1
Lipid disorders, diet in management of 51
Lipopolysaccharide (LPS) 342-3
Liver disease, anti-HCV in 94-5
Liver transplantation 75, 130-40
  contraindications 131
  evolution 130
  factors associated with poor prognosis
    132
  for malignant disease 134-5
  immunosuppression 138
  in alcoholic liver disease 137
  in children 132-3
    patient survival 133
    primary diagnoses in 132
  in fulminant hepatic failure 135
  in hepatitis B 136
  indications 131
  patient selection and timing 131-2
  rejection 138
  results 139
  risk factors 132
  technical developments 137-8
Long QT syndrome 229-30
Louse infection 202-7
Lovastatin 49
Low density lipoprotein (LDL) 49

Lumbosacral intervertebral disc disease,
  MRI 310
Lupus anticoagulant (LAC) test 62-3
Lupus erythematosus 188-93
Lymphocyte function associated antigen
  (LFA-1) 181-2
Lymphocytes, immunophenotyping of
  63-7

Magnetic resonance angiography (MRA)
  310-11
Magnetic resonance imaging (MRI) 304-10
  current indications 304-10
  fast scanning 311
  future developments 311
  pathological specificity 311
Major histocompatibility (MHC) Class I
  73-4
Major histocompatibility (MHC) Class II
  73-4, 180
Malathion
  in crab louse infection 206
  in head louse infection 203-4
  in scabies infection 210
Malignant melanoma 166-71
  clinicopathological subsets 168-70
  epidemiology 166-7
  incidence of 166
  management 170-1
  molecular biology 167-8
  personal risk factors 168
  prognosis 170
Marfan's syndrome 214
Mast cell inhibitors in ulcerative colitis
  150
Mast cells, degranulation of 233
Mesalazine
  adverse reactions 145-6
  in ulcerative colitis 144, 145
  renal toxicity 146
Messenger RNA 225
Metabolic acidosis 334
Metabolic fuels in blood 4-5
Methotrexate in primary biliary cirrhosis
  (PBC) 157
1-methyl-4-phenyl-1,2,3,6-tetrahydrapyridine
  (MPTP) 13
Mitochondrial dysfunction, diseases due to
  1-18
Mitochondrial fatty acid oxidation 1-6
  biochemistry of 1
  clinical features of defects of 3-4
  investigation of defects of 4-6
  treatment of disorders of 6
Mitochondrial respiratory chain 6-14
  biochemistry of 6-7
Mixed osteodystrophy 330

Molecular biology
  and the heart 225-7
  as basic science 225-6
  in cardiology 226-7
  in genetic disease 213-24
Molsidomine in portal hypertension 108
Monoclonal antibodies 60, 63, 80
Monosulfiram in scabies infection 209
Morphoea 191
Mosaicism 218-19
Motor neurone disease (MND), MRI in 308
mtDNA depletion syndrome 13
Mucosal antigen penetration 326
Multiple sclerosis, MRI in 305-7
Myocardial infarction 353
Myocardial revascularization 30
Myoclonus epilepsy with ragged red fibres (MERRF) 10-11
Myopathy, encephalopathy, lactic acidosis and stroke-like episodes (MELAS) 11

Nadolol in variceal bleeding 109
NADPH-oxidase system 76
NANB hepatitis 89, 92-6
Natural effector functions 80-2
Nephropathy in IDDM 250, 251
Nerve growth factors (NGF) 317-18
Nesidioblastosis, octreotide in 279
Neurodegenerative disease 13-14
Neurofibromatosis 215
Neutral endopeptidase (NEP) 257-62
  in hypertension 260
  inhibition in man 258-60
  pharmacological inhibition 258
Niacin 49
Nicotinamide dinucleotide (NADH) 1
Nitroglycerin 107
Nitrovasodilators 107-8
  combinations with beta-blockers 107-8
Non-A non-B (NANB) agents 89
Non-melanoma skin cancers (NMSC) 195-7
Non-steroidal anti-inflammatory drugs (NSAIDs) in ulcerative colitis 150
Norwegian scabies 210-11
Nuclear magnetic resonance (NMR) 304

Octreotide 272-84
  amino acid sequence 274
  antitumour activity of 281
  in acromegaly 276-7
  in acute gastrointestinal bleeding 280
  in AIDS-related diarrhoea 279
  in delayed dumping syndrome 280
  in diabetes mellitus 281

Octreotide, *continued*
  in gastrinoma 279
  in gastroenteropancreatic endocrine tumours 278-9
  in glucagonomas 279
  in hyperinsulinaemia 280
  in hypoglycaemia 280
  in insulinoma 279
  in nesidioblastosis 279
  in oncology 281
  in pancreatic fistulae 280
  in pancreatitis 280
  in pituitary disease 276-8
  in pituitary tumours 278
  in polycystic ovary syndrome (PCOS) 282
  in psoriasis 282
  in VIPoma 279
  in Zollinger-Ellison syndrome 279
  pharmacology of 274
  therapeutic uses 282
OKT3 81, 138
Olsalazine
  adverse reactions 145-6
  in ulcerative colitis 144, 145, 147
Oncogenesis 221-2
Oncology, octreotide in 281
Orbits and optic chiasm, MRI 310
Orthotopic liver transplantation (OLT)
  in primary biliary cirrhosis (PBC) 157-8
  in primary sclerosing cholangitis (PSC) 162
Osteoblast, role of 264
Osteogenesis imperfecta (OI) 218
Osteomalacia 330, 333
Osteoporosis 263-71
  disodium etidronate (EHDP) in 268
  future problems 269
  management recommendations 266
  prevention of 265-6
  research 263
22-Oxacalcitriol in hyperparathyroidism 335-6
Oxfordshire Community Stroke Project (OCSP) 285
Ozone depletion 197

Paget's disease 268
Pancreatic fistulae, octreotide in 280
Pancreatitis, octreotide in 280
Parathyroid hormone (PTH) 330-6
Parathyroidectomy in chronic renal disease 336
Parkinson's disease 14, 314, 316
Pediculus humanus capitis 202
Penicillamine in primary biliary cirrhosis (PBC) 157

Pentasa in ulcerative colitis 147
Percutaneous transluminal angioplasty 359
  blood pressure response to 361-2
  complications 365
  effect on renal function 363
  performance of 363-4
  prediction of blood pressure response 363
  role in management of renal artery stenosis 365
  technical aspects 364
  technical failure 364
Percutaneous transluminal balloon coronary angioplasty. See Coronary angioplasty
Permethrin in scabies infection 210
Phenobarbitone (PB) in epilepsy 295
Phenytoin (PHT)
  in epilepsy 294, 298-9
  in ulcerative colitis 150
Phosphate retention in renal osteodystrophy 331
Photoageing, changes of 194, 195
Phthirus pubis 206
Pituitary disease, octreotide in 276-8
Pituitary tumours, octreotide in 278
Plasma measurement 5
Platelet-activating factor (PAF) in ulcerative colitis 150
Polycystic ovary syndrome (PCOS), octreotide in 282
Polyethylene glycol (PEG-IL-2) 73
Polymerase chain reaction (PCR) 6, 9, 91
Polyposis coli, genetic markers for 240-8
Portal hypertension
  beta-blockers in 103-18
  drugs evaluated in 104
  future of long-term medical therapy 113-14
Portal hypertensive gastropathy, prevention of bleeding 111
Posterior fossa, MRI 309
Prader-Willi syndrome 215, 220
Prednisolone in ulcerative colitis 142
Pregnancy, diabetes in 249, 252
Premutation 216-18
Primary biliary cirrhosis (PBC) 154-8
  immunology 155-7
  M2 antigens 156
  medical treatment 157
  natural history 154-5
  orthotopic liver transplantation (OLT) 157
  recurrence in transplanted liver 158
Primary carnitine deficiency 4
Primary immunodeficiency 69-79
  principles of management 69-70

Primary sclerosing cholangitis (PSC) 159-63
  diagnosis of 159
  immunology 160-2
  natural history 159
  non-surgical treatment 162
  pathogenesis of 160
  prognostic models 159
Primidone (PRIM) in epilepsy 295
Prodrug and enzyme combinations 85
Programmed electrical stimulation 55-7
Proinsulin 22, 23
Propranolol 108
  effect on HVPG 105-6
  in variceal bleeding 109
Propranolol in gastric mucosal bleeding 111
Proteinuria
  and renal impairment 324
  in IDDM 250
Pseudomonas 83
Psoriasis
  octreotide in 282
  practical effects on daily life 174-5
  psychological impact 173-5
Psoriasis Disability Index 178
Pulmonary wedge pressure (PWP) 107
Pyrethroids
  in crab louse infection 206
  in head louse infection 205

Quality Adjusted Life Years (QALYs) 178

Radioimmunoconjugates 82
  potency 87
  principal forms of toxicity seen 85
Radioisotopes 82-3
Raynaud's phenomenon 192
Recombinant DNA techniques 60
Recombinant immunoblot assay (RIBA) 91
Renal artery stenosis 359-68
  clinical features 359-60
  diagnosis 360-1
  recurrence 364-5
  role of angioplasty in management of 365
  role of surgery 366
Renal disease
  hypertension in progression of 350-2
  in diabetes 251
Renal failure 348-58
  as cause of hypertension 349-50
  bone disease in 330-8
  hypertension as cause of 348-9
  in cardiovascular disease 352-4
Renal function, effect of angioplasty on 363

Renal osteodystrophy
  pathogenesis 331-4
  treatment 334-7
Renal transplantation 250
Renin-angiotensin system 257
Respiratory chain defects
  ageing studies 14
  biochemical studies 8-9
  clinical features 9-10
  clinical investigation 8
  clinical syndromes 10-14
  gastrointestinal involvement 12
  investigation of 8-9
  molecular studies 9
  morphological studies 8
  syndromes with non-neuromuscular presentation 12
  treatment 14
Restriction fragment length polymorphisms (RFLPs) 213, 227-9, 236
Retina, focal pigmentation of 240
Retinitis pigmentosa 214
Retinoblastoma 215, 221
Retinoic acid in UV-induced skin changes 198-9
Reverse genetics 238
Rhinitis 233
Riboflavine 6
Ricin 83, 84
Rifampicin in ulcerative colitis 150
RNA transcript 225
Roux hepatico-enterostomy 162
Rowell's syndrome 190

St Vincent Declaration 249
Salicylates
  dose response 146-7
  ulcerative colitis in 143-7
Sandostatin. See Octreotide
Sarcoidosis, MRI in 308
SAX 75
Scabies infection 207-11
  crusted scabies 210-11
  in pregnancy 210
  institutional outbreaks 211
  primary signs 207
  treatment of 208-10
    infants and young children 210
Scleroderma 191
Sclerotherapy in prevention of re-bleeding from varices 112-13
Seborrhoeic dermatitis 197
Senile dementia of Lewy body type (SDLT) 315-16
Severe combined immunodeficiency (SCID) 73-5

Shiga toxin 341-2
Shigella dysenteriae type 1 infection 340-2
Single strand conformational polymorphism (SSCP) 246
Sinorphan in hypertension 260
Skin
  and connective tissue diseases 188-93
  antimicrobial immune response 180
  immune function of 180
  UV-induced changes 198
Skin ageing 194-201
  intrinsic and extrinsic factors 194-5
  social impact 198-9
  ultraviolet light (UV) in 194-7
Skin cancer, non-melanoma (NMSC) 195-7
Skin disease
  clinical relevance 172
  current knowledge of psychological and disabling impact 173
  in the elderly 197-8
  measurement of psychological impact 176-8
  psychological impact 172-9
Sodium fluoride in bone formation 266
Sodium valproate (VPA) in epilepsy 294, 298
Somatostatin 272-84
  amino acid sequence 274
  hormones inhibited by 272
  organ distribution of 272-3
  pharmacology of 274
Sphincterotomy 125
Spinal cord
  imaging 311
  MRI 309-10
Spironolactone in portal hypertension 108-9
Splanchnic sphygmomanometer 114
Squamous cell carcinoma, UV-induced 198
Streptomyces tsukubaensis 138
Stroke 285
  management 289
  medical treatment 289-90
  prognosis 287-9
  randomized trials of medical therapies 290
  secondary prevention 290-1
  surgical treatment 290
Subacute necrotizing encephalomyelopathy 11
Subcutaneous immunoglobulin 72
Sudden infant death 3
Sulphasalazine
  in ulcerative colitis 147
  side-effects of 141, 144
Sulphonamides in ulcerative colitis 143-7
Superoxide dismutase (SOD) 90

Syndrome X 21, 23
Systemic lupus erythematosus (SLE) 62–3, 188–93
　antibody subsets in 191
　features of patients 189
　MRI in 307
Systemic sclerosis 188, 191–2
　classification of 191
　diffuse cutaneous 191
　limited cutaneous 191

T-cells 182, 184
Temporal lobes, MRI 308–9
Tetmosol in scabies infection 209–10
Tetrahydroaminoacridine (THA) 316
Thrifty phenotype hypothesis 24
Thrombotic thrombocytopenic purpura (TTP) 339
Tissue carnitine concentrations 5
Tixocortol pivalate in ulcerative colitis 142
Tolypocladium 148
Transforming growth factors (TGFβs) 227
Transient ischaemic attacks (TIAs) 285–7
　management 289
　prognosis 286–7
　secondary prevention 290–1
Trifunctional enzyme deficiency 4
Triple X syndrome 215
Tuberous sclerosis 218
Tumour necrosis factor (TNF) 342–3
　in malignant melanoma 171
Tumour necrosis factor alpha (TNF-α) 182, 184
Turner's syndrome 215

UK Sickness Impact Profile (UKSIP) 178
Ulcerative colitis 141–53
　corticosteroids in 142
　immunosuppressive drugs in 148–9

Ulcerative colitis, *continued*
　morbidity 141
　mortality rate 141
　outlook for 141
　potential drugs 150–1
　salicylates in 143–7
　sulphonamides in 143–7
Ultraviolet light (UV)
　in skin ageing 194–7
　in skin cancer 195–7
Ursodeoxycholic acid (UDCA) 162
　in primary biliary cirrhosis (PBC) 157

Vaccines 69–70
Varicella infection 197
Vascular disease, MRI in 305
Vasculitides 62
Vasculitis 61
VCAM-1 (vascular cell adhesion molecule) 182
Verapamil 55
Verocytotoxin (VT) 340–2
Vigabatrin (VGB), in epilepsy 295, 300
VIPoma, octreotide in 279
Vitamin D in bone mass 269

Warfarin in TIAs and stroke 291
Wedge hepatic venous pressure (WHVP) 104, 107, 108
Wegener's granulomatosis (WG) 61
White matter disease, MRI in 305–8
Wilms' tumour 215, 221, 222
Wolf's syndrome 215

X chromosome 216, 218, 221
Xeroderma pigmentosum (XP) 196

Zollinger–Ellison syndrome, octreotide in 279

This is what you receive each week when you subscribe to the *Journal*.

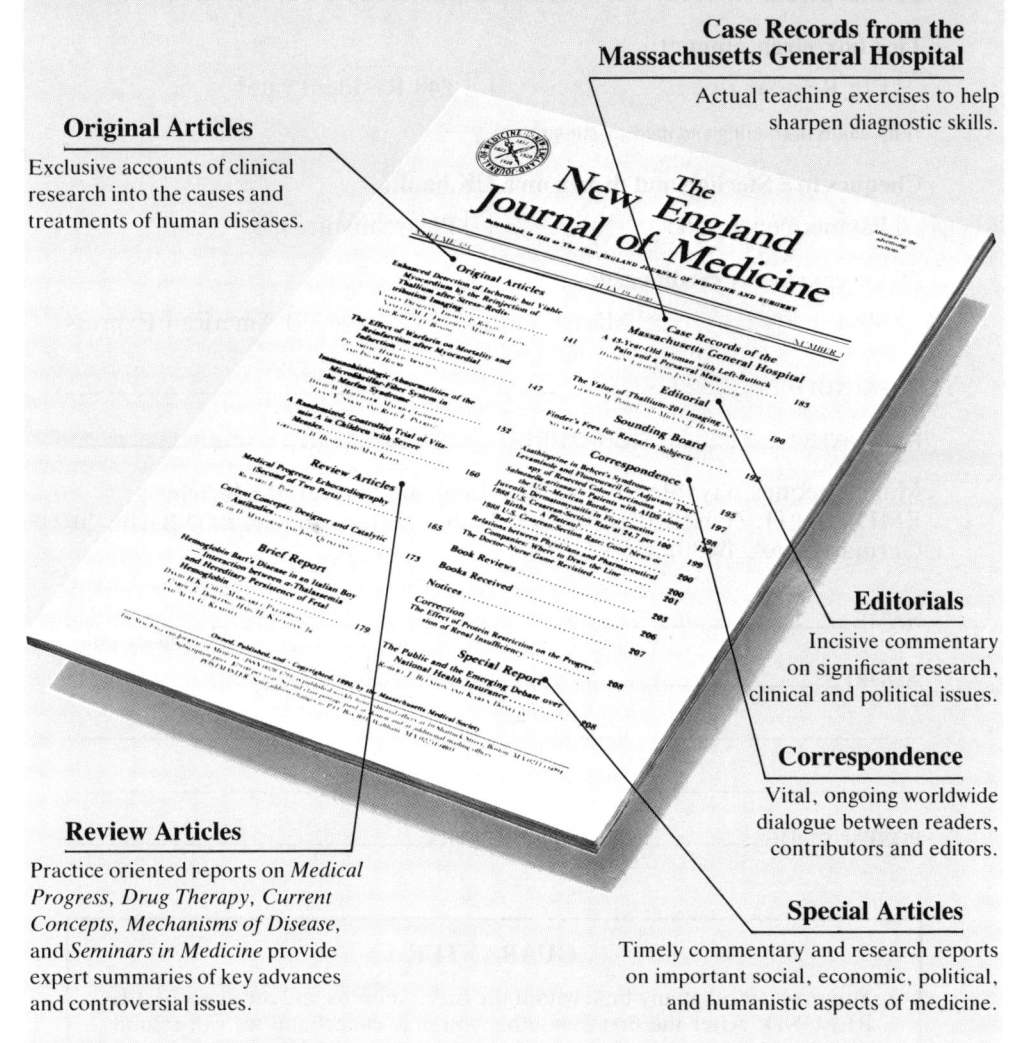

Original Articles
Exclusive accounts of clinical research into the causes and treatments of human diseases.

Case Records from the Massachusetts General Hospital
Actual teaching exercises to help sharpen diagnostic skills.

Editorials
Incisive commentary on significant research, clinical and political issues.

Correspondence
Vital, ongoing worldwide dialogue between readers, contributors and editors.

Review Articles
Practice oriented reports on *Medical Progress, Drug Therapy, Current Concepts, Mechanisms of Disease*, and *Seminars in Medicine* provide expert summaries of key advances and controversial issues.

Special Articles
Timely commentary and research reports on important social, economic, political, and humanistic aspects of medicine.

Don't miss this
NO RISK – SATISFACTION GUARANTEED Offer

To receive your own copy, photocopy and complete the enclosed Order Form and send today!

NO RISK – SATISFACTION GUARANTEED Offer

To receive your own copy, photocopy and complete this Order Form and send today!

☐ **Yes,** please enter my one year subscription (52 issues) to NEJM.

Tick box/circle amount:

☐ £75 Regular rate ☐ £48 Resident rate*

*Physicians in training and medical students

Cheques in £ Sterling and drawn on a UK bank.

☐ Payment enclosed ☐ Please invoice me

Please charge my credit card:

☐ Visa ☐ Master Card ☐ American Express

CARD NUMBER _____

EXP. DATE _____ / _____ SIGNATURE _____

Make cheques payable to: **The New England Journal of Medicine**
EMD GmbH, Zeitschriftenvertrieb, Hohenzollernring 96, 1000 Berlin 20, Germany Fax: 49(30) 336 9236

NAME _____
(Please print)
ADDRESS _____

_____

_____

POSTAL CODE _____ COUNTRY _____

GUARANTEE

You may cancel at any time within the first 3 months and receive a FULL REFUND. After the first 3 months, you may cancel and we will refund the unexpired portion of your subscription. Please allow 4–8 weeks for shipment of the first issue.

Rates include air-speeded delivery.
This offer valid through December 1993.